Nanofabrication
Enrapturing Cues and Prodigal Applications

Editors

Kamal Prasad

University Department of Physics
T.M. Bhagalpur University
Bhagalpur, India

Gajendra Prasad Singh

Department of Nanotechnology
Central University of Jharkhand
Ranchi, India

Anal Kant Jha

Department of Biotechnology
O.P. Jindal University
Raigarh, Chhattisgarh, India

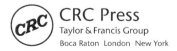

CRC Press
Taylor & Francis Group
Boca Raton London New York

CRC Press is an imprint of the
Taylor & Francis Group, an **informa** business

A SCIENCE PUBLISHERS BOOK

First edition published 2025
by CRC Press
2385 NW Executive Center Drive, Suite 320, Boca Raton FL 33431

and by CRC Press
4 Park Square, Milton Park, Abingdon, Oxon, OX14 4RN

Library of Congress Cataloging-in-Publication Data (applied for)

ISBN: 978-0-367-53785-2 (hbk)
ISBN: 978-0-367-53789-0 (pbk)
ISBN: 978-1-003-08335-1 (ebk)

DOI: 10.1201/9781003083351

Typeset in Times New Roman
by Prime Publishing Services

Preface

Nanotechnology is gaining vivid visibility among the scientific community due to its exponential promises and applications. People have been trying different novel green protocols using different means including carboxylic acids, biological cohorts, domestic and pharmaceutical wastes, etc. The sole purpose is to catch up with the worldwide emerging concept of circular economy and sustainability.

The procedure of synthesis, irrespective of the source; banks primarily upon the promises of participating molecule/metabolite that helps to accomplish the synthesis through its decomposition/dissociation/tautomerization/resonance at a given or optimized temperature and pH leading to the availability of required free energy that leads to the phase transformation. Different methods, though looking simple in the first place, has many enchanting yet challenging cues. Irrespective of the method being pursued or a potential source being hired, a restrict discipline of thermodynamics is always obeyed and this adds promising prodigality. This book touches on different aspects of nanofabrication techniques and their applications.

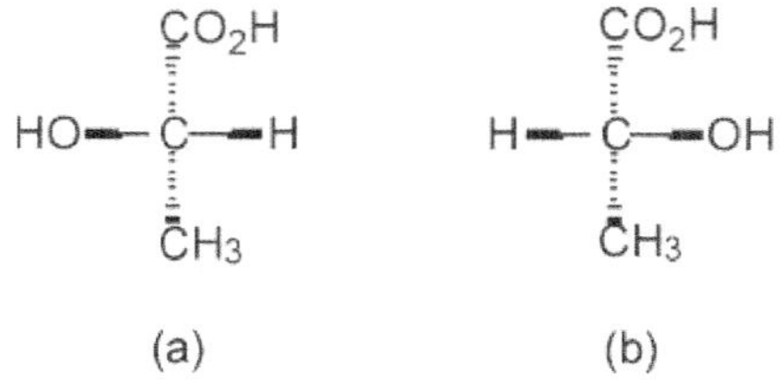

$$\begin{array}{ccc} & CO_2H & & CO_2H \\ & | & & | \\ HO-\!\!-C\!\!-\!\!H & & H\!\!-\!\!-C\!\!-\!\!OH \\ & | & & | \\ & CH_3 & & CH_3 \\ & (a) & & (b) \end{array}$$

Fig. 1. Pattern of reaction of glucose and molecular orientation of lactic acid.

3. Fungi (Eukaryotes)

The ambience of living cohorts tends to fluctuate; therefore, resilience to the shears of the environment is a must for organisms to persist. Chemical-stress-inducing factors like pollutants (organic or inorganic) might have different pattern of action but the annihilation remains the same. Along with this, certain natural shearing factors like radiation are also associated with oxidative damage in cells [5, 6]. Encountered by metal/metalloid toxicity, fungal members trigger a response at multiple levels originating from cell wall to nuclei that can be perceived in detail somewhere else [7]. The first line response of cellular defence is considered due to the quinones. Also, the reduction of nanoparticles using filamentous fungi has some influence over other organisms. Filamentous fungi are handy, want simple raw materials, and have high wall-binding capacity [8]. Members of fungi also harbour a good number of hydroxyl/methoxy derivatives of quinones such as benzoquinones and toluquinones, which are secreted especially by the members of the lower fungi (e.g., in *Penicillium* and *Aspergillus* species) in response to a potential metallic stress. Occurrence of these metabolites may start a redox reaction due to tautomerization leading to synthesis of a nanomaterial [9]. *Prototropic tautomerism*, defined by one of its early investigators as "the addition of a proton at one molecular site and its removal from another" [10], and hence clearly distinguished from ionization, is one of the most important phenomena in organic chemistry despite the relatively small proportion of molecules in which it can occur. On the other hand, the small differences in free energy between the components make them very useful. In biological systems, delicate and subtle control is needed for the organization of chains of reactions. Life is the controlled motion of electrons and protons. The thermodynamics and kinetics of electrons are to a large extent governed by redox centres, and the equally important motion of protons can be viewed as an extended series of tautomerization reactions. DNA is built from bases all of which have a number of different tautomers. There are even a few enzymes, called tautomerazes, that enable rapid tautomerization between keto and enol forms of molecules [11]. Tautomers are interesting for many reasons, technological as well as fundamental. Their optical properties make them suitable as signalling molecules in sensors, as they can rapidly switch between states. Many biologically important molecules have several tautomers. Adenine, for instance, an important moiety in DNA and adenosine triphosphate (ATP), comes in three varieties, the main one—according to some people—chosen by nature to avoid fluorescence. One of the more interesting and complicating properties is that tautomeric equilibria in the ground state are often vastly different from those in the excited states. In addition, tautomeric equilibria are easily shifted by the environment. Here, the pH modulation is the key factor that controls the procedure and leads to a successful and quick nanomaterial synthesis.

4. Plant Systems

Plants in different forms have proved their pivotal importance since inception of human life on this planet. While cyanobacteria are the pioneer oxygen generators, other cohorts irrespective of their systematic position have contributed towards our survival one way or the other. In the course of evolution, they have developed a plethora of promising metabolites in order to circumvent the environmental rigors and those metabolites have proven to be a boon for synthesizing different nanomaterials. An appreciably vast conglomerate of metabolites is synthesized and harboured among the different plant species such as flavones, ketones, aldehydes, amides terpenoids (citronellol and geraniol), and carboxylic acid. Water soluble compounds (metabolites) are really amenable in nanomaterials synthesis such as nano silver and the reduction is brought about by water soluble phytochemicals like flavones, quinones, soluble sugars, and organic acids (such as oxalic, malic, tartaric, protocatechuic, etc.). A long list of references is available on plant/plant part broth/extract mediated synthesis of silver, gold and platinum nanoparticles in which accountability lies over either the primary or the secondary metabolites and it continues to pour in. This in itself speaks of the scientific excitement being triggered among the workers.

Phyllanthin and hypophyllanthin (lignan) adjudicated synthesis of Ag and gold (Au) nanoparticles has been noted [12]. The fabrication of Ag nanoparticles using *Eclipta* leaf extract was achieved and the key phytochemical were assay to be flavonoids [13]. Cycas leaves contain Amentoflavone and Hinokiflavone, and biflavonyls, which have been found to synthesize Ag nanoparticles [14]. Synthesis of Au nanoparticles negotiated by Bael (*Aegle marmelos*) leaves has been noted in the past [15, 16]. Higher plants belonging to the xerophyte, mesophyte, and hydrophyte categories were assayed for their nanotransformation potential and all were found suitable for promoting nanosynthesis because of their inherent phytochemicals [17]. Earlier, by using *Geranium* [18], *Aloe vera* [19], Neem (*Azadirachta indica*) [20], *Emblica* [21], and *Avena* [22] leaf broth, metallic Ag was synthesized. The fabrication of Ag nanoparticles in the above reports highlight the reductive properties of water-soluble phytochemicals such as flavones, quinines, and organic acids that are abundant in the parenchyma cells of leaves [23]. Synthesis of nanoscale Ag was reported using mature chili fruit (*Capsicum annuum* L.) [24, 25] and orange juice [26, 27]. Majorly, the fabrication of nanoscale Ag resulted by dint of redox reactions, involving various phytochemicals like polyphenols, ascorbic acid, capsaicinoids, etc. Dissociation of citric acid also effectively contributed to the procedure by ensuring the presence of required free energy for nanotransformation. This leads to the conclusion that microbes like bacteria or fungi require a comparatively longer incubation in the growth media for reducing a metal ion, whereas plant extracts by virtue of containing water soluble phytochemicals bring nano-transformation almost in a jiffy. Therefore, in comparison to microbes, cells of the plants are handy and amenable

5. Animal Systems

The discipline of osmolarity is pivotal for any organism to survive under the normal conditions or under environmental stress. The ionic balance has to be maintained for maintaining a normal physiology and metabolism. Heavy metals are required by other animals, including insects in their metabolism; however, when its level reaches beyond detoxification efficiency, it results in toxicity shearing and the contention is that metals do have a role in the origin of life itself [34]. The internal homeostasis is conserved through regular diffusion and assembly of a distinct structure called spherocrystals-originating from the ER-Golgi complex where elements precipitate upon a glycosaminoglycan nucleus in a fragile peripheral stratum. Most of the spherocrystals may have minerals, most commonly phosphates, or else may store wastes such as urates. The presence of additional metals in abundance in the environment allows insects such as cockroaches and ants to stay alive and to trap the metals (e.g., Pb or Cd) in surrounding layers of spherocrystals; however, the biochemical composition of cytoplasm remains unaltered. The ability of arthropods to withstand elevated levels of toxic metals dwells in probably their odd habitats. Besides, the lysosomes have the potential to retain toxic heavy metals like Cd or Hg within metallothionein-like proteins [35]. The cockroach exoskeleton is comprised of chitin (polymeric N-acetylglucosamine). The simultaneous presence of amino and acetyl group culminates in mildly acidic behaviour in a biosynthetic medium, subject to amenable modulation during the experiments for obtaining the desired nanomaterial. Cells of the animal die or get completely diminished after heating, but the elaborated cell metabolites in the broth solution help in nanomaterials fabrication. In cockroaches, there are proteins identified as tropomyosin that initiate allergic alerts among humans. The thermodynamics of actin binding proteins have been less studied and control actin mechanics. It consists of four alpha helices—A, B, C, and D that together form a quaternary structure and is responsible for muscle contraction [36]. This protein, because of its inherent thermodynamic behaviour, is thought to assist the entrapment of nascent nanomaterials thus extending strength. It has further been suggested that an inclusive interrelation of Bla g2 with the structures of other well-known aspartic proteases, suggest that ligand binding could be involved in the activity of this allergen [34]. It has been proposed that the loss of balance of metals results from genetic impairments or environmental pollution and is associated with negative health effects worldwide. Various in-depth studies have highlighted that an appreciable number of genes and their regulatory cues are involved in maintaining heavy metal homeostasis involving the metals tested in the study, Cd, Cu and Zn, and initiates various responses including triggering of genes coding for metallothionein, transporters, glutathione-mediated detoxification pathway components, antimicrobial peptides, ubiquitin conjugating enzymes, heat shock proteins, and cytochrome P450 enzymes. The induction of metallothionein by the metals such as Cu, Zn, and Cd is well aligned with their role as metal scavenger and protective role against metal toxicity through the down regulation by copper depletion but remarkable variations in responses may be generated among metallothionein congeners. MtnA gets induced in response to a Cu assault, while MtnB and MtnC are more strongly induced by Zn and Cd, respectively. Recent studies have revealed that individual metallothioneins preferentially defend against specific metals, with MtnA playing an important role in defending against copper excess, MtnB during zinc and cadmium excess, while MtnC and MtnD play only smaller acts in defending against these three metals. Therefore, elaboration of MtnA is higher, compared to other metallothioneins, with an intense baseline level and consequently a fewer degree of fold-induction, and this is suggestive of the fact that MtnA is the major metal hunter in the larva of Drosophila [37, 38]. It has been speculated that ferritin is a metal detoxicant among mammals in general and is able to detoxify, store, and transport iron; it has also the ability to bind some other metal ion species. This has also been observed among Drosophila where an induction was observed under zinc assault. It is interesting to note that although the chemical properties of Zn and Cd are identical, they tend to trigger varied responses biologically. Consequently, regulatory chores to combat excess Zn exposures are also functional in Cd stress as well [37].

The exoskeleton of banana fly and household mosquito (Culex sp.) are built of chitin (a polymer of N-acetylglucosamine) [38]. It is mildly acidic due to the occurrence of both the amino group with the acetyl group, and this can be suitably manipulated to obtain desired nanomaterials (i.e., metals/oxides/chalcogenides). Cell death ensues upon boiling, but metabolites get disseminated in the broth mixture/solution and this aids in fabrication of nanomaterials. Furthermore, tropomyosin as previously mentioned initiates allergic alerts among humans and is an actin-bound protein moiety whose function is to ensure actin agility. Tropomyosin is pivotal for muscle contraction, among other things [39]. This protein might have played a fundamental role of encapsulation for the nascent nanomaterials. An inherent similarity of Bla g2 with the structures of other well-known aspartic proteases, and its homology to PAG, suggest that ligand binding could be participating in the act of this allergen [40]. Metal toxicity leads to stress once the organisms experience higher than their naturally bestowed capacity for detoxification. Besides, heavy metals are well known for their toxicity and ability to bioaccumulate in aquatic ecosystems. The requirement of heavy metals by fishes is in traces while most of them act as micronutrients for both plants and animals, which are important components of enzymes and hormones, hence making them indispensable for an array of metabolic reactions. The transport of metals among fishes occurs through the blood, where the metal ions are usually tagged to proteins. Further, when metals are brought into the vicinity of different organs and tissues of the fish, they get accumulated there [36]. Therefore, it is but obvious that metals are usually present in high concentrations in the organs like gills, intestines, and digestive glands. The intestines of fishes are seldom consumed; they usually accumulate more heavy metals and might be considered as good bio-monitors of metals occurring in the surrounding environment. Studies suggest that metallothionein genes get triggered under heavy metal stress by specific transcription factors like MTF-1, which attaches to MREs (metal response elements) that are short DNA sequences [41]. At the genomic level, the expression of MTs is regulated transcriptionally by metal responsive transcription factor 1 (MTF-1). MTF-1 binds to metal-response elements (MREs) in the MT promotor site upon metal assault, which are significant in mediating the transcriptional responses to heavy metals [42, 43]. Fish discards consisting primarily of fish intestines were taken into use for preparing Ag nanoparticles [39] and goat meat processing discards for fabricating ZnO nanoparticles [39], which contain promising metabolites that often end in wastes. Finally, the death of cells tends to liberate the potential metabolites that facilitate fabrication of the nanoscale materials. Inorganic elements carry out important and otherwise not guaranteed functions. They are listed below:

- structural function (Ca^{2+} and Mg^{2+} for DNA polyanion)
- charge carriers for fast information transfer (Na^+, K^+, Ca^{2+} for electrical impulses in nerves, muscles contraction)
- formation, metabolism and degradation of organic compounds. These functions often require Lewis acid/base catalysis (Zn^{2+} in hydrolytic enzymes)
- electron transfer for energy conversion. This function requires redox active metal centres ($Fe^{II}/Fe^{III}/Fe^{IV}$, Cu^I/Cu^{II}, Co^I/Co^{II}).

In metallothionein, the major protectant of most of the animals including insects, 30–35% of amino acids are cystein with soft –SH groups coordination of soft heavy metal ions such as Cd^{2+}, Hg^{2+}, Pb^{2+}, and Zn^{2+}. Biological function of metallothioneins, as stated earlier, is to protect cells from toxic heavy metals (Fig. 4). So, as and when an animal tissue broth is challenged with any metal ion solution, the molecules respond in a jiffy leading to a successful nanomaterial synthesis depending upon the modulation of the pivotal parameters like pH and temperature.

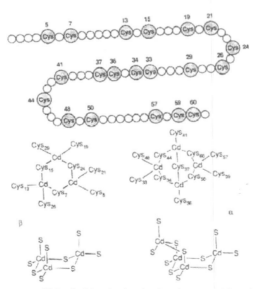

Fig. 4. Molecular structure of Metallothionein showing involvement of Cysteine in detoxification.

6. Soft Chemical Synthesis

The blind spree of industrialization in the past has indeed created many unhealing wounds over our environment and problems like global warming, green house effects are just to name a few. Every component of our ecosystem has been polluted. We generally forget that we have to transfer this environment to our coming generations. The world of chemistry has covered an appreciably long journey commencing from the 19th century as an era of classical organic chemistry when environment was virtually under little or no consideration and we created a huge dump of toxic chemicals in every component of the ecosystem. Light concern was displayed during the 20th century when materials were replaced in order to reduce emissions and the concept of environmental audit emerged. Energy and environment got integrated and things started changing globally. In 21st century, we realized the importance of green chemistry, sustainability and circular economy. Instead of exponentially strangling the existing resources, we realized that it is more sensible to realize the importance of recycling our existing ones by adopting clean and green procedures as well as by eliminating the toxic ingredients in our industrial procedures. The promulgation of WEEE and RoHS guidelines added an exemplary thrust to the above idea and an evolving approach towards Nanotechnology and Environmental Health and Safety (EHS) has been suggested in three phases by James Hutchison, director of the Safer Nanomaterials and Nanomanufacturing Initiative (SNNI) [44]:

1. Studies on significance of nanomaterials.
2. Research on significance and applications to be undertaken in a coordinated manner.
3. In order to eliminate hazards during the life cycle of materials, it would be necessary to emphasize on the green nanoscience approach during material and process designing steps.

The sole purpose of accomplishing a nanomaterial synthesis involving soft chemicals goes nicely along with above mentioned ideas. Green chemistry is "the utilization of a set of principles that reduces or eliminates the use or generation of hazardous substances in the design, manufacture, and application of chemical products". Nearly all of the principles of green chemistry can be readily applied to the design of nanoscale products, the development of nanosynthesis methods, and the application of nanomaterials.

The sole game proceeds as dissociation/ionization of metal salts, kinetics (first order, second order reaction), thermodynamics (principally free energy may be available through ionization/dissociation, decomposition due to heating, breaking of bonds, tautomerization, resonance, etc.), and phase transformation (by attaining the threshold in terms of available free energy- from micro to nano). The purpose is to achieve a high degree of super-saturation within narrow time and space. Along with this, suppression of aggregation/agglomeration, mono-disperse growth, diffusion controlled growth/Ostwald ripening are major stakes. At a given point of time, entire material will never get transformed; rather some will be transformed while others will be attaining the threshold, yet others will be at the interface of transformation. It is a procedure of slow graduation! In general, the synthetic strategies could be:

- Liquid Phase Synthesis
- Gas Phase Synthesis
- Vapour Phase Synthesis

Among these, the liquid phase synthesis is widely in use and is well developed due to the fact that it is amenable for higher compositions and sophisticated products; in addition to this, size control is also possible through modulation of the key parameters.

The soft chemical synthetic method was developed by our group as an off shoot of the sol-gel method where a lot of energy consuming and cumbersome steps were involved. We banked on the inherent chemical/thermodynamic potential of higher carboxylic acids such as citric, tartaric and/or stearic acid. Carboxylic acid, like citric acid, has an encouraging resonance energy of stabilization once dissolved in water and this helps in the procedure of synthesis. It helps in synthesizing metals, oxides/higher oxides, chalcognides, alloys, etc. Reaction conditions are required to be monitored carefully, very much amenable for synthesizing a variety of nanomaterials (Fig. 5).

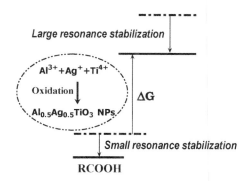

Fig. 5. Involvement of resonance energy in synthetic cue bestowed by citric acid.

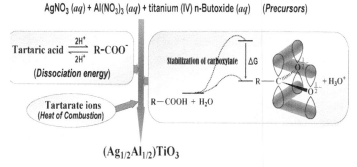

Fig. 6. Showing molecular level involvement of tartaric acid in synthetic cue.

Similarly, energy rich tartaric acid undergoes dissociation and under condition of heating at high temperature liberates sufficient amount of free energy for accomplishing synthesis of novel perovskites (e.g., $Ag_{1/2}Al_{1/2}TiO_3$) (Fig. 6).

7. Overall Thermodynamic Considerations

Cells are isothermal systems—they function at essentially constant temperature (and constant pressure). Heat flow is not a source of energy for cells because heat can work only as it passes to a zone or object at a lower temperature. The energy that cells can and must use is free energy, described by the Gibbs free-energy function G, which allows prediction of the direction of chemical reactions, their exact equilibrium position, and the amount of work they can, in theory, perform at constant temperature and pressure. Heterotrophic cells acquire free energy from nutrient molecules and photosynthetic cells acquire it from absorbed solar radiation. Both kinds of cells transform this free energy into ATP and other energy-rich compounds capable of providing energy for biological work at constant temperature.

Metal ions and biological ligands are important constituents of coordination complexes that are biologically pertinent: metal ions are Lewis acid sites that can accept lone pair of electrons of the ligand, which act as a Lewis base. This is well exemplified in metallothionein where 30–35% of its sulphur containing residue cysteine carries sulfhydryl groups. Metallothioneins protects the cells from toxic heavy metal assaults. Besides, the metal chelate complexes are stable due to release of non-chelating ligands. Additionally, the pKa values of coordinate ligands and alterations in the redox potentials also play significant role. The thermodynamic robustness of a metal centre is often affected by the biopolymers since it can regulate steric blockage of coordination sites and hydrogen bonding formation capability through its three-dimensional structure including its stereochemistry, available ligands for coordination, local hydrophilicity and/or hydrophobicity. Thermodynamic interaction/interdependence and its environment keeps molecules active and ensures nanomaterial formation. The mechanism of nanotransformation is based on the nucleation and growth theory to form a spherical particle in which the overall free energy change (ΔG) must be overcome. ΔG is the sum of the free energy due to the formation of a new volume and the free energy due to the new/novel surface being created [44]: $\Delta G = -\dfrac{4}{V}\, \pi r^3\, k_B\, T \ln(S) + 4\pi r^2\, \gamma$, here V, r, k_B, S and γ are the molecular volume of the precipitated species, radius of the nucleus, Boltzmann constant, saturation ratio, and surface free energy per unit surface area, respectively. What emanates from the above equation is that a decrease or increase in S helps in the formation of desired/targeted nanoparticles. The interactions of metabolites contained in the broth/culture medium with metal salt leads to concentration of metal ions surrounded by different metabolites like flavonoids, terpenoids, organic acids, proteins, etc., which get adhered to the metal nuclei and result in a lower surface energy of the crystal lattice. To summarize, the major metabolites along with the experimental cues determine the fate of fabrication of the type of nanomaterial and the source/mean/method, irrespective of the procedure whether chemical or biological, the crux always lies with the thermodynamic parameters. In addition, even in case of dead animal cells/tissues, its metabolites are not made ineffective, rather they engage in energy changes and are thermodynamically agile enough to pursue nano synthesis. The thermodynamic heat ensures phase transformation from microscale to the nanoscale.

Of the equal importance is yet another thermodynamic quantity, i.e., Partial Molar Volume (PMV) that decides the fate of a plant extract/animal tissue broth or a soft chemical mediated nanomaterials synthesis. The PMV is a thermodynamic quantity, which contains important information about the solute-solvent interactions as well as the solute structure in solution. Additionally, the PMV is the most essential quantity in the analysis of the pressure effect on chemical reactions. The PMV of a solute in solution Vu is defined as the volume change of solution when the solute is immersed into the solution: $Vu = (\partial V/\partial Nu)$. T, p, Nv; where V, T, and p are, respectively, the volume, temperature, and pressure of the solution system, and Nu and Nv are the numbers of solutes and solvents, respectively. Once we know the partial molar volume of two components of a binary mixture, we can calculate the total volume. The term activity is used in the description of the departure of the behaviour of a solution from ideality. In any real solution, interactions occur between the components which reduce the effective concentration of the solution. The activity is a way of describing this effective concentration. In an ideal solution or in a real solution at infinite dilution, there are no interactions between components and the activity equals the concentration. Non-ideality in real solutions at higher concentrations causes a divergence between the values of activity and concentration. The ratio of the activity to the concentration is called the activity coefficient, γ, that is γ = activity/concentration. Depending on the units used to express concentration, we can have either a molar activity coefficient, γm, a molar activity coefficient, γc, or, if mole fractions are used, a rational activity coefficient, γx. Properties such as volume, enthalpy, free energy and entropy, which depend on the quantity of substance, are called *extensive* properties. In contrast, properties such as temperature, density and refractive index, which are independent of the amount of material, are referred to as intensive properties. The quantity denoting the rate of increase in the magnitude of an extensive property with increase in the number of moles of a substance added to the system at constant temperature and pressure is termed a *partial molar quantity*. Partial molar quantities are of importance in the consideration of open systems, that is, those involving transference of matter as well as energy. Another partial molar property, already introduced, is the partial molar Gibbs function or the chemical potential. Of particular interest is the partial molar free energy, which is also referred to as the chemical potential, μ. So, the partial molar volumes provide useful information about various types of interactions occurring in solutions. It is particularly useful in nanomaterial synthetic protocols if we are pursuing the soft chemical route. These studies are of great help in characterizing the structure and properties of solutions. The solution structure is of great importance in understanding the nature of action of bioactive molecules in the body system. The addition of an organic solvent to water brings about a sharp change in the solvation of ions. The peculiarities of the aqueous–organic mixtures are well reflected in dramatic changes in the reaction rates. The medium effect or free energies of transfer of ions cannot be explained on the basis of change in the dielectric constants of the solvent mixtures alone. As partial molar volume of a solute reflects the cumulative effects of solute–solvent interactions, it would be of interest to study partial molar volumes of the organic acids viz. citric acid and tartaric acid in binary aqueous mixtures of ethanol. Such data are expected to highlight the role of organic acids in influencing the partial molar volumes in mixed solvent systems.

In a nutshell, the organic and inorganic systems show appreciable dynamism in terms of solvation, ionization and dissociation and this leads to the liberation of free energy. Their representation is broadly functional leading to a cascade of thermodynamic events. This area is largely unexplored and unreported in nanoscience and technology literatures and warrants further investigation in order to further thermodynamically details of free energy availability in different procedures.

References

[1] Gallegos, M.T., R. Schleif, A. Bairoch, K. Hofmann and J.L. Ramos. 1997. Arac/XylS family of transcriptional regulators. Microbiol. Mol. Biol. Rev. 61: 393.

[2] Hantke, K. 2001. Iron and metal regulation in bacteria. Curr. Opin. Microbiol. 4: 172.

[3] Hutkins, R.W. and N.L. Nannen. 1993. pH homeostasis in Lactic Acid bacteria. J. Dairy Sci. 76: 2354.

[4] http://www.lactic.com/index.php/lacticacid. (2009).

[5] Avery, S.V. 2001. Metal toxicity in yeasts and the role of oxidative stress. Adv. Appl. Microbiol. 49: 111.

[6] Limon-Pacheco, J. and M.E. Gonsebatt. 2009. The role of antioxidants and antioxidant-related enzymes in protective responses to environmentally induced oxidative stress. Mutat. Res. 674: 137.

[7] Jha, A.K. and K. Prasad. 2019. Biosynthetic methods for inorganic nanoparticles: Nature's silent pursuit. *In*: Nalwa, H.S. (ed.). Encyclopaedia of Nanoscience and Nanotechnology 26: 485.

[8] Jha, A.K., K. Prasad and K. Prasad. 2009. Biosynthesis of Sb_2O_3 nanoparticles: A low-cost green approach. Biotechnol. J. 4: 1582.

[9] Ray, S., S. Sarkar and S. Kundu. 2011. Extracellular biosynthesis of silver nanoparticles using the mycorrhizal mushroom *Tricholoma Crassum* (BERK.) SACC: Its antimicrobial activity against pathogenic bacteria and fungus, including multidrug resistant plant and human bacteria. Digest J. Nanomater. Biostruct. 6: 1289.

[10] Lapworth, A. and A. Hann. 1902. The mutarotation of camphorquinonehydrazone and mechanism of simple desmotropic change. J. Chem. Soc. 81: 1508.

[11] Poelarends, G., V. Veetuk and C. Whitman. 2008. Tautomerism: Introduction, history, and recent developments in experimental and theoretical methods. Cell. Mol. Life Sci. 65: 3606.

[12] Kasthuri, J., K. Kathiravan and N. Rajendiran. 2009. Phyllanthin assisted biosynthesis of silver and gold nanoparticles: A novel biological approach. J. Nanopart. Res. 11: 1075.

[13] Jha, A.K. and K. Prasad. 2014. Green synthesis of silver nanoparticles and its activity on SiHa cervical cancer cell line. Adv. Mater. Lett. 5: 501.

[14] Prasad, K.S., D. Pathak, A. Patel, P. Dalwadi, R. Prasad, P. Patel and K. Selvaraj. 2011. Biogenic synthesis of silver nanoparticles using *Nicotiana Tobaccum* leaf extract and study of their antibacterial effect. Afr. J. Biotechnol. 10: 8122.

[15] Rao, M.L. and N. Savithramma. 2011. Biological synthesis of silver nanoparticles using *Svensonia Hyderabadensis* leaf extract and evaluation of their antimicrobial efficacy. J. Pharm. Sci. Res. 3: 1117.

[16] Jha, A.K. and K. Prasad. 2011. Biosynthesis of gold nanoparticles using Bael (*Aegle marmelos*) leaf: Mythology meets technology. Int. J. Green Nanotechnol.: Phys. Chem. 3: 92.

[17] Das, S., J. Das, A. Samadder, S.S. Bhattacharyya, D. Das and A.R. KhudaBukhsh. 2013. Biosynthesized silver nanoparticles by ethanolic extracts of *Phytolacca decandra, Gelsemium*

sempervirens, *Hydrastis Canadensis* and *Thuja occidentalis* induce differential cytotoxicity through G2/M arrest in A375 cells. Colloids Surf. B: Biointerfaces 101: 325.

[18] Sathishkumar, M., S. Krishnamurthy and Y.S. Yun. 2010. Immobilization of silver nanoparticles synthesized using *Curcuma longa* tuber powder and extract on cotton cloth for bactericidal activity. Biores. Technol. 101: 7958.

[19] Chandran, S.P., M. Chaudhary, R. Pasricha, A. Ahmad and M. Sastry. 2006. Synthesis of gold nanotriangles and silver nanoparticles using *Aloe vera* plant extract. Biotechnol. Prog. 22: 577.

[20] Ghule, K., A.V. Ghule, J.Y. Liu and Y.C. Ling. 2006. Microscale size triangular gold prisms synthesized using Bengal gram beans (*Cicer arietinum* L.) extract and $HAuCl_{4x}3H_2O$: a green biogenic approach. J. Nanosci. Nanotechnol. 6: 3746.

[21] Narayanan, K.B. and N. Sakthivel. 2008. Coriander leaf mediated biosynthesis of gold nanoparticles. Mater. Lett. 62: 4588.

[22] Armendariz, V., I. Herrera, J. Peralta-Videa, M. Jose-Yacaman, H. Troiani and P. Santiago. 2004. Size controlled gold nanoparticle formation by *Avena sativa* biomass: use of plants in nanobiotechnology. J. Nanopart. Res. 6: 377.

[23] Ghule, K., A.V. Ghule, J.Y. Liu and Y.C. Ling. 2006. Microscale size triangular gold prisms synthesized using Bengal gram beans (*Cicer arietinum* L.) extract and $HAuCl_4$ $3H_2O$: A green biogenic approach. J. Nanosci. Nanotechnol. 6: 3746.

[24] Savithramma, N., M.L. Rao and P.S. Devi. 2011. Evaluation of antibacterial efficacy of biologically synthesized silver nanoparticles using stem barks of *Boswellia ovalifoliolata* Bal. and Henry and *Shorea tumbuggaia* Roxb. J. Biol. Sci. 11: 39.

[25] Jha, A.K. and K. Prasad. 2011. Green fruit of chili (*Capsicum annum* L.) synthesizes nano silver! Digest J. Nanomater. Biostruct. 6: 1717.

[26] Shankar, S.S., A. Rai, B. Ankamwar, A. Singh, A. Ahmad and M. Sastry. 2004. Biological synthesis of triangular gold nano prisms. Nat. Mater. 3: 482.

[27] Jha, A.K., V. Kumar and K. Prasad. 2011. Biosynthesis of metal and oxide nanoparticles using orange juice. J. Bionanosci. 5: 162.

[28] Awwad, A.M., N.M. Salem and A.O. Abdeen. 2013. Biosynthesis of silver nanoparticles using loquat leaf extract and its antibacterial activity. Adv. Mat. Lett. 4: 338.

[29] Rao, K.J. and S. Paria. 2013. Green synthesis of silver nanoparticles from aqueous *Aegle marmelos* leaf extract. Mater. Res. Bull. 48: 628.

[30] Singh, A., D. Jain, M.K. Upadhyay, N. Khandelwal and H.N. Verma. 2010. Green synthesis of silver nanoparticles using *Argemone mexicana* leaf extract and evaluation of their antimicrobial activities. Digest J. Nanomater. Biostruct. 5: 483.

[31] Pandey, S., G.K. Goswami and K.K. Nanda. 2013. Green synthesis of polysaccharide/gold nanoparticle nanocomposite: an efficient ammonia sensor. Carbohyd. Polym. 94: 229.

[32] Ghule, K., A.V. Ghule, B.J. Chen and Y.C. Ling. 2006. Preparation and characterization of ZnO nanoparticles coated paper and its antibacterial activity study. Green Chem. 8: 1034.

[33] Raut, W.R., J.R. Lakkakula, N.S. Kolekar, V.D. Mendhulkar and S.B. Kashid. 2009. Phytosynthesis of silver nanoparticle using *Gliricidia sepium* (Jacq.). Curr. Nanosci. 5: 117.

[34] Arruda, L.K., L.D. Vailes, B.J. Mann, J. Shannon, J.W. Fox, T.S. Vedvick, M.L. Haden and M.D. Chapman. 1995. Molecular cloning of a major cockroach (*Blattella germanica*) allergen, Bla g 2. Sequence homology to the aspartic proteases. J. Biol. Chem. 270: 19563.

[35] Ballan-Dufrançais, C. 2002. Localization of metals in cells of pterygote insects. Microsc. Res. Tech. 56: 403.

[36] Asturias, J.A., N. Gómez-Bayón, M.C. Arilla, A. Martínez, R. Palacios, F. Sánchez-Gascón and J. Martínez. 1999. Molecular characterization of American cockroach tropomyosin (*Periplaneta americana* allergen 7), a cross-reactive allergen. J. Immunol. 162: 4342.

[37] Yepiskoposyan, H., D. Egli, T. Fergestad, A. Selvaraj, C. Treiber, G. Multhaup, O. Georgiev and W. Schaffner. 2006. Transcriptome response to heavy metal stress in Drosophila reveals a new zinc transporter that confers resistance to zinc. Nucleic Acids Res. 34: 4866.

[38] Jha, A.K. and K. Prasad. 2016. Now the household mosquitoes (*Culex* Sp.) synthesize CdS nanoparticles! J. Chin. Adv. Mater. Soc. 4: 140.

[39] Egli, D., J. Domenech, A. Selvaraj, K. Balamurugan, H. Hua, M. Capdevila, O. Georgiev, W. Schaffner, and S. Atrian. 2006. The four members of the Drosophila metallothionein family exhibit distinct yet overlapping roles in heavy metal homeostasis and detoxification. Genes Cells 11: 647.

[40] Joshi, J.G. and A. Zimmerman. 1988. Ferritin: An expanded role in metabolic regulation. Toxicology 48: 21.

[41] Ayandiran, T.A., O.O. Fawole, S.O. Adewoye and M.A. Ogundiran. 2009. Bioconcentration of metals in the body muscle and gut of *Clarias gariepinus* exposed to sub lethal concentrations of soap and detergent effluent. J. Cell Animal Biol. 3: 113.

[42] Selvaraj, A., K. Balamurugan, H. Yepiskoposyan, H. Zhou, D. Egli, O. Georgiev, D.J. Thiele, and W. Schaffner. 2005. Metal-responsive transcription factor (MTF-1) handles both extremes, copper load and copper starvation, by activating different genes. Genes Dev. 19: 891.

[43] Cooper, A. 1999. Protein: A Comprehensive Treatise (Allen Geoffrey Ed.), Vol. 2, pp. 217–270, JAI Press, Inc., Greenwich, CT, USA.

[44] Stuart, G.W., P.F. Searle, H.Y. Chen, R.L. Brinster and R.D. Palmiter. 1984. A 12-base-pair DNA motif that is repeated several times in metallothionein gene promoters confers metal regulation to a heterologous gene. Proc. Natl. Acad. Sci. USA 81: 7318.

2

Biosynthesis of Silver Nanoparticles Using Leaf Extracts Characteristics

Zygmunt Sadowski, *Joanna Feder-Kubis* and *Anna Wirwis*

1. Introduction

Currently, the synthesis of nanoparticles might be performed by deploying a variety of techniques that are divided into three groups: physical, chemical and biological. The recommendations of "green chemistry" suggest employing biological methods that are environmentally friendly [1]. Biologically inspired methods of nanoparticles synthesis involve the application of bacteria [2], fungus [3], algae [4], yeasts [5], and plants [6]. Plants are the best candidate for nanoparticle biosynthesis due to their easy availability and the fact that they are readily available. Not all plants are suitable for the biosynthesis of nanoparticles. It turned out that plants that were previously applied as a therapeutic agent are most often used in biosynthesis. Plants offer this important advantage that it is simple to prepare desired extract for the ions' bioreduction. The substances extracted from plants, apart from reducing properties, also have the ability to stabilize the fabricated nanoparticles. Various parts of plant are fitting for the extraction (Fig. 1).

The most common are leaves, followed by flowers [7], stems [8], roots [9], and skins of fruit [10]. This chapter presents information on the biosynthesis of silver nanoparticles, with particular focus on the extract processes, where leaves are used as sources materials. Since ionic liquids are of importance in the extraction, the input in

Wroclaw University Science and Technology, Department of Process Engineering and Polymer and Carbon Materials, Wybrzeze Wyspianskiego 27, 50-370 Wroclaw, Poland.

* Corresponding author: zygmunt.sadowski@pwr.edu.pl

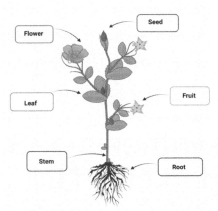

Fig. 1. Plant parts used in preparation of the extract (created with BioRender.com).

the synthesis of nanoparticles by the biological path using those ionic systems will be highlighted here. Silver nanoparticles are characterized by antibacterial properties, which is a sufficient reason why they can find application in the production of food packaging. Research on the production of this type of packaging is devoted to the BioNanoPolys program financed under the "Horizon 2020" program of the European Union.

2. Aqueous Extract of Leaves

Green leaves are collected, carefully washed with distilled water, then dried on the air in a sunny place and ground into powder which is the basis for extraction carried out at an elevated temperature, usually 60–90°C. Powder slurry is often briefly boiled (5–30 min) [11]. Filter Whatman No. 1 removes the biomass remaining after extraction from the suspension. Obtained in this manner, pure extract was next utilized for the synthesis of nanoparticles or should be stored in a refrigerator. The chemical composition of the extracts depends on the kind of plants from which they have been obtained. Different parts of plant have their own phytochemical compositions and potential bioreduction properties. Broadly, the extract consists of such groups of chemical compounds as: flavonoides, polyphenolics, reducing sugars, terpenoides, peptides, membrane proteins, and organic acids. These compounds have in turn such functional group as: amines, aldehydes, ketones, alcohols, carboxylic acid and sulfhydryl, that can actively participate in the silver ion bioreduction. Although bioreduction of silver ions using numerous type of plant extract still is ambiguous, the following phyto-reduction reaction can be predicted Fig. 2.

a) Flavonoids

b) Terpenoids

c) Saponins

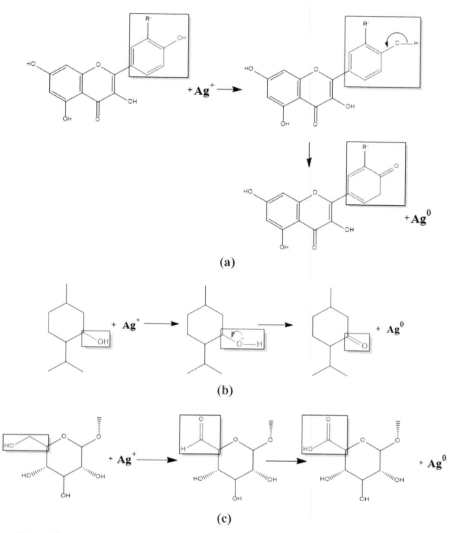

Fig. 2. Phyto-reduction of Ag+ ions to AgNPs by (a) flavonoids, (b) terpenoids, and (c) saponins.

3. Silver Nanoparticles Biosynthesis

It was about 20 years ago that the first information on the biosynthesis of silver nanoparticles with the use of aqueous leaf extract emerged. The extract was prepared by means of *Azardirachta indica* (Neen) [12], alfalfa [13], and *Pelargonium graveolens* Geranium [12]. This method of nanoparticle biosynthesis soon won popularity. Review published ten and more years later reveal dozens of examples of various plants suitable for the synthesis of nanoparticles [14, 15]. Table 1 shows the list of plants whose leaves were a source material for silver nanoparticles' biosynthesis in the period 2020–2022.

Table 1. List of plants used for AgNPs biosynthesis in the period 2020–2022.

Plant	Family	AgNP size [nm]	Shape	References
Brillantaisia patula	Acanthaceae	45–110	spherical	[16]
Caesalpinia digyna	Fabaceae	11.3–45.4	spherical	[17]
Cannabis sativa	Cannabaceae	26.52 (average)	uniformity	[18]
Carica papaya	Caricaceae	10–20	smooth and spherical	[19]
Carissa carandas	Caricaceae	35 (for 25°C) 30 (for 60°C)	spherical	[20]
Crossoptery febrifuga	Rubiaceae	45–110	spherical	[16]
Cucumis prophetarum	Cucurbitaceae	30–50	spherical	[21]
Delonix regia	Fabaceae	43.5 (average)	oval	[22]
Elytraria acaulis (Lindau)	Acanthaceae	5–100	spherical	[23]
Eryngium caucasicum	Apiaceae	10–20 17.5 (average)	spherical	[24]
Eucalyptus camaldulensis	Myrtaceae	28 (SEM) 68 (DLS)	spherical	[11]
Hagenia abyssinica	Rosaceae	22.2 (SEM)	spherical	[25]
Ixora brachypoda	Rubiacea	18–50 27.76 (average)	spherical	[26]
Juglans negia	Juglandaceae	6.93 and 7.16 (ultrasound)	oval	[27]
Juniperus excelsa	Cupressaceae	16.08–24.42	hexagonal spherical	[28]
Lotus lalambebsis	Fabaceae	6–26	oval	[29]
Melia azedarach	Melaiaceae	18–30 23 (average)	spherical	[30]
Mentha aquatica	Lamiaceae	14 8 (ultrasound)	spherical	[31]
Mentha pulegium	Lamiaceae	17.7 (average)	spherical	[32]
Musa paradisiaca	Musaceae	80–100	bed	[33]
Naringi crenulate	Rutaceae	20–40	spherical	[34]
Oryza sativa	Poeceae	36–107	spherical	[35]
Platycladus orientalis	Cupressaceae	8 (average)	spherical	[36]
Quercus coccifera	Fagaceae	50–70	spherical	[37]
Salanum surattense	Solanceae	52.27 (average)	spherical	[38]
Salvia coccinea	Lamiaceae	24–28.4	spherical	[39]
Senna siamea	Fabaceae	45–110	spherical	[16]
Syngonium podophyllum	Araceae	2–47 25 (average)	spherical	[40]

carried out at a temperature of 40°C with a 1:1 ratio of IL to water. The results of saponins and polyphenols extraction with the ILs were 30% better than those from reactions based on ethanol-water mixture. ILs can play various roles in the synthesis of silver nanoparticles, including stabilizing properties and functionalizing agents. Additionally, imidazolium salts possess weak reducing properties and have been shown to be the way for silver nanoparticle nucleation. The stability of nanoparticles is contingent on capping reagents and ILs, like surfactants, are able to prevent aggregation. Generally, there is electrostatic and steric stability. The charge located on the surface of nanoparticles is of the essence in electrostatic stability. The multiplicity of zeta potential is an indicator of nanoparticles' stability. The steric stability is a result of protective layer formatted around nanoparticle that prevents aggregation. The formation of the hydrogen bond is one of the factor determining the occurring of a layer of ionic liquid molecules around the nanoparticle. The most common ionic liquids serving as stabilizing agents include imidazolium base ILs [56]. These liquids have a long alkyl chain that functions like a surfactant that sterically stabilizes AgNPs. This means that the structure of the IL molecule plays an important role on the morphology of tested AgNPs.

Acknowledgement

This chapter was supported by the H2020 project (grant agreement no. 953206) Open innovation test bed for developing safe nano-enabled bio-based materials and polymer bionanocomposites for multifunctional and new advanced applications "BioNanoPolys" (2021–2024).

References

[1] Saravanan, A., P.S. Kumar and S. Karishma. 2021. A review on biosynthesis of metal nanoparticles and its environmental application. Chemosphere 264: 128580.

[2] Narayanan, K.B. and N. Sakthivel. 2010. Biological synthesis of metal nanoparticles by microbes. Adv. Colloid Interface Sci. 156: 1.

[3] Mukherjee, P., S. Senapati, D. Mandal, D. et al. 2002. Extracellular synthesis of gold nanoparticles by the fungus *Fusariun oxysporum*. Chem. Bio. Chem. 3: 461.

[4] Sarayaraj, K., S. Rajesh, and M.J. Rathi. 2012. Silver nanoparticles biosynthesis using marine alga *Padina pavonic* and its microbial activity. Dig. J. Nanometer. Biostructure 7: 1557.

[5] Kowshik, M., S. Ashtaputre, S. Kharrazi et al. 2003. Extracellular synthesis of silver nanoparticles by a silver-tolerant yeast strain MKY3. Nanotechnology 14: 95.

[6] Ahmed, S., Saifullah, M. Ahmad, L.B. Swami and S. Ikram. 2016. Green synthesis of silver nanoparticles using *Azadirachta indica* aqueous leaf extract. J. Radiat. Res. Appl, Sci. 9: 1.

[7] Babu, A.S. and G.H. Prabu. 2011. Synthesis of AgNPs using the extract of *Colotropis procera* flower at room temperature. Mater. Lett. 65: 1675.

[8] Veeramani, S., E. Ravindran, P. Ramodoss, C. Joseph, K. Shanmugan and S. Renganathans. 2018. Silver nanoparticles – Green synthesis with aq. extract of stems *Ipomoea Pes-Caprae*. characterization, antimicrobial and anti-cancer potential. Int. J. Med. Nano Res. 5: 24.

[9] Arokiyaraj, S., S. Vincent, M. Saravanan, Y. Lee, K.Y. Oh and H.K. Kim. 2017. Green synthesis of silver nanoparticles using *Rheum palmatum* root extract and their antibacterial activity against *Staphylococcus aurelus* and *Pseudomonas aeruginosa*. Artif. L. Cell, Nanomed. Biotechnol. 45: 372.

[10] Bankar, A., B. Joshi, R.A. Kumar and S. Zinjarde. 2010. Banana peel extract mediated novel rout for the synthesis of nanoparticles. Colloids Surf. A Physicochem. Eng. Asp. 368: 58.

[11] Alghorai, I., Ch. Soukkaich, R. Zein, A. Alahamad, J-G. Walter and M. Daghestani. 2020. Aqueous extract of *Eucalyptus camaldulensis* leaves as reducing and capping agent in biosynthesis of silver nanoparticles. Inorg. Nano-Mat. Chem. 50: 895.

[12] Shankar, S.S., A. Ahmed and M. Sastry. 2003. Geranium leaf assisted biosynthesis of silver nanoparticles. Biotechnol. Prog. 19: 1627.

[13] Gardea-Torresday, L.J., E. Gomez. R.J. Peralta-Videa, G.J. Parsons, H. Troiani and M. Jose-Yacaman. 2003. Alfalfa sprouts: A natural source for the synthesis of silver nanoparticles. Langmuir 19: 1357.

[14] Shah, M., D. Fawcett, S. Sharma, K.S. Tripathy and J.E.G. Poinern. 2015. Green synthesis of metallic nanoparticles via biological entities. Materials 8: 7278.

[15] Ahmed, S., M. Ahmed, L.S. Swami and S. Ikaram. 2016. A review on plants extract mediated synthesis of silver nanoparticles for antimicrobial applications: A green expertise. J. Adv. Res. 7: 17.

[16] Kambale, EK.E., I.C. Nkanga and B-P. Mutonkole. 2020. Green synthesis antimicrobial nanoparticles using aqueous leaf extract from three congolese plant species. Heliyon. 6: e4493.

[17] Niloy, S.M., M. Hossain and M. Takikawa. 2020. Synthesis of silver nanoparticles using *Caesalpinia digyna* and investigation of their antimicrobial activity an *in vivo* biocompatibility. ACS Appl. Bio. Mater. 3: 7722.

[18] Chouhan, S. and S. Guleria. 2020. Green synthesis of AgNPs using *Cannabis sativa* leaf extract: Characterization, antibacterial, anti-yeast and α-amylaz inhibitory activity. Mater. Sci. Energy. Technol. 3: 536.

[19] Singh, P.S., A. Mishra, K.R. Shyanti, R.P. Singh and A. Acharya. 2021. Silver nanoparticles synthesized using *Carica papaya* leaf extract, AgNPs-PEL causes cell cycle arrest and apoptosis in human prostate (DU 145) cancer cells. Biol. Trace Elem. Res. 199: 1316.

[20] Singh, R., C. Hano, G. Nath and B. Sharma. 2021. Green biosynthesis of silver nanoparticles using leaf extract of *Carissa carandas* L. and their antioxidant and antimicrobial activity against human pathogenic bacteria. Biomolecules 11: 299.

[21] Hemlata, R.P. Meena, P.A. Singh and K.K. Tejavath. 2020. Biosynthesis of silver nanoparticles using *Cucumis prophetarium* aqueous leaf extract and their antibacterial and antiproliferative activity against cancer cell lines. ACS Omega 5: 5520.

[22] Siddiquee, A., M. Uddin Parray and H.S. Mehdi. 2020. Green synthesis of silver nanoparticles from *Delonix regia* leaf extract: *In-vitro* cytotoxicity and interaction studies with bovine serum albumin. Mat. Chem. Phys. 242: 122493.

[23] Rangayasami, A., K. Kannan, S. Jashi and M. Subban. 2020. Bioengineered silver nanoparticles using *Elytraria acaulis* (L.f) Lindau leaf extract and its biological applications. Biocatal. Agric. Biotechnol. 27: 101690.

[24] Azizi, M., S. Sedaghat, K. Tahvildari, P. Derakhshi and A. Ghaemi. 2020. Green biosynthesis of silver nanoparticles with *Eryngium caucasicum Trautv* aqueous extract. Inorg. Nano-Mat. Chem. 50: 429.

[25] Melkamu, W.W. and T.L. Bitew. 2021. Green synthesis of silver nanoparticles using *Hagenia abyssinica* (Bruce) *J.F Gmel* plant leaf extract and their antibacterial and anti-oxidant activities. Heliyon. 7: e08459.

[26] Bhat, M., B. Chakraborty and S.R. Kumar. 2021. Biogenic synthesis, characterization and antimicrobial activity of *Ixora brachypoda* (DC) leaf extract mediated silver nanoparticles. J. King Saud Univ. Sci. 33: 101296.

[27] Hosseini, A.A., H. Djahaniani and F. Nabati. 2021. Ultrasound-assisted biosynthesis of Ag nanoparticles using *Juglans negia* L. leaves extract. Main Group Chem. 20: 1.

[28] Good El-Rab, F.M.S., M.E. Halawan and S.S.S. Alzahrani. 2021. Biosynthesis of silver nano-drug using *Juniperus excelsa* and its synergistic antibacterial activity against multidrug-resistant bacteria for wound dressing application. Biotech. 11: 255.

[29] Abdallah, M.B. and M.E. Ali. 2021. Green synthesis of silver nanoparticles using *Lotus lalambensis* aqueous leaf extract and their anti-candidal activity against oral candidiasis. ACS Omega 6: 8151.

[30] Jebril, S., B.K.R. Janana and C. Dridi. 2020. Green synthesis of silver nanoparticles using *Melia azedarach* leaf extract and their antifungal activities. *In vitro* and *in vivo*. Mater. Chem. Phys. 248: 122898.

[31] Nouri, A., T.M. Yaraki, A. Lajevarch, Z. Rezaei, M. Gharbanpour, and M. Tanzifi. 2020. Ultrasonic-assisted green synthesis of silver nanoparticles using *Mentha aquatica* leaf extract for enhanced antibacterial properties and catalytic activity. Colloid Interface Sci. Commun. 36: 100252.

[32] Wang, Y. and S. Wei. 2021. Green fabrication of bioactive silver nanoparticles using *Mentha pulegium* extract under alkaline: An enhanced anticancer activity. ACS Omega 10: 16267.

[33] Narasimha, R., V.L. Hublikar, M.S. Patil and P. Bhat. 2021. Microwave assisted biosynthesis of silver nanoparticles using banana leaves extract. J. Water Environ. Nanotechnol. 6: 49.

[34] Vallinayagam, S., K. Rajendran and V. Sekar. 2021. Green synthesis and characterization of silver nanoparticles using *Naringi crenulate* leaf extract: Key challenges for anticancer activities. J. Mol. Struct. 1243: 130829.

[35] Saha, I., M. Hasanuzzaman, D. Sibhas, C.S. Debnath and K.M. Adak. 2021. Silver-nanoparticle and abscisic acid modulate sub 1A submergence tolerance in rice (*Oryza sativa* L.). Environ. Exp. Bot. 181: 104276.

[36] Anshiba, J., M. Poonkothai, P. Karthika and R. Mythili. 2022. Green route a novel and eco-friendly phytosynthesis of silver nanoparticles using *Platycladus orientalis* L. leaf extract. Mater. Lett. 309: 131347.

[37] Kocazorbaz, K.E., H. Moulahoum and E. Tut. 2021. Kermes oak (*Quercus coccifera* L.) extract for a biogenic and eco-benign synthesis of silver nanoparticles with efficient biological activities. Environ. Technol. Innov. 24: 102067.

[38] Moni, M., H.J. Chano and D.A. Gandhi. 2020. Environmental and biomedical application of AgNPs synthesized using the aqueous extract of *Solanum surattense* leaf. Inorg. Chem. Commun. 121: 108228.

[39] Shanmugan, G., A. Sundaramoorthy and N. Shanmugan. 2021. Biosynthesis of silver nanoparticles from leaf extract of *Salvia coccinea* and its effects anti-inflammatory potential in tuman monocytic THP-cells. ACS App. Bio Mater. 4: 8433.

[40] Naaz, R., U.V. Siddiqui, U.S. Qadrir and A.W. Siddiqi. 2021. Green synthesis of silver nanoparticles using *Syngonium podophyllum* leaf extract and its antibacterial activity. Mater. Today: Proc. 46: 2353.

[41] Prathna, C.T., N. Chandrasekaran, M.A. Raichu and A. Nukherjee. 2011. Kinetic evolution studies of silver nanoparticles in bio-based green synthesis process. Colloids Surf. A Physicochem. Eng. Asp. 377: 212.

[42] Li, G., D. He, Y. Qian et al. 2012. Fungus – mediated green synthesis of silver nanoparticles using *Aspergillus terneus*. Int. J. Mol. Sci. 13: 466.

[43] Khan, Z., I.J. Hussan and A.A. Hashmi. 2012. Shape-directing role of cetyltrimethylammonium bromide in green synthesis of Ag-nanoparticles using Neem (*Azadirachta indica*) leaf extract. Colloids Surf. B. 95: 229.

[44] Joseph, S. and B. Mathew. 2015. Microwave-assisted green synthesis of silver nanoparticles and the study on catalytic activity in the degradation of dyes. J. Mol. Liq. 204: 181.

[45] Joseph, S. and B. Mathew. 2014. Microwave assisted biosynthesis of silver nanoparticles using the rhizome extract of *Alpinia galanga* and evaluation of their catalytic and antimicrobial activities. J. Nanopart. 9: 967802.

[46] Anjana, N.V., M. Joseph, S. Francis, A. Joseph, E. Koshy and B. Mathew. 2021. Microwave assisted green synthesis of silver nanoparticles for optical, catalytic, biological and electrochemical applications. Artif. Cells, Nanomed. Biotechnol. 49: 438.

[47] Huang, J., L. Lin, Q. Li et al. 2008. Continuous-flow biosynthesis of silver nanoparticles by lixivium of sundried *Cinnamomum camphora* leaf in turbular microreactor. Ind. Eng. Chem. Res. 47: 6081.

[48] Liu, H., J. Huang, D. Sun et al. 2012. Microfluidic biosynthesis of silver nanoparticles: Effect of process parameters on size distribution. Chem. Eng. J., 209: 568.

[49] Cushing, L.B., L.V. Kolesnichenko and J. O'Connor. 2004. Recent advances in the liquid-phase syntheses of inorganic nanoparticles. Chem. Rev. 104: 3893.

[50] Anju, R.T., S. Parvathy, V.M. Veettil, J. Rosemary, H.T. Ansalna and M.M. Shahzabanu. 2021. Green synthesis of silver nanoparticles from *Aloe vera* extract and its antimicrobial activity. Mater. Today: Proc. 43: 3956.

[51] Kanawaria, K.S., A. Sankhla and K.P. Jatav. 2018. Rapid biosynthesis and characterization of silver nanoparticles: an assessment of antibacterial and antimycotic activity. Appl. Phys. A. 124: 320.

[52] Rashidipour, M. and H. Rouhollah. 2014. Biosynthesis of silver nanoparticles using extract of olive leaf synthesis and *in vitro* cytotoxic effect on MCF7 cells. J. Nanostruct. Chem. 4: 112.

[53] Jin, R., L. Fan, X. An et al. 2011. Microwave assisted ionic liquid pretreatment of medicinal plant for fast solvent extraction of active ingredients. Sep. Purif. Technol. 83: 45.

[54] Patil, V., S. Mahajn, M. Kulkarni et al. 2020. Synthesis silver nanoparticles colloids in imidazolium halide ionic liquids and their antibacterial activity for gram-positive and gram-negative bacteria. Chemosphere 2020: 125302.

[55] Ribeiro, D.B., Z.A.M. Coelho, N.P.L. Rebelo and M.I. Marrucho. 2013. Ionic liquids as additives for extraction of saponin and polyphenols from Mate and tea (*Camellia sinensis*). Ind. Eng. Chem. Res. 32: 12146.

[56] Verma, C., E.E. Ebensa and A.M. Quraishi. 2019. Transition metal nanoparticles in ionic liquids synthesis and stabilization. J. Mole. Liq., 276: 826.

3

Nanofabrication Using Natural Cohorts

Shushay Hagos Gebre

1. Introduction

The physical and chemical approaches are used extensively and effectively to synthesize the nanomaterials. However, these approaches employed harsh environmental conditions, rigorous energy, and toxic byproducts. Physical processes are performed without toxic reducing reagents, and narrow size distribution of the nanoparticles (NPs) are formed. However, physical techniques such as ball milling and laser ablation demand high energy consumption, tedious procedures and instrumentations and stringent conditions [1–3]. The chemical method is also popular, and most of its protocol depends on using toxic reducing agents like *N, N*-dimethylformamide (DMF), celyltriethylammonium chloride (CTAC), sodium borohydride, hydrazine, and organic solvents. The chemicals employed during the production of the nanomaterials are highly reactive, release undesirable byproducts and cause potential environmental and biological threats [4, 5]. The nanomaterials may not used directly for clinical application due to the toxic chemical absorbed on their surface [6]. In this context, researchers have developed a lucrative, environmentally benign strategy that provides a superior platform to fabricate various nanomaterials with well-defined morphology. The bionanofabrication of nanomaterials using living entities of plants and microorganisms has opened a new frontier for the biosynthesis of nanomaterials. Since this strategy does not require further stabilizing or capping chemical agents, the plant and microorganism constituents are used as capping and stabilizing agents [7]. Nature can also synthesize biocompatible nanomaterials,

College of Natural and Computational Science, Department of Chemistry, Jigjiga University, P.O. Box 1020, Jigjiga, Ethiopia.
Email: shushayhagos@gmail.com

for example, magnetite nanostructures are obtained in magnetotactic bacteria as a part of their magnetic navigation devices which alludes to studying another microorganism [8].

Furthermore, microbes naturally detoxify metal ions into nanomaterials. The detoxifying mechanism may vary from one microorganism to another; some export them using efflux pumps, changing their solubility and altering their redox state. Other organisms may reduce the metal ions to their elemental forms. Then researchers harnessed the latter to redox the mechanism for synthesizing various nanomaterials using microbial cells like bacteria, fungi, yeast, and algae. Nowadays, the nanofabrication of nanomaterials with the help of microorganisms is popular and has incredible capability in non-toxic solvents (H_2O) under mild conditions [9].

Thus, the biological or green method is environmental friendly in which the primary and secondary metabolites are used as natural biological agents during the biosynthesis procedure. The functional groups of the proteins or enzymes and phytochemicals are synergistically used as reducing, capping, and stabilizing agents. The plant system is straightforward and advantageous to the microorganism due to the devoid of complex and multi-step procedures like culturing and isolation [10]. The biosynthesis of the NPs with the help of plant extract includes the basic sequential steps of bio-reduction, nucleation, growth, coarsening, and aggregation [11] (Fig. 1a).

The nanofabrication is not limited to metal or metal oxide nanoparticles (MoNPs) [12, 13]. Hence, metallic nanocomposites, bimetallic, trimetallic [14], quadrometallic nanostructures (QMNs), and hybrid are also promoted using the green route [15]. The nanomaterials are manipulated to various forms of multicomponent systems to improve their stability and performance. Due to the synergistic consequence among the metals, the ternary materials showed better performance in energy conversion than the bimetallic and monometallic systems. Organic nanomaterials like reduced graphene oxide (rGO), the effective supporting material for the metal NPs, are also synthesized using the plant array system. Leave extracts of *Cynodon dactylon*, *Azadirachta indica*, and *Juglans regia* plants have been used to synthesize metal-free carbon nanotube [16].

The functional groups of the biomolecules are synergistically or collectively used as capping agents to stabilize the NPs. Especially the plant and food-related derived NPs can be used for clinical applications without fear since they are free from toxic chemicals that probably adsorbs on their surface. Water extract *Citrus macroptera* fruit peel promotes the formation of 11 nm average size and face-centered cubic crystals and spherical morphology Ag NPs for catalytic degradation of organic dyes [17]. Similarly, an aqueous extract of *Caesalpinia bonducella* seeds were used to derive rice-shaped CuO NPs. The plant is known for its antioxidant activity since it contains citrulline, phytosterinin, β-carotene, and flavonoids which act as reducing, stabilizing, and capping agents. The obtained CuO NPs was utilized as a sensor and appeared to have good reproducibility and stability for 120 days [18]. Ethanol extracted embelin from *Embelia tsjeriam-cottam* fruit was successfully converted salt solution of Ag^+ and Au^{+3} to their corresponding quasi-spherical and nanostars. Embelin was used as a reducing and capping agent,

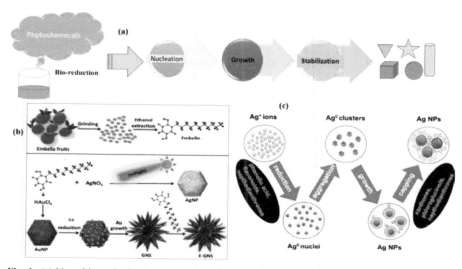

Fig. 1. (a) Nano biosynthesis steps using plant phytochemical (b) extraction of embelin from the fruits of *Embelia tsjeriam-cottam* and synthesis of embelin stabilized silver nanoparticles (Ag NP), gold nanoparticles (AuNP) and gold nanostars (E-GNS) using embelin reducing and stabilizing agent [19], (c) Putative model for the *H. perforatum* extract-mediated green synthesis of Ag NPs [20], Reproduced with permission from American Chemical Society.

which was able to used to grow the NPs via nucleation and their subsequent growth, as shown in Fig. 1b. The mall sizes of 3–15 nm of Ag and 12–15 nm of Au NPs are formed, respectively. The embelin stabilized gold nanostars (E-GNS), Au, and Ag NPs were created at a pH of 12 [19]. In another recent study, aerial part of *Hypericum perforatum*, which is also known as St. John's wort, has been used for the fabrication of Ag NPs. The medicinal plant has unique bioactive compounds such as xanthones, phloroglucinols, and naphthodianthrones used as reducing and capping agents. When the plant extract is added, the Ag^+ ion is rapidly reduced to Ag^0. The atomic nuclei form a cluster of NPs until the maximum size is reached. The hydrophobicity nature of the Ag NPs allows binding with the capping agents on their surface to stabilize the surface energy, as demonstrated in Fig. 1c [20].

2. Microbial Based Nanofabrication

2.1 Fungi Mediated Nanofabrication

The use of fungal biomass for the fabrication of nanomaterials is a recent interest due to its ready availability, simple culturing process, bioaccumulation ability to uptake metals, and its secretion of higher amount of proteins than the other microorganisms [21]. Fungi have enzymes and reducing components on their surface capable of bio-reduction of the metal ions to the nanoscale [22]. Further, fungi cell walls are rich in glycoproteins and carbohydrates made from glucan and chitin, which can react with the metal ions in the extra or intracellular systems [23]. The extracellular synthesis is better than the intracellular one since additional purification and extraction methods are required for the intracellular system, which may reduce the yield and quality of the final product [24]. To date, various fungi strains, namely *Rhizopus Oryzae, Neurospora crassa, Trichoderma harzianum, Aspergillus oryzae, Helminthosporum solani, Cladosporium* sp., *Fusarium* sp., *Penicillium* sp., *Fusarium semitectum,* and *Candida albicans* are reported for the biosynthesis of MNPs, MoNPs, and nanocomposites [25, 26].

Biomolecules obtained from fungi extracts also serve as a capping agent during the synthesis of the NPs, which protects the NPs from agglomerations. Biologically (fungi *Pycnoporus* sp. templated) synthesized Ag NPs were carried out against Gram-positive and negative bacteria using the agar well diffusion method. The microbial-mediated Ag NPs exhibited a zone inhibition of 24, 25, 26, and 22 mm for *aureus, B. subtilis, E. coli,* and *Klebsiella pneumonia,* respectively. However, the chemically synthesized Ag NPs showed 20, 19, 20, and 18 mm corresponding to *aureus, B. subtilis, E. coli,* and *Klebsiella pneumonia* [27]. Different shapes of Au NPs were synthesized using cell-free extract of the fungal strain *Rhizopus oryzae* at room temperature. The operating parameters (reaction time, metal ion concentration, and pH) greatly affect the formation of different shapes of Au, namely hexagonal, pentagonal, triangular, spherical, spheroidal, urchinlike, two-dimensional nanowires, and nanorods. The Au NPs were obtained using $HAuCl_4$ (1500 mg/L and pH 5.0) after 24 hrs reaction time. Then, the triangles, hexagons, pentagons, and star-shaped Au NPs are formed at a concentration and pH of (1000 mg/L and pH 8.0), (1500 mg/L and pH 3.0), (2000 mg/L and pH 6.0), and (2000 mg/L and pH 10.0) after 24 h reaction time, respectively. As the gold ion concentration increases to 2500 mg/L at pH 9.0, a quasi-spherical shape resembling sea urchin is formed. Further increasing the gold ion concentration to 4000 mg/L, pH 10.0 lead to the formation of long wire Au NPs after 20 hrs, increasing the reaction time to 30 hrs to form single nanorods [28].

2.2 Bacteria Mediated Nanofabrication

Bacteria are another potential source for the fabrication of nanomaterials through extracellular or intracellular pathways. Bacterial reducing enzymes such as NADH-dependent reductase or nitrate-dependent reductase play an essential role to reduce the metal ions into NPs [29]. The extracellular protocol is straightforward as it does not use complex downstream procedures [30]. *Proteus vulgaris* cultured mediated iron oxide NPs is synthesized using 10 mL of 3 mM $FeCl_3$ solution with 90 mL of bacterial supernatant extracellularly. The mixture was shaken for 5 days. A spherical shape with 19.23–30.51 nm size was obtained. Further, the NP was stable for two months without any deterioration while using as antioxidant and antibacterial activities [31]. The bacteria-assisted biosynthesis is more challenging than the fungi or plant sources due to cell culturing and isolation procedures.

The nanofabrication mechanism may vary from bacteria to bacteria due to the varieties of bioactive macromolecules. The oxidation of NADH-dependent reductase enzyme to NAD^+ involves an electron transfer used for the bio-reduction of the metal ions to specific NPs [32]. The nanofabrication has been taking place in the cell wall of the bacteria. The metal ions enter the cytoplasm and are transported via the wall meshwork for extracellular delivery. Peptidoglycans of the cell wall

Table 2. Biosynthesis of nanomaterials using plant part extracts.

Plants	Parts	NPs	Metal ion source	Size (nm)	Shape	Reaction conditions	References
Buddleja globosa	leave	Ag	$AgNO_3$	16	Spherical	5% extract, r.t., 5 h, 10 mM $AgNO_3$	[90]
Silybum marianum	seed	Pd	$PdCl_2$	5	Spherical	10^{-1} M $PdCl_2$, 4 mL extract, r.t., 2 h	[91]
Pongamia pinnata	bark	Ag	$AgNO_3$	5–55	Spherical	10 mL extract, 1 mM $AgNO_3$, r.t.,	[92]
Tagetes erecta	flower	Ag	$AgNO_3$	10–90	Spherical	1 mM $AgNO_3$, 6 mL extract, r.t., 24 h	[93]
Carica papaya	latex	Ag	$AgNO_3$	12 ± 6	Spherical	2% extract, 2 mM $AgNO_3$, 37°C, 72 h	[94]
Cocos nucifera L.	-	Pd	$Pb(OAC)_2$	47 ± 2	Spherical	1 mM $Pb(OAC)_2$, 20 mL extract, r.t.	[95]
Limonia acidissima	fruit	Ag	$AgNO_3$	25–45	Spherical	1 mM $AgNO_3$, 10 mL extract	[96]
Centella asiatica	-	Ce	$(NH_4)_2Ce(NO_3)_6$	1–100	Spherical	4.5 mM salt, 5 mg/mL extract, 10 min	[97]
Azadirachta indica	leave	Ag	$AgNO_3$	34	Dispersed and Spherical	1 mM $AgNO_3$, 1–5 mL extract, r.t., 24 h	[98]
Murraya koenigii	leave	Fe	$FeSO_4.7H_2O$	59	Spherical	0.10 M metal precursor, r.t.	[99]
Gleichenia pectinata	leave	Ag	$AgNO_3$	7.51	Spherical	5 mM $AgNO_3$, 10 mL extract, 30 min	[100]
Punica granatum	seed	α-Fe_2O_3	$FeCl_3 6H_2O$	26.53	Irregular	150 mL $FeCl_3 6H_2O$, 75°C, 15 min, 50 mL extract	[101]
Emblica officinalis	fruit	Se	Na_2SeO_3	20–60	Spherical	2 mL extract, 10 mM Na_2SeO_3, 27 ± 2°C, 24 h	[102]
Ficus hispida Linn	leave	Ag	$AgNO_3$	20	Spherical	4 mM $AgNO_3$, 10 mL extract, 60 min, 90°C	[103]
Annona muricata	leave	Au	$AuCl_3$	25.5	Spherical	1 mL extract, 1 mM $AuCl_3$, 22 h	[104]
Coptidis rhizome	rhizome	Ag	$AgNO_3$	26.42	Spherical	1 mM $AgNO_3$, 40°C	[105]
Ziziphus zizyphus	leave	Au	$HAuCl_4.3H_2O$	50	Spherical	5 mL extract, 1 mM $HAuCl_4$	[106]
Origanum vulgare L.	-	Ag	$AgNO_3$	2–25	Spherical	1 mL extract, 0.5 mM $AgNO_3$, 2 h, 85–90°C	[107]

Table 2 contd. ....

...Table 2 contd.

Plants	Parts	NPs	Metal ion source	Size (nm)	Shape	Reaction conditions	References
Withania coagulans	leave	$Pd/RGO/Fe_3O_4$	$FeCl_3.6H_2O$, $PdCl_2$	7–13	-	6 h, 100°C, 15 mL extract	[108]
Astragalus tribuloides	root	Ag	$AgNO_3$	34.2	Spherical	10 mL extract, 1 mmol/L $AgNO_3$, r.t.	[109]
Alternanthera sessilis	leave	Ag	$AgNO_3$	23.44	Spherical	1 mM $AgNO_3$, 5–10 mL extract, 60 min	[110]
Capsicum baccatum L.	fruit	Au	$HAuCl_4.xH_2O$	23.9 ± 9.7	Spherical	3 mL extract, 0.5 mM $HAuCl_4$, r.t., 60 min	[111]
Catharanthus roseus	leave	Au	$HAuCl_4$	25–35	Sphere-shaped	1 mM $HAuCl_4$, 1 mL extract, 24 h	[112]
Colocasia esculenta and Mesua ferrea L.	leave, peel	rGO	Graphite	5.3	Sheet	10 mL extract, 60 mg GO	[113]
Phoenix dactylifera	root	Ag	$AgNO_3$	15–40	Spherical	5 mL root extract, 0.1 mM $AgNO_3$	[114]
Phoenix dactylifera	leave	Pd	$PdCl_2$	13	Irregular	0.003 M $PdCl_2$, 10 mL extract, 10 min	[115]
Alysicarpus monilifer	leave	Ag	$AgNO_3$	15 ± 2	Spherical	150 mL extract, 1 mM $AgNO_3$, 10 min	[116]
Cocos nucifera	-	Pb	$Pb(OAC)_2$	47 ± 2	Spherical	20 mL, 80 mL lead acetate, r.t.	[95]
Sphaeranthus indicus	leave	Au	$HAuCl_4.3H_2O$	25	Spherical	1 mM $AuCl_4$, 10 mL extract, 30 min, pH = 5.4	[117]
Nerium oleander	leave	Au	$HAuCl_4$	2–10	Spherical	10 mL, 3×10^{-2} M $HAuCl_4$, 2 h	[118]
Zanthoxylum chalybeum	root	Ag	$AgNO_3$	50–100	Spherical	10 mL of 2.5 mg/mL root extract, pH = 9, 60°C, 18 h, 0.5–5.0 mM $AgNO_3$	[119]
Ramunculus laetus	leave	Ag	$AgNO_3$	24.125	Spherical	0.1 M $AgNO_3$, 10 mL extract, 24 h	[120]

Ocimum sanctum	leave	Ag	$AgNO_3$	14	Spherical	60°C, 10 min, 2 mM $AgNO_3$	[121]
Amentotaxus assamica	leave	Au	$HAuCl_4$	16	Spherical	0.01 M $HAuCl_4$, 55°C	[122]
Cacumen platycladi	leave	Au-Pd	$HAuCl_4/PdCl_2$	7.4	Spherical	0.25 mM of $HAuCl_4$, $PdCl_2$, 20 mL extract	[123]
Ocimum tenuiflorum	leave	ZnO	$Zn(NO_3)_2$	38		45 min, 130°C, 50 mL extract, 5 g $Zn(NO_3)_2$	[124]
Eryngium campestre	leave	Cu/Cr/Ni	$CuSO_4.5H_2O$, $Cr(NO_3)_3.9H_2O$, $Ni(NO_3)_2.6H_2O$	100–104	Irregular	3.5 min, *r.t.*, pH = 7	[125]
Origanum vulgare	leave	Cu/Co/Ni	$Cu(NO_3)_2 \cdot 3H_2O$, $Co(NO_3)_2 \cdot 6H_2O$, $Ni(NO_3)_2 \cdot 6H_2O$	28.25	Irregular	20 mL extract, 0.01 M of each metal precursors, 40°C	[126]

catechins, and co-enzymes are responsible reducing agents. Similarly, live plants can also reduce the metal ions to nanostructuré [75]. Plant-based polyphenols are known as natural antioxidants with potential drug, and food additives are largely studied mainly as possible biological reducing agents in the biosynthesis [5].

Small size NPs are obtained using the plant extracts than the chemical methods; for example, 11–21 nm size ZnO NPs were obtained using Avocado fruit extract. However, 30–40 nm size of the NP was produced using precipitation synthesis methods. The activity of the bioinspired ZnO NPs was also 15–24 mm of a zone of inhibition against *Bacillus subtilis, Staphylococcus aureus,* and *Salmonella,* which is nearer to the standard drug (25 mm), while a 7–15 mm zone of inhibition was registered for the chemically synthesized ZnO [76]. In another study, *Bixa orellana* seed-extract derived TiO_2 NPs and sol-gel-mediated TiO_2 NPs were used for photovoltaic applications. The seed-mediated NP was a pure anatase phase, whereas the chemically synthesized one was a mixed phase of brookite and anatase. The formation of the pure anatase enhanced the surface area of the NPs and exhibited better performance than the conventionally obtained TiO_2 NPs. The seed-derived TiO_2 showed 1.97% photovoltaic conversion efficiencies; however, the sol-gel-mediated one possessed only 1.03% [77].

Aqueous leave extracts of *Gardenia jasminoides* promoted Ag–Fe bimetallic NP have been obtained. The spherical shape and 13 nm (± 6.3 nm) average diameter size magnetic NP exhibited better bactericidal activity against gram-positive and gram-negative bacteria than the monometallic NP due to the synergistic effect between Ag and Fe [78]. NPs such as CuO, Fe_3O_4, and Fe are successfully fabricated for catalytic applications using *Stachys Lavandulifolia* flowers, *Pisum sativum* peels, and *Trigonella foenum-graecum* seeds, respectively [79–81]. Recent studies witnessed that multi-metallic NPs showed superior biological, environmental, and energy conversion activities due to the electronic effect among the metals. A novel Au/Pt/Ag trimetallic nanoparticle (TNPs) is obtained from an aqueous extract of *Lamii albi flos* and 5 mM of $AgNO_3$, $HAuCl_4$, and K_2PtCl_6 in a 1:1:1 ratio after string for 24 h at 70°C. The TNPs with 35–40 nm particle size showed promising results in the bactericidal activities [82]. In another study, 20 nm size, spherical, triangular, and hexagonal shaped *Meliloti officinal* derived Au/ZnO/Ag TNP is prepared from 5 mM of each $HAuCl_4$, $ZnCl_2$, and $AgNO_3$ solution in the same ratio at 70°C for 24 h [83]. A simple bioinspired method synthesizes Ag NPs using *Rhodiola rosea* Rhizome extract. A regular spherical shape with a small size (10 nm) of the NPs is obtained. The rhizome-mediated Ag NPs exhibited better performance in antioxidant and catalytic degradation of hazardous organic dyes. The NPs also used for fluorescence enhancer at a minimum concentration [84]. Polyphenols, gamma sterol, and n-hexadecanoic acid-rich *Curculigo orchioides* rhizome extracts are used for the biosynthesis of spherical morphology with 15–18 nm size of Ag NPs. The as-synthesized NPs showed promising results in antibacterial, larvicidal, and anticancer activities [85].

Various shape-controlled nanomaterials are fabricated using seed and fruit extracts, for example, stable rice-shaped Cu NPs are obtained using *Caesalpinia bonducella* seed extract assisted biosynthesis (Fig. 3a, b) [18]. *Xanthium strumarium*

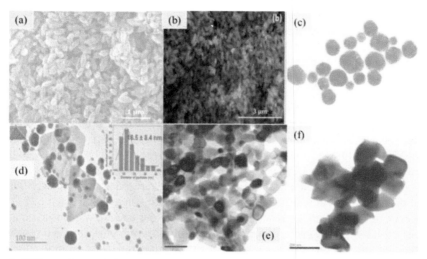

Fig. 3. Different shapes of plant part extract-mediated NPs (a, b) rice-shaped Cu NPs [18], Reproduced with permission from American Chemical Society (c) pentagonal, spherical, and hexagonal shaped Au NPs [86], (d) triangular shaped Au NPs [87], (e) TEM image of ZnO NPs synthesized using water extract of *Artocarpus gomezianus* fruit [88], (f) TEM image of CuO NPs synthesized using water extracts of *Tinospora cordifolia* leaves [89], (c–e) Reproduced with permission from Elsevier.

L. fruit isolated (caffeoylxanthiazonoside) is reported for the biosynthesis of 25 nm average size and pentagonal, spherical, and hexagonal shaped Au NPs (Fig. 3c) [86]. Similarly, triangular and hexagonal shaped Au NPs are produced using *Diospyros Kaki* L. fruits rich in polyphenols, flavonoids and sugars biomolecules (Fig. 3d). At various reaction temperatures, 99.45 ± 0.14%, 99.74 ± 0.02%, and 97.99 ± 0.02% of Au^{3+} ions were successfully converted into Au NPs applying 0.5, 1.0 and 1.5 mM of $HAuCl_4.4H_2O$, respectively, after centrifugal ultrafiltration [87]. Highly porous nature ZnO NPs with an energy bandgap of 3.3 eV and 370 nm UV-Visible absorbance is obtained using water extract *Artocarpus gomezianus* fruit (Fig. 3e). It was found that 17.16% of polyphenols and 22% of flavonoids were the secondary metabolites responsible for reducing of the $Zn(NO_3)_3.6H_2O$ to ZnO NPs [88]. Furthermore, water extract *Tinospora cordifolia* was also reported for the fabrication of large surface area, small size (6–8 nm), and sponge-like structure CuO NPs (Fig. 3f). Plant extracts of 0.3, 0.4, and 0.5 g were mixed with 1.205 g of $Cu(NO_3)_2.3H_2O$ to yield CuO NPs with higher bandgap energy than the bulk CuO [89].

5. Factors Influencing the Nanofabrication of Nanomaterials

Various factors are considered during the biosynthesis of the nanomaterials to control the shape, size, surface area, and yield of the particles, such as reaction time, temperature, pH, plant/microbes' extract volume, and precursor concentration [127]. The reaction time is primarily short minutes, and the reactions are carried out at average temperatures [90]. A calcination temperature is carried out after the NPs have grown to increase the crystallinity, aggregation, and to remove impurities.

Still, the size of the particles rises as the temperature increases. The calcination temperature also affects the phase transformation among the NPs, for example, the transformations from anatase to brookite or rutile and vice versa in TiO_2 NPs [128].

Most findings suggested that aggregated and large particle size NPs have resulted in lower pH (< 2); however, at a high pH value, the accessibility of the functional groups of the plant extract is available for the NPs' nucleation resulting in the formation of small sized nanoparticles [129]. The effect of banana peel extract (BPE) volume was reported during the synthesis of Ag NPs. Intensive color (dark reddish-brown) and maximum surface plasmon resonance (SPR) peak was observed when 3 mL of BPE was used, but light reddish-brown color was observed when 0.25, 0.5, and 0.75 mL of the BPE extracts were applied. This implies all available silver ions were reduced when enough phytochemicals were present. Similarly, highly monodispersed Ag NP was obtained at a pH of 11 with an average size of 23.7 nm. However, at a pH of 2.0, no reaction occurred and color change was observed at pH values of 4.5–6.5. The biomolecules are probably inactive or protonated under the acidic medium, and electrostatic repulsion between the protonated biomolecules and Ag^+ ion occurred, whereas under neutral or basic conditions, the biomolecules are negatively charged, which enables them to transfer the electrons to the Ag^+, which reduces Ag(0) [130].

Biomass of *Cacumen Platycladi* extracts (CPE) was reported for Pt NPs synthesis. The reaction temperature for converting Pt(II) to Pt NP was studied. The conversion rate was 81.2% at 90°C, whereas 27% conversion was obtained at 30°C; the particle size of the Pt NPs was 2.0 ± 0.4, 2.6 ± 0.4, and 2.9 ± 0.7 nm at 30, 60, and 90°C, respectively. Regarding the effect of the salt concentration (Na_2PtCl_4), 86.5% and 64.7% conversion of Pt NPs has been exhibited using 0.5 and 2 mM Na_2PtCl_4, respectively. The CPE concentration also affects the conversion rate and size of the NPs. Greater than 95% conversion and 2.4 ± 0.8 nm particle size of Pt NPs were recorded using 70% CPE at 25 h reaction time, whereas 3.7 ± 0.7, 3.1 ± 0.7, and 2.9 ± 0.7 nm particle size of the NPs exhibited CPE percentages of 10, 30, and 50%, respectively [131]. The shape and size of the nanomaterials can be controlled by adjusting the solution temperature. If the reaction temperature is too high, it increases the reaction kinetics. However, if the kinetics of responses is fast, it is difficult to control the growth of the nanomaterials and poor bio-reduction process, uncontrolled, large size, and fast aggregations occur. In this regard, most biosynthesis reactions are carried out at a low temperature, which helps to control the reaction easily [132].

6. Possible Reaction Mechanisms

Without a clear understanding, diverse primary and secondary metabolites cooperatively reduce the metal ions to nanoscale forms. The metabolites that act as a defense mechanism or chemical transformations of the plants to control various acute diseases are synergistically employed as reducing and capping agents. The functional groups of the phytochemical, mostly polar groups such as amine, hydroxy, carboxylic acids, thiol, and carbonyl groups, react with the electron-deficient metal ions, which are reduced via electrons that flow from the phytochemicals to the metal to activate the nucleation process. The plant phytochemicals are used as donors of electrons to the metal ion to convert into nanostructures. The formation of high surface area in the NPs allows for accommodating the phytochemical functional groups and a potential chelating site to form stable nanostructures. All the phytochemicals may not participate in reducing the ions, but they also showed outstanding tenacity against agglomeration [133–136].

Aqueous leave extracts of *Plantago asiatica* have been reported for the nanofabrication of Cu NPs. The Cu NPs are produced in a 20 mL solution of 3 mM $CuCl_2.2H_2O$ with 100 mL of the leave extract with vigorous shaking at 80°C. The changing of color to dark within 5 min indicates the formation of Cu NPs. The antioxidant polyphenolic (quercetin) compound of the leave extract is used as a reducing agent, which oxidizes itself to ketone groups as shown in the proposed reaction mechanism (Fig. 4a) [137]. In another study, *Cocos nucifera* L. methanol extract was used to fabricate Pd NPs for photocatalytic application. 20 mL of methanol extract was mixed with 80 mL of lead acetate solution and was allowed to stir at room temperature. The extract contained phenolic compounds with a major constituent of 3-methoxy cinnamic acid as determined by Gas chromatography-mass spectrometry (GC-MS). The 3-methoxy cinnamic acid has been dehydrated while reacting with the salt solution to yield Pb-NPs (Fig. 4b) [95].

The transformation of the bioactive constituents of the plant extracts is confirmed by comparing the plant extracts before and after the synthesis of the nanomaterials, mostly via the FTIR spectra. For example, *Anacardium occidentale* testa, known in catechin, epicatechin, and epigallocatechin compounds, was used for the nanofabrication of Ag NPs. As shown in Fig. 4c, the spectra (green) of the plant extract showed both hydroxy and carbonyl groups; similarly, the plant-derived Ag NPs showed both groups (orange spectra) in the FTIR, but additional sharp spectra at 1384 cm^{-1} is shown for nitrate ion [138].

In most of the reported studies, the peaks of the common functional groups are present even after calcination at a higher temperature. Once the phytochemicals can stabilize the nanomaterials, they are expected to decompose to CO_2, O_2, H_2O, and NO_2 gases after calcination; this needs deeper investigation since the peaks that appeared in the FTIR spectra may result from the adsorption of the gases on the surface of the nanomaterials. For example, *Gloriosa superba* L. leaf extract-derived CeO_2 NPs calcined at 400°C for 2 h confirmed the presence of the main functional groups almost similar to the uncalcined CeO_2 and the plant extract spectrum as shown in Fig. 4d. The Ce-OH, water, and CO_2 absorption peaks may be due to the trapped air from ambience [139]. Similarly, the *Cissus quadrangularis* leaf extract mediated CuO NPs (30 ± 2 nm) calcined at 300–400°C in a furnace showed the presence of organic functional groups such as O-H, C=O, and C-O stretching peaks in both the leaf extracts and the calcined NPs [140] (Fig. 4e). Calcination temperature affects the size, shape, and performance of the biosynthesized NPs. For example, *Bacillus subtilis* mediated Ag NPs showed potent inhibition against pathogenic bacteria; however, after calcination at 300°C, it does not show any inhibition. Similarly, the size of the uncalcined NPs was 18–100 nm; however, after calcination, it becomes 49–253 nm [141]. If the plant or microbe extracts themselves have antimicrobial

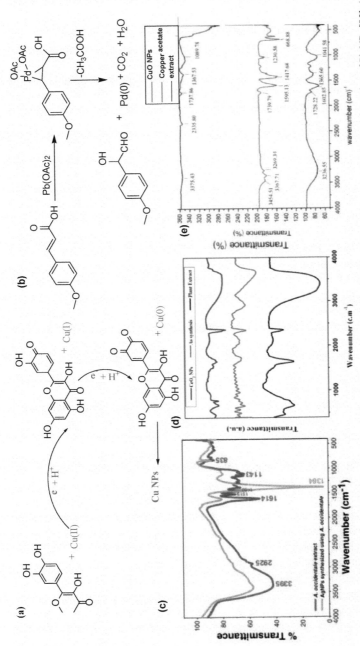

Fig. 4. (a) Green synthesis of Cu NPs using the aqueous extract of the *Plantago asiatica* leave [137], (b) Possible mechanism behind formation of Pb-NPs [95], (c) FT-IR spectra of *A. occidentale* testa extract and synthesized Ag NPs [138], (d) FTIR spectra of *G. superba* plant extract, as-prepared sample and CeO$_2$ NPs [139], (e) FT-IR spectroscopy of CuO NPs [140], Reproduced with permission from Elsevier.

activity, the capped NPs pertain to a synergistic effect. The NPs obtained without calcination (dried at oven) clearly show the presence of the bioactive molecules of the plant extract in the FTIR spectra.

7. Conclusion and Future Prospects

The green synthesis of the nanomaterials is a simple and one-step method, an economically feasible and environmentally benign approach, and an efficient alternative to the chemical methods. The green chemistry approach receives researchers' attention for synthesizing various forms of nanomaterials using extracts of plant parts and microbes as reducing, stabilizing or capping agents for biomedical, agricultural, and environmental applications. The biosynthesized nanoparticles are biocompatible and showed promising activities against antibacterial, antioxidant, anticancer, biosensors and drug delivery. They also reduce environmental hazards, wastes, generate energy, etc. Though the green synthesis has all the advantages above, some limitations must be dealt with in the future. The yield and reproducibility of the green approach must be explored. The bio-reduction reaction mechanism between the salt metal ions and phytochemicals should be investigated well. The concentration of the phytochemicals responsible for the bio-reduction of the metals may vary due to seasonal and environmental uncertainties, which may limit the effectiveness of the bio-reduction process. Finally, the toxicity and side effects of the nanomaterials/nanoparticles should be considered and investigated since some reports showed that the metal nanoparticles are toxic to human and aquatic systems.

References

[1] Gebre, S.H. 2021. Recent developments in the fabrication of magnetic nanoparticles for the synthesis of trisubstituted pyridines and imidazoles: A green approach. Synth. Commun. 51: 1669. https://doi.org/10.1080/00397911.2021.1900257.

[2] Kora, A.J. 2018. Plant and tree gums as renewable feedstocks for the phytosynthesis of nanoparticles: a green chemistry approach. *In*: Kanchi, S. and S. Ahmed (eds.). Green Metal Nanoparticles Microwave, 79. Scrivener Publishing LLC, Hyderabad.

[3] Souza, T.A.J., L.R.R. de Souza and L.P. Franchi. 2019. An integrated view of green synthesis methods, transformation in the environment, and toxicity. Ecotoxicol. Environ. Safety 171: 691. https://doi.org/10.1016/j.ecoenv.2018.12.095.

[4] Fakhari, S., M. Jamzad and H.K. Fard. 2019. Green synthesis of zinc oxide nanoparticles: a comparison. Green Chem. Lett. Rev. 12: 19. https://doi.org/10.1080/17518253.2018.1547925.

[5] Yadi, M., E. Mostafavi, B. Saleh, S. Davaran, R. Khalilov, M. Nikzamir and M. Milani. 2018. Current developments in green synthesis of metallic nanoparticles using plant extracts: a review. Artificial Cells, Nanomed., Biotechnol. 46: S336. https://doi.org/10.1080/21691401.2018.1492931.

[6] Naika, H.R., K. Lingaraju, K. Manjunath, D. Kumar, G. Nagaraju, D. Suresh and H. Nagabhushana. 2015. Green synthesis of CuO nanoparticles using *Gloriosa superba* L. extract and their antibacterial activity. J. Taibah Uni. Sci. 9: 7. https://doi.org/10.1016/j.jtusci.2014.04.006.

[7] Akhtar, M.S., J. Panwar and Y. Yun. 2013. Biogenic synthesis of metallic nanoparticles by plant extracts. ACS Sustain. Chem. Eng., 1: 591. https://doi.org/10.1021/sc300118u.

[8] Stankic, S., S. Suman, F. Haque and J. Vidic. 2016. Pure and multi metal oxide nanoparticles: synthesis, antibacterial and cytotoxic properties. J. Nanobiotechnol. 14: 73. https://doi.org/10.1186/s12951-016-0225-6.

[9] Choi, Y. and S.Y. Lee. 2020. Biosynthesis of inorganic nanomaterials using microbial cells and bacteriophages. Nature Rev. Chem. 4: 638. https://doi.org/10.1038/s41570-020-00221-w.

[10] Lade, B.D. and A.S. Shanware. 2020. Phytonanofabrication: Methodology and factors affecting biosynthesis of nanoparticles. *In*: Bochenkov, V. and T. Shabatina (eds.). Smart Nanosystems for Biomedicine, Optoelectronics and Catalysis, 1, IntechOpen, Nagpur.

[11] Chugh, H., D. Sood, I. Chandra, V. Tomar, G. Dhawan and R. Chandra. 2018. Role of gold and silver nanoparticles in cancer nano-medicine. Artificial Cells, Nanomed., Biotechnol. 46: S1210. https://doi.org/10.1080/21691401.2018.1449118.

[12] Gebre, S.H. 2021. Recent developments of supported and magnetic nanocatalysts for organic transformations: an up-to-date review. Appl. Nanosci. 13: 15. https://doi.org/10.1007/s13204-021-01888-3.

[13] Gebre, S.H. and M.G. Sendeku. 2019. New frontiers in the biosynthesis of metal oxide nanoparticles and their environmental applications: an overview. SN Appl. Sci. 1: 928. https://doi.org/10.1007/s42452-019-0931-4.

[14] Gebre, S.H. and M.G. Sendeku. 2022. Trimetallic nanostructures and their applications in electrocatalytic energy conversions. J. Energy Chem. 65: 329. https://doi.org/10.1016/j.jechem.2021.06.006.

[15] Flak, D., E. Coy, M. Jarek, O. Ivashchenko, Ł. Przysiecka, B. Peplin and S. Jurga. 2021. Organic-inorganic hybrid nanoparticles synthesized with *hypericum perforatum* extract: potential agents for photodynamic therapy at ultra-low power light. ACS Sustain. Chem. Eng. 9: 1625. https://doi.org/10.1021/acssuschemeng.0c07036.

[16] Tripathi, N., V. Pavelyev and S. Islam. 2017. Synthesis of carbon nanotubes using green plant extract as catalyst: unconventional concept and its realization. Appl. Nanosci. 7: 557. https://doi.org/10.1007/s13204-017-0598-3.

[17] Saha, P., Mahiuddin, A.B.M.N. Islam and B. Ochiai. 2021. Biogenic synthesis and catalytic efficacy of silver nanoparticles based on peel extracts of *Citrus macroptera* fruit. ACS Omega 6: 18260. https://doi.org/10.1021/acsomega.1c02149.

[18] Sukumar, S., A. Rudrasenan and D.P. Nambiar. 2019. Green-synthesized rice-shaped copper oxide nanoparticles using *Caesalpinia bonducella* seed extract and their applications. ACS Omega 5: 1040. https://doi.org/10.1021/acsomega.9b02857.

[19] Sasidharan, S., R. Poojari, D. Bahadur and R. Srivastava. 2018. Embelin mediated green synthesis of quasi-spherical and star-shaped plasmonic nanostructures for antibacterial activity, photothermal therapy and computed tomographic imaging. ACS Sustain. Chem. Eng. 6: 10562. https://doi.org/10.1021/acssuschemeng.8b01894.

[20] Pradeep, M., D. Kruszka, P. Kachlicki, D. Mondal and G. Franklin. 2022. Uncovering the phytochemical basis and the mechanism of plant extract-mediated eco-friendly synthesis of silver nanoparticles using ultra-performance liquid chromatography coupled with a photodiode array and high-resolution mass spectrometry. ACS Sustain. Chem. Eng. 10: 562. https://doi.org/10.1021/acssuschemeng.1c06960.

[21] Nagajyothi, P.C., S.V.P. Vattikuti, K.C. Devarayapalli, K. Yoo, J. Shim and T.V.M. Sreekanth. 2019. Green synthesis: Photocatalytic degradation of textile dyes using metal and metal oxide nanoparticles-latest trends and advancements. Critical Rev. Environ. Sci. Technol. 50: 2617. https://doi.org/10.1080/10643389.2019.1705103.

[22] Virkutyte, J. and R.S. Varma. 2013. Green synthesis of nanomaterials: environmental aspects. *In*: Sharma, S. (ed.). Sustainable Nanotechnology and the Environment: Advances and Achievements, 11. American Chemical Society, Washington DC.

[23] Matussin, S., M.H. Harunsani, A.L. Tan and M.M. Khan. 2020. Plant-extract-mediated SnO_2 nanoparticles: Synthesis and applications. ACS Sustain. Chem. Eng. 8: 3040. https://doi.org/10.1021/acssuschemeng.9b06398.

[24] Wang, N., H.Y.J. Fuh, S.T. Dheen and A.S. Kumar. 2021. Synthesis methods of functionalized nanoparticles: a review. Bio-Des. Manufact. 4: 379. https://doi.org/10.1007/s42242-020-00106-3.

[25] Bakshi, M., S. Mahanty and P. Chaudhuri. 2017. Fungi-mediated biosynthesis of nanoparticles and application in metal sequestration. *In*: Das, S. and H.R. Dash (eds.). Handbook of Metal–Microbe Interactions and Bioremediation, 423. https://doi.org/10.1201/9781315153353.

[26] Shi, C., N. Zhu, Y. Cao and P. Wu. 2015. Biosynthesis of gold nanoparticles assisted by the intracellular protein extract of *Pycnoporus sanguineus* and its catalysis in degradation of 4-nitroaniline. Nanoscale Res. Lett. 10: 1478. https://doi.org/10.1186/s11671-015-0856-9.

[27] Gudikandula, K., and S.C. Maringanti. 2016. Synthesis of silver nanoparticles by chemical and biological methods and their antimicrobial properties. J. Experiment. Nanosci. 11: 714. https://doi.org/10.1080/17458080.2016.1139196.

[28] Das, S.K., A.R. Das and A.K. Guha. 2010. Microbial synthesis of multishaped gold nanostructures. Small 6: 1012. https://doi.org/10.1002/smll.200902011.

[29] Duan, H., D. Wang and Y. Li. 2015. Green chemistry for nanoparticle synthesis. Chem. Soc. Rev. 44: 5778. https://doi.org/10.1039/C4CS00363B.

[30] Ovais, M., A.T. Khalil, M. Ayaz, I. Ahmad, S.K. Nethi and S. Mukherjee. 2018. Biosynthesis of metal nanoparticles via microbial enzymes: A mechanistic approach. Internat. J. Mol. Sci. 19: 1. https://doi.org/10.3390/ijms19124100.

[31] Majeed, S., M. Danish, M.N.M. Ibrahim, S.H. Sekeri, M.T. Ansari, A. Nanda and G. Ahmad. 2021. Bacteria mediated synthesis of iron oxide nanoparticles and their antibacterial, antioxidant, cytocompatibility properties. J. Cluster Sci. 32: 1083. https://doi.org/10.1007/s10876-020-01876-7.

[32] Gahlawat, G. and A.R. Choudhury. 2019. A review on the biosynthesis of metal and metal salt nanoparticles by microbes. RSC Adv. 9: 12944. https://doi.org/10.1039/c8ra10483b.

[33] Saravanan, M., S.K. Barik, D. MubarakAli, P. Prakash and A. Pugazhendhi. 2018. Synthesis of silver nanoparticles from *Bacillus brevis* (NCIM 2533) and their antibacterial activity against pathogenic bacteria. Microb. Pthogen. 116: 221. https://doi.org/10.1016/j.micpath.2018.01.038.

[34] Grasso, G., D. Zane and R. Dragone. 2020. Microbial nanotechnology: Challenges and prospects for green biocatalytic synthesis of nanoscale materials for sensoristic and biomedical applications. Nanomater. 10: 11.

[35] Khan, A.A., S. Khan, S. Khan, S. Rentschler, S. Laufer and H. Deigner. 2021. Biosynthesis of iron oxide magnetic nanoparticles using clinically isolated *Pseudomonas aeruginosa*. Sci. Rep. 11: 20503. https://doi.org/10.1038/s41598-021-99814-8.

[36] Ebadi, M., M.R. Zolfaghari, S.S. Aghaei, M. Zargar, M. Shafie, H.S. Zahiri and K.A. Noghabi. 2019. A bio-inspired strategy for the synthesis of zinc oxide nanoparticles (ZnO NPs) using the cell extract of *Cyanobacterium Nostoc* sp. EA03: from biological function to toxicity evaluation. RSC Adv. 9: 23508. https://doi.org/10.1039/c9ra03962g.

[37] Jayaseelan, C., A.A. Rahuman, A.V. Kirthi, S. Marimuthu, T. Santhoshkumar, A. Bagavan and K.V.B. Rao. 2012. Novel microbial route to synthesize ZnO nanoparticles using *Aeromonas hydrophila* and their activity against pathogenic bacteria and fungi. Spectroch. Acta Part A: Mol. Biomol. Spectros. 90: 78. https://doi.org/10.1016/j.saa.2012.01.006.

[38] Jayaseelan, C., A.A. Rahuman, S.M. Roopan, A.V. Kirthi, J. Venkatesan, S.K. Kim and C. Siva. 2013. Biological approach to synthesize TiO_2 nanoparticles using *Aeromonas hydrophila* and its antibacterial activity. Spectroch. Acta Part A: Mol. Biomol. Spectros. 107: 82. https://doi.org/10.1016/j.saa.2012.12.083.

[39] Al-namil, D.S., E. El Khoury and D. Patra. 2019. Solid-state green synthesis of Ag NPs: Higher temperature harvests larger Ag NPs but smaller size has better catalytic reduction reaction. Sci. Rep. 9: 1. https://doi.org/10.1038/s41598-019-51693-w.

[40] Siddiqi, K.S. and A. Husen. 2016. Fabrication of metal and metal oxide nanoparticles by algae and their toxic effects. Nanoscale Res. Lett. 11: 1. https://doi.org/10.1186/s11671-016-1580-9.

[41] Chugh, D., V.S. Viswamalya and B. Das. 2021. Green synthesis of silver nanoparticles with algae and the importance of capping agents in the process. J. Genetic Eng. Biotechnol. 19: 126. https://doi.org/10.1186/s43141-021-00228-w.

[42] Arya, A., V. Mishra and T.S. Chundawat. 2019. Green synthesis of silver nanoparticles from green algae (*Botryococcus braunii*) and its catalytic behavior for the synthesis of benzimidazoles. Chem. Data Collections 20: 100190. https://doi.org/10.1016/j.cdc.2019.100190.

[43] Al-radadi, N.S., T. Hussain, S. Faisal, S. Ali and R. Shah. 2022. Novel biosynthesis, characterization and bio-catalytic potential of green algae (*Spirogyra hyalina*) mediated silver nanomaterials. Saudi J. Biol. Sci. 29: 411. https://doi.org/10.1016/j.sjbs.2021.09.013.

[44] González-ballesteros, N., S. Prado-López, J.B. Rodríguez-González, M. Lastra and M.C. Rodríguez-Argüelles. 2017. Green synthesis of gold nanoparticles using brown algae *Cystoseira baccata*: Its activity in colon cancer cells. Colloids Surf. B: Biointerfaces 153: 190. https://doi.org/10.1016/j.colsurfb.2017.02.020.

[45] Liu, B., J. Xie, J.Y. Lee, Y.P. Ting and J.P. Chen. 2005. Optimization of high-yield biological synthesis of single-crystalline gold nanoplates. J. Phys. Chem. B 109: 15256.

[46] Chellapandian, C., B. Ramkumar, P. Puja, R. Shanmuganathan, A. Pugazhendhi and P. Kumar. 2019. Gold nanoparticles using red seaweed *Gracilaria verrucosa*: Green synthesis, characterization and biocompatibility studies. Process Biochem. 80: 58. https://doi.org/10.1016/j.procbio.2019.02.009.

[47] Jiamboonsri, P. and S. Wanwong. 2021. Photoassisted synthesis of silver nanoparticles using riceberry rice extract and their antibacterial application. J. Nanomater. 2021: 1. https://doi.org/10.1155/2021/5598924.

[48] Koli, R.R., M.R. Phadatare, B.B. Sinha, D.M. Sakate, A.V. Ghule, G.S. Ghodake and V.J. Fulari. 2019. Gram bean extract-mediated synthesis of Fe_3O_4 nanoparticles for tuning the magneto-structural properties that influence the hyperthermia performance. J. Taiwan Inst. Chem. Eng. 95: 357. https://doi.org/10.1016/j.jtice.2018.07.039.

[49] Lee, K., S. Park, M. Govarthanan, P. Hwang, Y. Seo, M. Cho and B.-T. Oh. 2013. Synthesis of silver nanoparticles using cow milk and their antifungal activity against phytopathogens. Mater. Lett. 105: 128. https://doi.org/10.1016/j.matlet.2013.04.076.

[50] Pandey, S., C. De Klerk, J. Kim, M. Kang and E. Fosso-Kankeu. 2020. Ecofriendly approach for synthesis, characterization and biological activities of milk protein stabilized silver nanoparticles. Polymers 12: 1418. https://doi.org/10.3390/polym12061418.

[51] Balasooriya, E.R., C.D. Jayasinghe, U.A. Jayawardena, R. Weerakkodige, D. Ruwanthika, R.M. De Silva and P.V. Udagama. 2017. Honey mediated green synthesis of nanoparticles: New era of safe nanotechnology. J. Nanomater. 2017: 1.

[52] Philip, D. 2010. Honey mediated green synthesis of silver nanoparticles. Spectroch. Acta Part A 75: 1078. https://doi.org/10.1016/j.saa.2009.12.058.

[53] Venu, R., T.S. Ramulu, S. Anandakumar, V.S. Rani and C.G. Kim. 2011. Bio-directed synthesis of platinum nanoparticles using aqueous honey solutions and their catalytic applications. Colloids Surf. A: Physicochem. Eng. Aspects 384: 733. https://doi.org/10.1016/j.colsurfa.2011.05.045.

[54] Philip, D. 2009. Honey mediated green synthesis of gold nanoparticles. Spectroch. Acta Part A 73: 650. https://doi.org/10.1016/j.saa.2009.03.007.

[55] Cai, Y., Y. Shen, A. Xie, S. Li and X. Wang. 2010. Green synthesis of soya bean sprouts-mediated superparamagnetic Fe_3O_4 nanoparticles. J. Mag. Mag. Mater. 322: 2938. https://doi.org/10.1016/j.jmmm.2010.05.009.

[56] Dhand, V., L. Soumya, S. Bharadwaj, S. Chakra, D. Bhatt and B. Sreedhar. 2016. Green synthesis of silver nanoparticles using *Coffea arabica* seed extract and its antibacterial activity. Mater. Sci. Eng. C 58: 36. https://doi.org/10.1016/j.msec.2015.08.018.

[57] Rajesh, S., V. Dharanishanthi and A.V. Kanna. 2015. Antibacterial mechanism of biogenic silver nanoparticles of *Lactobacillus acidophilus*. J. Experimen. Nanosci. 10: 1143. https://doi.org/10.10 80/17458080.2014.985750.

[58] Lateef, A., I. Adelere, E.B. Gueguim-Kana, T. Asafa and L.S. Beukes. 2014. Green synthesis of silver nanoparticles using keratinase obtained from a strain of *Bacillus safensis* LAU 13. Int. Nano Lett. 5: 29. https://doi.org/10.1007/s40089-014-0133-4.

[59] Abirami, M. and K. Kannabiran. 2016. *Streptomyces ghanaensis* VITHM1 mediated green synthesis of silver nanoparticles: Mechanism and biological applications. Front. Chem. Sci. Eng. 10: 542. https://doi.org/10.1007/s11705-016-1599-6.

[60] Gowramma, B., U. Keerthi, M. Raf and D.M. Rao. 2015. Biogenic silver nanoparticles production and characterization from native stain of *Corynebacterium* species and its antimicrobial activity. Biotech. 5: 195. https://doi.org/10.1007/s13205-014-0210-4.

[61] Rajeshkumar, S. 2016. Anticancer activity of eco-friendly gold nanoparticles against lung and liver cancer cells. J. Genetic Eng. Biotechnol. 14: 195. https://doi.org/10.1016/j.jgeb.2016.05.007.

[62] Elamawi, R.M., R.E. Al-harbi and A.A. Hendi. 2018. Biosynthesis and characterization of silver nanoparticles using *Trichoderma longibrachiatum* and their effect on phytopathogenic fungi. Egyptian J. Bio. Pest Control 28: 1. https://doi.org/10.1186/s41938-018-0028-1.

[63] Balakumaran, M.D., R. Ramachandran, P. Balashanmugam, D.J. Mukeshkumar and P.T. Kalaichelvan. 2016. Mycosynthesis of silver and gold nanoparticles: Optimization, characterization and antimicrobial activity against human pathogens. Microbiol. Res. 182: 8.

[64] Arya, A., K. Gupta, T.S. Chundawat and D. Vaya. 2018. Biogenic synthesis of copper and silver nanoparticles using green alga *Botryococcus braunii* and its antimicrobial activity. Bioinorg. Chem. Appli. 2018: 1. https://doi.org/10.1155/2018/7879403.

[65] Sharma, G., A.R. Sharma, R. Bhavesh, J. Park, B. Ganbold, J. Nam and S. Lee. 2014. Biomolecule-mediated synthesis of selenium nanoparticles using dried *Vitis vinifera (Raisin)* extract. Molecules 19: 2761. https://doi.org/10.3390/molecules19032761.

[66] Ramkumar, V.S., A. Pugazhendhi, S. Prakash, N.K. Ahila, G. Vinoj, S. Selvam and R.B. Rajendran. 2017. Synthesis of platinum nanoparticles using seaweed *Padina gymnospora* and their catalytic activity as PVP/PtNPs nanocomposite towards biological applications. Biomed. Pharmacother. 92: 479. https://doi.org/10.1016/j.biopha.2017.05.076.

[67] Othman, A.M., M.A. Elsayed, N.G. Al-balakocy, M.M. Hassan and A.M. Elshafei. 2020. Biosynthesis and characterization of silver nanoparticles induced by fungal proteins and its application in different biological activities. J. Genetic Eng. Biotechn. 17: 1.

[68] Salem, D.M.S.A., M.M. Ismail and M.A. Aly-eldeen. 2019. Biogenic synthesis and antimicrobial potency of iron oxide (Fe_3O_4) nanoparticles using algae harvested from the Mediterranean Sea, Egypt. Egyptian J. Aquatic Res. 45: 197. https://doi.org/10.1016/j.ejar.2019.07.002.

[69] Mahdavi, M., F. Namvar, M. Bin Ahmad and R. Mohamad. 2013. Green biosynthesis and characterization of magnetic iron oxide (Fe_3O_4) nanoparticles using seaweed (*Sargassum muticum*) aqueous extract. Molecules 18: 5954. https://doi.org/10.3390/molecules18055954.

[70] Ishwarya, R., B. Vaseeharan, S. Kalyani, B. Banumathi, M. Govindarajan, N.S. Alharbi and G. Benelli. 2018. Facile green synthesis of zinc oxide nanoparticles using *Ulva lactuca* seaweed extract and evaluation of their photocatalytic, antibio film and insecticidal activity. J. Photochem. Photobiol., B: Biology 178: 249. https://doi.org/10.1016/j.jphotobiol.2017.11.006.

[71] Abdel-raouf, N., N.M. Al-enazi, M.B.I. Ibraheem, M.R. Alharbi and M.M. Alkhalaifi. 2019. Biosynthesis of silver nanoparticles by using of the marine brown alga *Padina pavonia* and their characterization. Saudi J. Biol. Sci. 26: 1207. https://doi.org/10.1016/j.sjbs.2018.01.007.

[72] Vanlalveni, C., S. Lallianrawna, A. Biswas, M. Selvaraj, B. Changmai and S.L. Rokhum. 2021. Green synthesis of silver nanoparticles using plant extracts and their antimicrobial activities: a review of recent literature. RSC Adv. 11: 2804. https://doi.org/10.1039/d0ra09941d.

[73] Chung, I., I. Park, K. Seung-hyun, M. Thiruvengadam and G. Rajakumar. 2016. Plant-mediated synthesis of silver nanoparticles: their characteristic properties and therapeutic applications. Nanoscale Res. Lett. 11: 40. https://doi.org/10.1186/s11671-016-1257-4.

[74] Metz, K.M., S.E. Sanders, J.P. Pender, M. Dix, D.T. Hinds, S.J. Quinn, and P.E. Colavita. 2015. Green synthesis of metal nanoparticles via natural extracts: the biogenic nanoparticle corona and its effects on reactivity. ACS Sustainable Chem. Eng. 3: 1610. https://doi.org/10.1021/acssuschemeng.5b00304.

[75] Mohammadinejad, R., S. Karimi, S. Iravani and R.S. Varma. 2016. Plant-derived nanostructures: types and applications. Green Chem. 18: 20. https://doi.org/10.1039/C5GC01403D.

[76] Bekele, B., A. Degefa, F. Tesgera, L.T. Jule, R. Shanmugam, L.P. Dwarampudi and K. Ramasamy. 2021. Green versus chemical precipitation methods of preparing zinc oxide nanoparticles and investigation of antimicrobial properties. J. Nanomater. 2021: 1.

[77] Chandra, I., S. Singh, S. Senapati, P. Srivastava and L. Bahadur. 2019. Green synthesis of TiO_2 nanoparticles using *Bixa orellana* seed extract and its application for solar cells. Solar Energy 194: 952. https://doi.org/10.1016/j.solener.2019.10.090.

[78] Padilla-Cruz, A.L., J.A. Garza-Cervantes, X.G. Vasto-Anzaldo, G. García-Rivas, A. León-Buitimea and J.R. Morones-Ramírez. 2021. Synthesis and design of Ag-Fe bimetallic nanoparticles as antimicrobial synergistic combination therapies against clinically relevant pathogens. Sci. Rep. 11: 5351. https://doi.org/10.1038/s41598-021-84768-8.

[79] Prasad, C., G. Yuvaraja and P. Venkateswarlu. 2017. Biogenic synthesis of Fe_3O_4 magnetic nanoparticles using *Pisum sativum* peels extract and its effect on magnetic and methyl orange dye degradation studies. J. Mag. Mag. Mater. 424: 376. https://doi.org/10.1016/j.jmmm.2016.10.084.

[80] Radini, I.A., N. Hasan, M.A. Malik and Z. Khan. 2018. Biosynthesis of iron nanoparticles using *Trigonella foenum-graecum* seed extract for photocatalytic methyl orange dye degradation and antibacterial applications. J. Photochem. Photobiol., B: Biol. 183: 154. https://doi.org/10.1016/j.jphotobiol.2018.04.014.

[81] Veisi, H., B. Karmakar, T. Tamoradi, S. Hemmati, M. Hekmati and M. Hamelian. 2021. Biosynthesis of CuO nanoparticles using aqueous extract of herbal tea (*Stachys Lavandulifolia*) flowers and evaluation of its catalytic activity. Sci. Rep. 11: 1983. https://doi.org/10.1038/s41598-021-81320-6.

[82] Dlugaszewska, J. and R. Dobrucka. 2019. Effectiveness of biosynthesized trimetallic au/pt/ag nanoparticles on planktonic and biofilm *Enterococcus faecalis* and *Enterococcus faecium* forms. J. Cluster Sci., 30: 1091. https://doi.org/10.1007/s10876-019-01570-3.

[83] Dobrucka, R. 2019. Biogenic synthesis of trimetallic nanoparticles Au/ZnO/Ag using *Meliloti officinalis* extract. Int. J. Environ. Anal. Chem. 100: 981. https://doi.org/10.1080/03067319.2019.1646736.

[84] Hu, D., X. Yang, W. Chen, Z. Feng, C. Hu, F. Yan and Z. Chen. 2021. *Rhodiola rosea* rhizome extract-mediated green synthesis of silver nanoparticles and evaluation of their potential antioxidant and catalytic reduction activities. ACS Omega 6: 24450. https://doi.org/10.1021/acsomega.1c02843.

[85] Kayalvizhi, T., S. Ravikumar and P. Venkatachalam. 2016. Green synthesis of metallic silver nanoparticles using *Curculigo orchioides* rhizome extracts and evaluation of its antibacterial, larvicidal, and anticancer activity. J. Environ. Eng. 142: 1. https://doi.org/10.1061/(ASCE)EE.1943-7870.0001098.

[86] Peng, Q. and R. Chen. 2019. Biosynthesis of gold nanoparticles using caffeoylxanthiazonoside, chemical isolated from *Xanthium strumarium* L. fruit and their anti-allergic rhinitis effect—a traditional Chinese medicine. J. Photochem. Photobiol., B: Biol. 192: 13. https://doi.org/10.1016/j.jphotobiol.2018.12.015.

[87] Huo, C., M. Khoshnamvand, P. Liu, C. Liu and C. Yuan. 2019. Rapid mediated biosynthesis and quantification of AuNPs using persimmon (*Diospyros Kaki* L.f) fruit extract. J. Mol. Struct. 1178: 366. https://doi.org/10.1016/j.molstruc.2018.10.044.

[88] Suresh, D., R.M. Shobharani, P.C. Nethravathi, M.A. Pavan Kumar, H. Nagabhushana and S.C. Sharma. 2015. *Artocarpus gomezianus* aided green synthesis of ZnO nanoparticles: Luminescence, photocatalytic and antioxidant properties. Spectrochim. Acta Part A: Mol. Biomol. Spectros. 141: 128. https://doi.org/10.1016/j.saa.2015.01.048.

[89] Udayabhanu, P.C. Nethravathi, M.A.P. Kumar, D. Suresh, K. Lingaraju, H. Rajanaika and S. Sharma. 2015. *Tinospora cordifolia* mediated facile green synthesis of cupric oxide nanoparticles and their photocatalytic, antioxidant and antibacterial properties. Mater. Sci. Semicond. Process. 33: 81. https://doi.org/10.1016/j.mssp.2015.01.034.

[90] Carmona, E.R., N. Benito, T. Plaza and G. Recio-sánchez. 2017. Green synthesis of silver nanoparticles by using leaf extracts from the endemic *Buddleja globosa* hope. Green Chem. Lett. Rev. 10: 250. https://doi.org/10.1080/17518253.2017.1360400.

[91] Gopalakrishnan, R., B. Loganathan, S. Dinesh and K. Raghu. 2017. Strategic green synthesis, characterization and catalytic application to 4-nitrophenol reduction of palladium nanoparticles. J. Cluster Sci. 28: 2123. https://doi.org/10.1007/s10876-017-1207-z.

[92] Rajeshkumar, S. 2016. Synthesis of silver nanoparticles using fresh bark of *Pongamia pinnata* and characterization of its antibacterial activity against gram positive and gram negative pathogens. Resource Efficient Technol. 2: 30. https://doi.org/10.1016/j.reffit.2016.06.003.

[93] Padalia, H., P. Moteriya and S. Chanda. 2015. Green synthesis of silver nanoparticles from marigold flower and its synergistic antimicrobial potential. Arabian J. Chem. 8: 732. https://doi.org/10.1016/j.arabjc.2014.11.015.

[94] Chandrasekaran, R., S. Gnanasekar, P. Seetharaman, R. Keppanan, W. Arockiaswamy and S. Sivaperumal. 2016. Formulation of *Carica papaya* latex-functionalized silver nanoparticles for its improved antibacterial and anticancer applications. J. Mol. Liq. 219: 232. https://doi.org/10.1016/j.molliq.2016.03.038.

[95] Elango, G. and S.M. Roopan. 2015. Green synthesis, spectroscopic investigation and photocatalytic activity of lead nanoparticles. Spectrochem. Acta Part A: Mol. Biomol. Spectros. 139: 367. https://doi.org/10.1016/j.saa.2014.12.066.

[96] Pawar, O., N. Deshpande, S. Dagade, S. Waghmode and P.N. Joshi. 2016. Green synthesis of silver nanoparticles from purple acid phosphatase apoenzyme isolated from a new source *Limonia acidissima*. J. Exper. Nanosci. 11: 28. https://doi.org/10.1080/17458080.2015.1025300.

[97] Sankar, V., P. Salinraj, R. Athira, R.S. Soumya, and K.G. Raghu. 2015. Cerium nanoparticles synthesized using aqueous extract of *Centella asiatica*: characterization, determination of free

radical scavenging activity and evaluation of efficacy against *cardiomyoblast hypertrophy*. RSC Adv. 5: 21074. https://doi.org/10.1039/c4ra16893c.

[98] Ahmed, S., Saifullah, M. Ahmad, B.L. Swami and S. Ikram. 2016. Green synthesis of silver nanoparticles using *Azadirachta indica* aqueous leaf extract. J. Rad. Res. Appl. Sci. 9: 1. https://doi.org/10.1016/j.jrras.2015.06.006.

[99] Devatha, C.P., A.K. Thalla and S.Y. Katte. 2016. Green synthesis of iron nanoparticles using different leaf extracts for treatment of domestic waste water. J. Cleaner Prod. 139: 1425. https://doi.org/10.1016/j.jclepro.2016.09.019.

[100] Femi-adepoju, A.G., A.O. Dada, K.O. Otun, A.O. Adepoju and O.P. Fatoba. 2019. Green synthesis of silver nanoparticles using terrestrial fern (*Gleichenia Pectinata* (Willd.) C. Presl.): characterization and antimicrobial studies. Heliyon 5: 1. https://doi.org/10.1016/j.heliyon.2019.e01543.

[101] Ahmed, A., M. Usman, B. Yu, Y. Shen and H. Cong. 2021. Sustainable fabrication of hematite (α-Fe$_2$O$_3$) nanoparticles using biomolecules of *Punica granatum* seed extract for unconventional solar-light-driven photocatalytic remediation of organic dyes. J. Mol. Liq. 339: 116729. https://doi.org/10.1016/j.molliq.2021.116729.

[102] Gunti, L., R.S. Dass and N.K. Kalagatur. 2019. Phytofabrication of selenium nanoparticles from *emblica officinalis* fruit extract and exploring its biopotential applications: antioxidant, antimicrobial, and biocompatibility. Front. Microbiol. 10: 1. https://doi.org/10.3389/fmicb.2019.00931.

[103] Ramesh, A.V., D.R. Devi, G. Battu and K. Basavaiah. 2018. A Facile plant mediated synthesis of silver nanoparticles using an aqueous leaf extract of *Ficus hispida* Linn. f. for catalytic, antioxidant and antibacterial applications. South Afri. J. Chem. Eng. 26: 25. https://doi.org/10.1016/j.sajce.2018.07.001.

[104] Folorunso, A., S. Akintelu, A. Kolawole, S. Ajayi, B. Abiola, I. Abdusalam and A. Morakinyo. 2019. Biosynthesis, characterization and antimicrobial activity of gold nanoparticles from leaf extracts of *Annona muricata*. J. Nanostruct. Chem. 9: 121. https://doi.org/10.1007/s40097-019-0301-1.

[105] Sharma, G., J. Nam, A.R. Sharma and S. Lee. 2018. Antimicrobial potential of silver nanoparticles synthesized using medicinal herb *Coptidis rhizome*. Molecules 23: 1. https://doi.org/10.3390/molecules23092268.

[106] Aljabali, A.A.A., Y. Akkam, M. Salim, A. Zoubi, K.M. Al-batayneh, B.A. Id and D.J.E. Id. 2018. Synthesis of gold nanoparticles using leaf extract of *Ziziphus zizyphus* and their antimicrobial activity. Nanomater. 8: 1. https://doi.org/10.3390/nano8030174.

[107] Rafi, M., S. Id, M. Khan, M.K. Id, A. Al-warthan, A. Mahmood and S.F. Adil. 2018. Plant-extract-assisted green synthesis of silver nanoparticles using *Origanum vulgare* L. extract and their microbicidal activities. Sustainability 10: 1. https://doi.org/10.3390/su10040913.

[108] Atarod, M., M. Nasrollahzadeh and S.M. Sajadi. 2016. Green synthesis of Pd/RGO/Fe$_3$O$_4$ nanocomposite using *Withania coagulans* leaf extract and its application as magnetically separable and reusable catalyst for the reduction of 4-nitrophenol. J. Colloid Interf. Sci. 465: 249. https://doi.org/10.1016/j.jcis.2015.11.060.

[109] Sharifi-rad, M., P. Pohl, F. Epifano and J.M. Álvarez-Suarez. 2020. Green synthesis of silver nanoparticles using *Astragalus tribuloides* delile. root extract: characterization, antioxidant, antibacterial, and anti-inflammatory activities. Nanomater. 10: 2383. https://doi.org/10.3390/nano10122383.

[110] Selvaraj, V., S. Sagadevan, L. Muthukrishnan, R.M. Johan and J. Podder. 2019. Eco-friendly approach in synthesis of silver nanoparticles and evaluation of optical, surface morphological and antimicrobial properties. J. Nanostruct. Chem. 9: 153. https://doi.org/10.1007/s40097-019-0306-9.

[111] Kumar, B., K. Smita and L. Cumbal. 2015. Phytosynthesis of gold nanoparticles using Andean Ají' (*Capsicum baccatum* L.). Cogent Chem. 1: 1. https://doi.org/10.1080/23312009.2015.1120982.

[112] Ke, Y., M. Saleh, A. Aboody, W. Alturaiki, S.A. Alsagaby, F.A. Alfaiz and S. Mickymaray. 2019. Photosynthesized gold nanoparticles from *Catharanthus roseus* induces caspase-mediated apoptosis in cervical cancer cells (HeLa). Artificial Cells, Nanomed. Biotechnol. 41: 1938. https://doi.org/10.1080/21691401.2019.1614017.

[113] Thakur, S. and N. Karak. 2012. Green reduction of graphene oxide by aqueous phytoextracts. Carbon 50: 5331. https://doi.org/10.1016/j.carbon.2012.07.023.

[114] Oves, M., M. Aslam, M.A. Rauf, S. Qayyum, H.A. Qari, M.S. Khan and I.M. Ismail. 2018. Antimicrobial and anticancer activities of silver nanoparticles synthesized from the root hair extract of *Phoenix dactylifera*. Mater. Sci. Eng. C 89: 429. https://doi.org/10.1016/j.msec.2018.03.035.

[115] Tahir, K., S. Nazir, A. Ahmad, B. Li, S. Asim, A. Shah and F.U. Khan. 2016. Biodirected synthesis of palladium nanoparticles using *Phoenix dactylifera* leaves extract and their size dependent biomedical and catalytic. RSC Adv. 6: 85903. https://doi.org/10.1039/c6ra11409a.

[116] Kasithevar, M., M. Saravanan, P. Prakash, H. Kumar, M. Ovais, H. Barabadi and Z.K. Shinwari. 2017. Green synthesis of silver nanoparticles using *Alysicarpus monilifer* leaf extract and its antibacterial activity against MRSA and CoNS isolates in HIV patients. J. Interdiscip. Nanomed. 2: 131. https://doi.org/10.1002/jin2.26.

[117] Balalakshmi, C., K. Gopinath, M. Govindarajan, R. Lokesh, A. Arumugam, N.S. Alharbi and G. Benelli. 2017. Green synthesis of gold nanoparticles using a cheap *Sphaeranthus indicus* extract: Impact on plant cells and the aquatic *Crustacean Artemia nauplii*. J. Photochem. Photobiol., B: Biol. 173: 598. https://doi.org/10.1016/j.jphotobiol.2017.06.040.

[118] Tahir, K., S. Nazir, B. Li, A. Ullah, Z. Ul, H. Khan and A. Ahmad. 2015. *Nerium oleander* leaves extract mediated synthesis of gold nano- particles and its antioxidant activity. Mater. Lett. 156: 198. https://doi.org/10.1016/j.matlet.2015.05.062.

[119] Mahamadi, C. and T. Wunganayi. 2018. Green synthesis of silver nanoparticles using *Zanthoxylum chalybeum* and their antiprolytic and antibiotic properties. Cogent Chem. 4: 1. https://doi.org/10.1080/23312009.2018.1538547.

[120] Khalid, S., S.A. Majid and M.A. Akram. 2019. The prophylactic effect of *Ranunculus laetus* (wall)-mediated silver nanoparticles against some gram-positive and gram-negative bacteria. Bull. Nat. Res. Centre 43: 1.

[121] Jain, S. and M.S. Mehata. 2017. Medicinal plant leaf extract and pure flavonoid mediated green synthesis of silver nanoparticles and their enhanced antibacterial property. Sci. Rep. 7: 15867. https://doi.org/10.1038/s41598-017-15724-8.

[122] Phukan, S., P. Bharali, A.K. Das and H. Rashid. 2016. Phytochemical assisted synthesis of size and shape tunable gold nanoparticles and assessment of their catalytic activities. RSC Adv. 6: 49307. https://doi.org/10.1039/c5ra23535a.

[123] Zhan, G., J. Huang, M. Du, I. Abdul-Rauf, Y. Ma and Q. Li. 2011. Green synthesis of Au-Pd bimetallic nanoparticles: Single-step bioreduction method with plant extract. Mater. Lett. 65: 2989. https://doi.org/10.1016/j.matlet.2011.06.079.

[124] Upadhyay, P.K., V.K. Jain, A.K. Shrivastav, S. Sharma and R. Sharma. 2020. Green and chemically synthesized ZnO nanoparticles: A comparative study. Adv. Mater. Appl. 798: 012025. https://doi.org/10.1088/1757-899X/798/1/012025.

[125] Vaseghi, Z., A. Nematollahzadeh and O. Tavakoli. 2019. Plant-mediated Cu/Cr/Ni nanoparticle formation strategy for simultaneously separation of the mixed ions from aqueous solution. J. Taiwan Inst. Chem. Eng. 96: 148. https://doi.org/10.1016/j.jtice.2018.10.020.

[126] Alshehri, A.A. and M.A. Malik. 2020. Facile one-pot biogenic synthesis of Cu-Co-Ni trimetallic nanoparticles for enhanced photocatalytic dye degradation. Catalysts 10: 1138.

[127] Jadoun, S., R. Arif, N.K. Jangid and R.K. Meena. 2021. Green synthesis of nanoparticles using plant extracts: a review. Environ. Chem. Lett. 19: 355. https://doi.org/10.1007/s10311-020-01074-x.

[128] Kim, M.G., J.M. Kang, J.E. Lee, K.S. Kim, K.H. Kim, M. Cho and S.G. Lee. 2021. Effects of calcination temperature on the phase composition, photocatalytic degradation, and virucidal activities of TiO_2 nanoparticles. ACS Omega 6: 10668. https://doi.org/10.1021/acsomega.1c00043.

[129] Nasrollahzadeh, M., M. Atarod, M. Sajjadi, S.M. Sajadi and Z. Issaabadi. 2019. Plant-mediated green synthesis of nanostructures: mechanisms, characterization, and applications. Interface Sci. Technol. 1st Ed. 28: 199. https://doi.org/10.1016/B978-0-12-813586-0.00006-7.

[130] Ibrahim, H.M.M. 2019. Green synthesis and characterization of silver nanoparticles using banana peel extract and their antimicrobial activity against representative microorganisms. J. Rad. Res. Appl. Sci. 8: 265. https://doi.org/10.1016/j.jrras.2015.01.007.

[131] Zheng, B., T. Kong, X. Jing, T. Odoom-wubah, X. Li, D. Sun and Q. Li. 2013. Plant-mediated synthesis of platinum nanoparticles and its bioreductive mechanism. J. Colloid Interf. Sci. 396: 138. https://doi.org/10.1016/j.jcis.2013.01.021.

[132] Malek, F. and M. Nahid. 2018. Influence of temperature and concentration on biosynthesis and characterization of zinc oxide nanoparticles using cherry extract. J. Nanostruct. Chem. 8: 93. https://doi.org/10.1007/s40097-018-0257-6.

[133] Ahmed, R.H. and D.E. Mustafa. 2020. Green synthesis of silver nanoparticles mediated by traditionally used medicinal plants in Sudan. Int. Nano Lett. 10: 1. https://doi.org/10.1007/s40089-019-00291-9.

[134] Behravan, M., A.H. Panahi, A. Naghizadeh, M. Ziaee, R. Mahdavi and A. Mirzapour. 2019. Facile green synthesis of silver nanoparticles using *Berberis vulgaris* leaf and root aqueous extract and its antibacterial activity. Int. J. Biol. Macromol. 124: 148. https://doi.org/10.1016/j.ijbiomac.2018.11.101.

[135] Marslin, G., K. Siram, Q. Maqbool, R.K. Selvakesavan, D. Kruszka, P. Kachlicki and G. Franklin. 2018. Secondary metabolites in the green synthesis of metallic nanoparticles. Materials 11: 1. https://doi.org/10.3390/ma11060940.

[136] Ocsoy, I., D. Tasdemir, S. Mazicioglu, C. Celik, A. Kati and F. Ulgen. 2018. Biomolecules incorporated metallic nanoparticles synthesis and their biomedical applications. Mater. Lett. 212: 45. https://doi.org/10.1016/j.matlet.2017.10.068.

[137] Nasrollahzadeh, M., S.S. Momeni and S.M. Sajadi. 2017. Green synthesis of copper nanoparticles using *Plantago asiatica* leaf extract and their application for the cyanation of aldehydes using $K_4Fe(CN)_6$. J. Colloid Interf. Sci. 506: 471. https://doi.org/10.1016/j.jcis.2017.07.072.

[138] Edison, T.N.J.I., R. Atchudan, M.G. Sethuraman and R.Y. Lee. 2016. Reductive-degradation of carcinogenic azo dyes using *Anacardium occidentale* testa derived silver nanoparticles. J. Photochem. Photobiol., B: Biol. 162: 604. https://doi.org/10.1016/j.jphotobiol.2016.07.040.

[139] Arumugam, A., C. Karthikeyan, A.S.H. Hameed, K. Gopinath, S. Gowri and V. Karthika. 2015. Synthesis of cerium oxide nanoparticles using *Gloriosa superba* L. leaf extract and their structural, optical and antibacterial properties. Mater. Sci. Eng. C 49: 408. https://doi.org/10.1016/j.msec.2015.01.042.

[140] Devipriya, D. and S.M. Roopan. 2017. *Cissus quadrangularis* mediated ecofriendly synthesis of copper oxide nanoparticles and its antifungal studies against *Aspergillus niger*, *Aspergillus flavus*. Mater. Sci. Eng. C 80: 38. https://doi.org/10.1016/j.msec.2017.05.130.

[141] Mathivanan, K., R. Selva, J.U. Chandirika, R.K. Govindarajan, R. Srinivasan, G. Annadurai and P.A. Duc. 2019. Biologically synthesized silver nanoparticles against pathogenic bacteria: Synthesis, calcination and characterization. Biocatal. Agricul. Biotechnol. 22: 101373. https://doi.org/10.1016/j.bcab.2019.101373.

4

Nanofabrication Using Common Kitchen/Domestic Wastes

An Approach Towards Sustainability and Circular Economy

Manisha Mishra,[1] *Anal K. Jha*[2] *and K. Prasad*[3,*]

1. Introduction

The focus on green synthesis of nanomaterials transcribes and modernizes each new day into innovative Green Nanotechnology approaches that has shifted global efforts by the scientific community into a more synergistic inter- and cross disciplinary endeavor to reduce hazardous wastes. Recently, with the emergence and catastrophe caused by Covid-19 pandemic, the world has experienced variation in the load of the municipal solid waste (MSW) that is majorly accounted for by the top three MSW producers—the United States, the Chinese Republic, and India, in terms of volume and variety, and has also influenced the sources of waste generation and its management [1, 2]. According to Gao et al. [3], kitchen wastes comprise a major proportion of MSW, and whether they can be engineered or not depends on the extent of deterioration and original content. These wastes contribute a major

[1] University Department of Botany, T.M. Bhagalpur University, Bhagalpur 812007, India.
[2] Department of Biotechnology, O.P. Jindal University, Raigarh, Chhattisgarh 496109, India.
[3] University Department of Physics, T.M. Bhagalpur University, Bhagalpur 812007, India.
* Corresponding author: k.prasad65@gmail.com

chunk of the MSW as demand for food remains perpetual. The menace caused by these wastes is further aggravated due to population explosion and gets compounded as industrialization, urbanization and economic development sets in [4]. In homes, restaurants, and hotels, the left-over organic matter is referred to as kitchen waste [5]. The fundamental problem in waste management lies in competent sorting and the kitchen wastes when effectively sorted from MSW can enhance the treatment process [6, 7]. Although the kitchen wastes are rich in organic content, their elevated moisture content and heterogeneity pose serious threat to their effective conversion into valuable resources [8].

Sustainability is the new buzz word across the nations, ever since people have realized that environment is greatly at stake due to anthropogenic activities, and therefore, protecting the environment is of paramount concern for one and all. Besides this, as Industry 4.0 context is emerging, the concept of green chemistry needs to be made more sustainable. Nanotechnology can provide technological solutions that can accelerate and align efforts raised by the international scientific community to consummate the United Nations Sustainable Development Goals through interdisciplinary knowledge and skills [9]. Goal 9 of the Sustainable Development Goals of the United Nations emphatically maintains that manufacturing, and hence fabrication, is a key to global economic development [10]. This can be achieved by emphasizing the circular economy concept that can generate resources and leave zero waste. Nanotechnology was initially put up by Norio Taniguchi and it is expected that this technology can buttress the circular economy concept and its immense popularity in various applications such as in medical imaging, textile industry, tissue engineering, nanocomposites, biomedicine, and bioremediation has indeed proved that [11]. The research on synthesis of nanomaterials using kitchen wastes and their applications rests on the fabrication of nontoxic nanosized materials that are monodispersed and of various sizes and shapes. Synthesis of nanomaterials with high monodispersity is possible due to abundance of glutathione and phytochelatins in plants that aid in metal sequestration, and hence define dimension of nanomaterial [12]. The fabrication protocols should aim to produce nanoparticles with uniform size and shape, and unless this criterion is met along with limited or no toxicity to biological systems, their applications in addressing human health and the environmental concerns remains a challenge. The nanomaterials can be biomineralized in protein cages and can generate nanoparticles with controlled morphology and this approach is considered safe for biological applications [13]; however, as regards their application aspect, their antimicrobial, anticancer and anthelminthic features have to be carefully confirmed upon synthesis.

The fabrication of nanomaterials is now considered as a major driver of industrial revolution and is majorly undertaken for their role in various sectors that emerges out of their unique surface area to volume ratio at the nanoscale level and promises solutions to several problems [14]. For fabrication, green protocol is preferred over chemical and other methods, because the former utilizes kitchen wastes and is relatively simple and cheap, reduces waste in the environment and is eco-friendly too [15]. The kitchen wastes are a kind of agro-waste and may contain lignin, cellulose, chitin, and polyphenolic compounds. When utilized, pyrolysis of kitchen wastes can yield carbon dots while the remaining components in plant tissues can serve as reducing, stabilizing, and capping agents in the synthesis of nanoparticles. The extracts made out of these kitchen and other agro wastes can yield metals, metal oxides, and nanocomposites, whereas nanosilica, nanocellulose, and carbon nanodots can be obtained directly from the agro-wastes [16]. The rich diversity of plant life, a faster reaction rate, and affordability makes kitchen wastes a valuable material for nanofabrication. The kitchen wastes in developing countries contain large quantities of water and nonhollo cellulose degradable organics [17]. Vegetable and fruit peels, seeds, tubers, and other chopped parts contained in the kitchen wastes are rich in phytochemicals like flavanols, terpenoids, coumarins, hesperidin, etc. and also contain co-enzymes, enzymes, proteins, phenolic compounds, alkaloids, sugars, and terpenoids. Besides this, fruit and vegetable wastes possess elevated carbohydrate content and various organics, multifunctional groups and polymeric proteins that can be harnessed to generate high-value products for nanomaterial fabrication by clean manufacturing technologies [18, 19]. The phytochemistry and biochemical composition of the plant extract can be obtained by LC-MS and these phytochemicals act as reducing and capping agents of metal ions during synthesis of nanosized materials. Figure 1 highlights the schema depicting the role of phytochemicals in nanomaterial fabrication.

There are several disadvantages of physical and chemical methods of nanomaterial fabrication including production of several toxins that are hazardous (and adsorb on the nanomaterial surface), have enormous amount of energy requirement and involvement of reducing agents that are harsh, low yield, high cost,

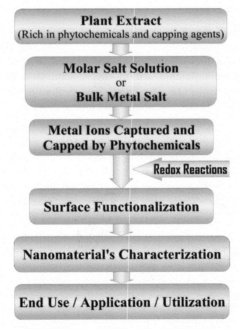

Fig. 1. The schematic highlights role of phytochemicals in nanomaterial fabrication.

and lead to environmental damage [20]. As compared to this, using kitchen wastes makes use of relatively benign phytochemicals and are hence preferred over the physical and chemical methods. The enormous applications of metal nanoparticles in various fields are achieved by their fabrication using noble metals like Ag, Au, Fe, Cu, Pt, Zn, Pd, and their oxides and involves reduction of metal salts to metal nanoparticles by phytochemicals present in the plant extract [21].

Nanomaterials fabricated by the green synthesis protocols are advantageous as compared to the physicochemical methods and as science becomes more application-oriented, the novelty of nanomaterials lures environmentalists as they find a haven to manage kitchen wastes and generate value-added products to meet the demand for sustainable and economically viable processes that are safe, effective, and applicable in agriculture, medicine, etc. The higher reactivity and elaborated surface area of these nanosized materials can effectively reduce air and water pollution [22]. It has been noted that although scale-up of nano-conversion carried out in the laboratory is not efficient, the fabrication of nanomaterials from garbage, combustible waste ash, pharmaceutical waste, agricultural waste, and microbial biomass is not uncommon [23]. Thus, nanotechnology involves science and engineering at the nanoscale and finds application in fabric manufacturing, food and agricultural processing industries, and medical and medicinal applications and as antimicrobials, of which the last one is the most popular of all [24]. This chapter has been divided into two parts. The first part discusses the fabrication protocol whereas the second part delves into the types of nanomaterials—metals, metal oxides, carbon dots and porous nanocarbon spheres.

2. Fabrication Protocol

The fabrication of nanomaterials is undertaken by two approaches, namely, top-down and bottom-up. The former involves synthesis of nanomaterials from bulk materials and involves techniques like lithography, sputtering, etching, etc. The bottom-up approach involves growing nanomaterials through self-assembly and supramolecular chemistry. It involves fabrication from simple molecules to bulk materials and can be either combined with the top-down approach or used on its own [25, 26]. Structurally, the nanomaterial consists of a core, that is surrounded by a shell and it is the latter that determines the properties of the ultimate material. Surrounding the shell is the surface layer that can be functionalized using metals, metal oxides, surfactants, polymers like poly lactic acid, etc. and functionalization is usually undertaken depending on the final outcome or desired purpose. Structurally, the shell and the core are different and the name of the nanoparticle derives from its core [25]. Functionalization is also done to prevent particle agglomeration which may be undesirable for ultimate applications. In general, the protocol for nanomaterial fabrication involves collection and sorting of kitchen wastes. It is imperative to carefully determine the solvent used for extraction of phytochemicals, capping agent and the reducing agent, and the procedure is initiated by extract preparation, screening for phytochemicals and precursor preparation. Plant extracts are rich in polyphenols that are bio-reductive and need an organic solvent to solubilize. Often important parameters such as pH, temperature, and incubation time need to be optimized. After

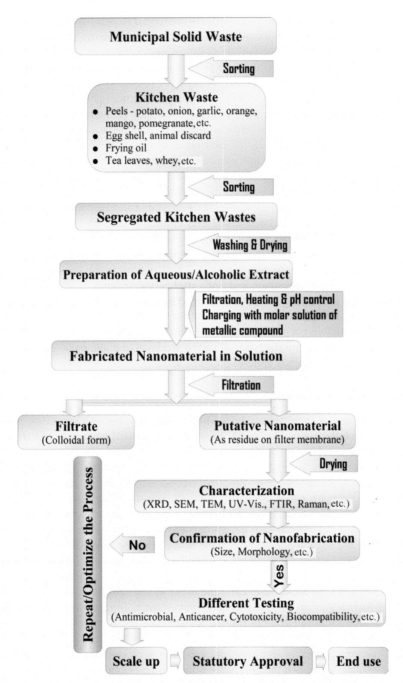

Fig. 2. The schematic highlights of the various steps involved in nanomaterial fabrication utilizing kitchen wastes, right from their sorting from municipal solid waste until the end use.

fabrication step, nanoparticles have to be characterized for various field applications by suitable techniques like SEM and TEM for determination of their optical, thermal and physicochemical properties [27, 14]. The schematic highlights of various steps involved in nanomaterial fabrication utilizing kitchen wastes have been illustrated in Fig. 2.

3. Fabrication of Metal Nanoparticles

Metallic nanoparticles are nanostructured materials, and the fabrication and application of nobel metal nanoparticles is gaining immense popularity as an active research theme nowadays [28]. Often chemicals like $NaBH_4$, hydrazine, and formaldehyde that are used to reduce noble metal salt precursors poses toxicity during fabrication and hence concerns are always raised over their use in biological applications. However, nanofabrication using biological reduction process is considered safer and non-toxic. The enhanced surface area including large surface to volume ratio, improved stability, and easy functionalization provides exclusivity to noble metal nanoparticles and they find immense application in various fields [29].

Of the various noble metal NPs, the fabrication of AgNPs by the green protocol have been attempted by various research groups utilizing kitchen wastes like grape pomace, pomegranate peels, watermelon, banana peel extract, mango peel extract, *Terminalia chebula*, pine apple, cauliflower wastes, waste tea leaves, garlic, etc. The green synthesis bestows AgNPs with unique physicochemical and biological properties. Besides, the protocol abstains from the use of hazardous solvents and chemicals, and instead mostly utilizes fruit waste valorization. By adjusting the experimental parameters, the shape, size and concentration of nanoparticles can be altered. However, brows are still raised over their large-scale production and quality control as suggested by Ali et al. [30]. Besides, the process is eco-friendly, cost-effective, and fabricated nanoparticles are biocompatible [31]. Their biocompatibility allows them to be used as antimicrobial, antifungal, antiviral, and anticancer agents, in the treatment of diabetes-related complications, and wound healing properties and also for the degradation of pollutants. AgNPs fabrication was achieved by utilizing grape pomace, which itself is rich in tannins, and these phytochemicals acted as reducing and capping agents during synthesis. The characteristic peak obtained at 420 nm in UV-vis spectroscopy confirmed the fabrication of AgNPs, and from the application perspective, it was found that the synthesized nanoparticles showed exceptional antibacterial activity against selected pathogenic strains [32]. Utilizing the green method, Saad et al. [33] fabricated AgNPs that were effective in controlling larva of *Spodoptera littoralis,* from the extracts of pomegranate peels and watermelon, and the phytochemicals responsible for fabrication were identified as polyphenols. By using neem leaf and banana peel extract, AgNPs were fabricated and it was used in dye removal, wastewater treatment, and also as an anti-microbial agent [34]. Enhanced antimicrobial activity of AgNPs was observed when fabricated from banana peel extract [35]. Yet another application could be in packaging films for food items and to achieve this, PLA/MPE/AgNPs (poly lactic acid/mango peel extract/silver nanoparticles) were fabricated using mango peel extract by Cheng et al. [36]. The fabrication of AgNPs and AuNPs have also been done using potato peel extract [37]. Biocompatible AgNPs were fabricated using *Ipomea batatas* (L.) *Lam* peels containing various phenolic and bioactive compounds [38]. The extracts of fruits of *Terminalia chebula* or black- or chebulic myrobalan were used to fabricate AgNPs that could be used for the reduction of methylene blue [39]. Gold NPs have also been fabricated using *Terminalia chebula* using the green protocol [40]. Research has shown that the ratio of silver ion precursor versus peel extract of *Ananas comosus* (Pineapple) and pH determines whether monodispersed and stable AgNPs will form or not and the authors have also reported the fabrication of AgNPs sized between 14–20 nm, without addition of any reducing or stabilizing agents [41]. Extracts obtained from cauliflower wastes were used to fabricate AgNPs and the synthesized nanoparticles were used in photocatalytic degradation of methylene blue (MB) dye and sensing Hg^{2+} ions [42]. In yet another report, green synthesis of AgNPs using waste tea leaves was done [43]. By utilizing milk whey proteins as a reducing agent, Verma et al. [44] fabricated silver nanoparticles and suggested that this was an economical and also environmentally amenable approach. By utilizing extract from garlic as a reducing agent and post-synthesis stabilizing ligands, AgNPs were fabricated, that were both monodisperse and stable [45].

AuNPs with desirable shape and dimensionality can be made using the green chemistry of kitchen wastes; for example, onion peels contain various soluble phenolic compounds and carry cysteine derivatives that aid in stabilizing and reducing AuNPs [46]. Members of the Brassica family comprise the most consumed vegetables and they contain phenolic compounds (which confer them with anti-oxidant properties) and these phytochemicals act as capping and reducing agents during the fabrication of AuNPs from *Brassica oleracea*. The synthesis of spherical AuNPs, having an average diameter of 25.08 ± 3.73 nm was confirmed and characterization was done by UV-vis and FTIR. This method was found to be a better alternative for the revalorization of *Brassica* by-products and synthesis of nanomaterials [47]. AuNPs also find many applications including health care; however, chemically synthesized AuNPs are toxic which deters their use in biological applications. Another application of AuNPs can be in the eradication of 4-nitrophenol and as insecticidal agents in industrial wastewaters [48].

4. Fabrication of Metal Oxide Nanomaterials

Metal oxide nanoparticles are fabricated for their bactericidal activity against a range of microorganisms and the most commonly fabricated ones include those based on CuO, ZnO, CoO, MgO, NiO, Al_2O_3, In_2O_3, Cr_2O_3, Ni_2O_3, Mn_2O_3, TiO_2, ZrO_2, SiO_2, Co_3O_4, etc. The antimicrobial and antibacterial property of these nanomaterials depends on various factors like shape, surface charge, nanomaterial concentration, material type, medium components and pH, dispersion and contact of nanomaterial to the bacterial cell, physicochemical properties, presence of active oxygen, liberation of antimicrobial ions, size, specific surface-area-to-volume ratios, role of biofilm formation, role of growth rate, cell wall of bacteria, and effect of UV illumination. The conventional antibacterial agents often display reduced efficiency due to long production–consumption cycle. Besides, more pervasive and widespread use of counterfeited medicines in undeveloped and developing economies further aggravates the problem. This challenge is usually addressed by effective nanostructure synthesis to deliver the antimicrobial agent for efficient targeting of the bacterial community. The potency of the said method reduces the chances of resistance development in microbial pathogens. Besides, at concentration effective enough for killing microbial pathogens, most of the metal oxide NPs have no toxicity towards humans and at least, at the research level, studies by Hoseinzadeh et al. [24] have suggested that NPs are excellent antibacterial agents.

Metal oxide nanoparticles can be put to tremendous use because of their large surface area to volume ratio, coupled with reduced size, antimicrobial activity, photocatalytic and semiconducting properties. Several of these features facilitate the use of ZnONPs as anticancer drugs in new generation physical therapies, nanoantibiotics, and osteoinductive agents for bone tissue regeneration [49]. ZnO is currently listed as a generally recognized as safe (GRAS) material by the Food and Drug Administration (FDA) and also finds application as a food additive. The incorporation of ZnO in polymeric matrices improves antimicrobial activity and packaging properties [50]. The incorporation of metal oxide NPs in fuels can improve thermal efficiency and decrease specific fuel consumption. Besides, they enhance the cetane number, viscosity, and heating values of test fuels; however, they cause no appreciable change in noise and vibration [51]. For the conversion of solid kitchen waste into biofuel, cobalt and nickel oxide nanoparticles were fabricated using bread fungus and coriander leaves [52]. Recently, pursuant to the popular trend among the scientific community regarding the use of biologically active plant materials for nanofabrication that is sustainable, Chauhan et al. [53] fabricated ZnONPs using peels of water chestnut. The phytochemicals in water chestnut acted as both stabilizing and reducing agent, ensuring an economically viable option that was nontoxic and environmentally benign. Banana peel extract is rich in polyphenols and by utilizing it as stabilizing and reducing agent, iron oxide nanoparticles (IONPs) of size around 60 nm were synthesized via the green synthesis protocol [54]. The triglycerides present in waste frying oil were converted to biodiesel via esterification and the process utilized magnetic graphene oxide modified with three basic metal cations of cerium, zirconium, and strontium oxides to produce heterogeneous MGO@MMO nanocatalyst [55]. Silver and silver oxide nanoparticles were fabricated using powder from eggshell, and poultry waste and those were then used as materials for the fabrication of hybrid nanocomposites to make cheap polymer matrices made of antibacterial filler [56].

Green synthesis of TiO_2 nanoparticles from remnant water, a kitchen waste, that was used to soak Bengal gram beans (*Cicer arietinum* L.) was made to react with $TiCl_4$. Upon nanomaterial characterization, it was shown that uniformly sized TiO_2 nanoparticles were synthesized that did not aggregate even upon calcination and this was attributed to the stabilizing molecules naturally present in the extract [57]. Rueda et al. [58] carried out a fast and low-cost green synthesis method of Titanium Dioxide Nanocrystals (TiO_2-NCs) in which two volumetric ratios of tangerine peels, an organic waste, as bio-mediator of chemical reactions, were used to transform Titanium Dioxide (TiO_2) precursor into TiO_2-NCs. This approach could effectively bring down the environmental impact caused due to peels that eventually ended up in landfills and also it also demonstrated that a relatively large concentration of phytochemicals is crucial for the growth and formation of TiO_2-nanocrystals. By utilizing waste cooking oil, methyl ester sulfonate (MES) surfactant was prepared. MES along with TiO_2 nanoparticles were used to generate nanofluid detergent [59]. TiO_2 NPs were fabricated from aqueous extract of *Laurus nobilis* (bay leaf) and the fabricated TiO_2 NPs revealed a strong antioxidant activity when compared with the ascorbic acid standard. The process could be scaled up for large-scale industrial production, which would be eco-friendly, and economically viable with high productivity [60]. The fabrication of TiO_2 NPs by green synthesis shows immense potential when compared to physical and chemical fabrication protocols and the fabricated particles find application in electronics, energy generation devices, batteries, and sensor manufacturing and also find immense use in photodynamic cancer therapy, as antileishmanial agents, and antibacterial medicines [61]. The removal of As(III) and As(V) from contaminated waste waters was performed using novel zirconium hydroxide nanoparticle encapsulated magnetic biochar composite (ZBC) fabricated from kitchen rice residue. ZBC displayed acceptable magnetic separation ability and its surface was encapsulated with lots of hydrous zirconium oxide nanoparticles [62].

5. Fabrication of Carbon Dots

Carbon dots are immensely getting popular these days as unique class of nanomaterials that display unique optical properties, low toxicity, high biocompatibility, and economical fabrication process. These functionalities facilitate their applications in bioimaging, catalysis, sensing, and drug delivery and they are basically of two types—graphene and carbon quantum dots. Graphene quantum dots (GQDs) are anisotropic, circular, or elliptical-shaped and crystalline having few graphene layers connected via chemical groups, whereas carbon quantum dots (CQDs) are of two types based on the absence or presence of a crystal lattice and are strictly spherical shaped [63]. Although both types of CDs—synthesized by chemical methods and the green protocol—are fluorescent materials, CDs resulting from green synthesis protocols are pocket friendly, water-soluble, and non-toxic, with adjustable luminescence, and are highly biocompatible. CDs are excellent nanomaterials that can be used for the delivery of drugs, bioimaging, fluorescent inks, catalysis, and also detection of heavy metal ions [64]. Various researchers have fabricated carbon dots by utilizing the rich diversity of kitchen wastes. Green synthesis of CQDs was attempted using carbonized biomass peels of garlic, taro and sugarcane bagasse, and the researchers have highlighted that CQDs fabricated from taro peel waste showed maximum fluorescence quantum yield and was utilized to make fluorescence-based nanoprobes. These nano-based probes showed excellent photoluminescence, biocompatibility and enhanced stability and could be used as sensors for the detection of fluorides in water [65]. Another group of workers have used cooked food wastes for the fabrication of CQDs to detect additives and heavy metal ions in food and in addition to being cost effective, this fabrication procedure also addresses the environmental pollution problem [66].

The waste frying oil is an important kitchen waste and serious concern emerges due to lack of its proper disposal. The possession of distinct pH sensitivity and the linear enhancement of the intensity of photoluminescence in 3–9 pH range leads to the use of waste frying oil for fabrication of sulfur-doped carbon dots (S-C-dots). These carbon dots are photostable, possess fascinating optical properties with reduced toxicity and find immense applications as fluorescent probes for cell imaging [67]. In yet another instance, sweet potato peels were used to fabricate carbon dots (CDs) that were found to be superior fluorophores and possessed lowered toxicity and superb photostability [68]. The preparation of gelatin based functional filler for food packaging films with low cytotoxicity was achieved by incorporation of carbon dots, fabricated from potato peels, and it was found that the said packaging film was biocompatible and demonstrated strong antioxidant and antimicrobial activities [69]. Thus, CDs emerge as value added products of immense potential and their incorporation into gelatin films can provide for low-cost and functional nanofiller for the preparation of gelatin film for use in packaging applications, with various advantages including enhanced transparency, antibacterial efficacy, appreciable permeability to water vapor and hydrophobicity without affecting its tensile strength [70]. Waste tea powder was used to fabricate carbon dots (CDs) by simple carbonization and it was then grafted on TiO_2 by sol-gel method to produce nanocomposite in the range of 20 nm and was used as an active photocatalyst for the photodegradation of methyl orange [71]. Potato peels were used to fabricate catalytic magnetic microbots upon functionalization of iron oxide nanoparticles with carbon dots (C-Dots). These magnetic microbots could be reused without compromising with their performance in large-scale water treatment. This application showed synergistic effect of carbon dots and iron oxide nanoparticles in dye removal from water [72]. Recently, it has been reported that heteroatom doping enhanced optical and electronic properties of CDs by altering the structure and composition of CDs. Electrodes that are efficient and economical with improved capacity to store charge have been developed from potato peel that were doped with sulfur and phosphorus to generate co-doped porous activated carbon. The supercapacitor electrode material had large specific surface area and was porous—the latter feature was beneficial in reducing adsorption of ions and also enlarging the contact area [73]. Nitrogen functionalized carbon dots coated on zinc oxide nanoparticles (N-CDs/ZnONPs) were developed for the detection of latent DNA fingerprints in investigation of crimes, wherein the nanocomposite were fabricated using melamine, potato peel waste and zinc acetate dehydrate as precursors and showed improved efficiency, non-toxicity and excellent optical properties for the detection of freshly applied fingerprints [74]. In yet another set of experiments, carbon dots co-doped with S and N were synthesized by using water chestnut and onion and they were used as an off–on fluorescent probe for the quantification and imaging of coenzyme A [75]. Carbon dots were fabricated using garlic that is usually rich in C, N and S, is also used as a condiment in our kitchens and contain carbohydrates, proteins, and thiamine. In the presence of ferric ions, the fluorescence of these CDs showed quenching and therefore, they could be used as luminescent probes [76]. Soaked Bengal gram bean (*Cicer arietinum* L.) were used to fabricate Ni-doped SnO_2 nanoparticles and coated onto glass to form thin films that could find application as promising biosensors [77]. Earnest et al. [5] fabricated iron nanoparticles doped kitchen waste charcoal from rotten or expired pulses and rice spent tea leaves, fruits, and vegetable peels that could be used for arsenic and fluoride removal from potable water. By using kitchen wastes like grape peel, fluorescent carbon nanodots that were dispersible in water were fabricated and they showed excellent Fe^{3+} selectivity based on fluorescence quenching between nanodots and metal ions [78].

6. Fabrication of Porous Nanocarbon Spheres (PNCSs)

Porous nanocarbon spheres (PNCSs) can be produced by the valorization of kitchen wastes and they can be utilized as pocket friendly catalysts for bulk chemical transformation. An immensely cost-effective catalyst for use as bulk scale chemical transformation was produced by the valorization of kitchen wastes to the sustainable PNCSs [79]. As an example, onion peels upon pyrolysis at 1000°C yielded porous nanocarbon spheres that found application in the azo dye degradation, and the resulting corresponding amines were utilized for the synthesis of different azo compounds. It is expected that valorization of wastes would be beneficial for the environment and help in the upsurge and development of novel technologies, more in consonance with the concept of circular economy and sustainability and convert residues from different food sectors into valuable bio(nano)materials and it would also boost livelihoods and jobs [80]. The fabrication of carbon dot @ silver nanohybrids was done by utilizing peels of orange, mango and Colocasia (Taro), and these nanohybrids were larvicidal to mosquito vectors like *Aedes albopictus*, *Anopheles stephensi* and *Culex quinquefasciatus* that often bred in stagnant waters, municipal wastes and sewage water [81]. In yet another instance, kitchen wastes rich in starchy wastes were utilized to fabricate bacterial cellulose (BC) loaded with carbonaceous compounds that found application in the removal of cationic dyes [82].

7. Conclusion

The text clearly highlights the biogenic fabrication of nanosized materials from various kitchen wastes and their far-reaching applications in every aspect of human lives and touches on the pervasive concept of sustainability and circular economy highlighted therein. However, getting nanomaterials of uniform size and morphology and process scale up needs to be addressed. The green synthesis protocols have many advantages; however, they get largely confined upon fabrication due to various perils such as [83] –

i) Selection of suitable solvent system for plant extract preparation that is safe

ii) Careful optimization of process parameters affecting the fabrication process

iii) Ascertaining cytotoxicity of the fabricated nanomaterials

iv) Bulk synthesis

v) Generation of materials with controlled morphology, their upkeep and covering knowledge gaps.

Working out more rational fabrication protocols will depend on understanding the chemistry behind fabrication and the desired material characteristics that can be tailored to synthesize nanomaterials that are environmentally benign, biocompatible, and can have applications in biomedical science, environmental remediation, and consumer industries. Scaling up is definitely required as with other technologies and that would require extensive research on understanding synthesis mechanisms that would help in selection and identification of nontoxic biological and chemical agents, making the greener approach more practical industrially, and optimization of the factors that affect green synthesis process. It is expected that with these maneuvers, modern technologies including nanotechnology and Artificial Intelligence, drones, 3-D printing and Robotics can revolutionize present day industry, and business models by fundamentally revamping them [84]. As evident from the latest literature, the technology at the nanoscale can definitely be benefitted by Artificial Intelligence and mathematical modeling, however much needs to be worked out on this platform [85]. Persistent and collaborative global efforts by the researchers and scientific community can definitely serve to rule out the above challenges and make the technology more viable and amenable.

References

[1] Nanda, S. and F. Berruti. 2021. Municipal solid waste management and landfilling technologies: a review. Environ. Chem. Lett. 19: 1433–1456.

[2] Yousefi, M., V. Oskoei, A.J. Jafari, M. Farzadkia, M.H. Firooz, B. Abdollahinejad and J. Torkashvand. 2021. Municipal solid waste management during COVID-19 pandemic: effects and repercussions. Environ. Sci. Pollut. Res. 28: 32200–32209.

[3] Gao, W., Y. Chen, L. Zhan and X. Bian. 2015. Engineering properties for high kitchen waste content municipal solid waste. J. Rock Mech. Geotech. Eng. 7: 646–658.

[4] Nanda, S. and F. Berruti. 2021. A technical review of bioenergy and resource recovery from municipal solid waste. J. Hazard. Mater. 403: 123970.

[5] Earnest, I., R. Nazir and A. Hamid. 2021. Quality assessment of drinking water of Multan city, Pakistan in context with Arsenic and Fluoride and use of Iron nanoparticle doped kitchen waste charcoal as a potential adsorbent for their combined removal. Appl. Water Sci. 11: 1–15.

[6] Meng, X., X. Tan, Y. Wang, Z. Wen, Y. Tao and Y. Qian. 2019. Investigation on decision-making mechanism of residents' household solid waste classification and recycling behaviors. Resour. Conserv. Recycl. 140: 224–234.

[7] Yu, Q. and H. Li. 2020. Moderate separation of household kitchen waste towards global optimization of municipal solid waste management. J. Clean. Prod. 277: 123330.

[8] Sindhu, R., E. Gnansounou, S. Rebello, P. Binod, S. Varjani, I.S. Thakur, R.B. Nair and A. Pandey. 2019. Conversion of food and kitchen waste to value-added products. J. Environ. Manage. 241: 619–630.

[9] Pokrajac, L., A. Abbas, W. Chrzanowski, G.M. Dias, B.J. Eggleton, S. Maguire, E. Maine, T. Malloy, J. Nathwani, L. Nazar and A. Sips. 2021. Nanotechnology for a sustainable future: addressing global challenges with the international network 4 sustainable nanotechnology. ACS Nano. 15: 18608–18623.

[10] Akinaga, H. 2019. Sens. Mater. Nanofabrication technologies for All. Sens. Mater. 31: 2477–2480.

[11] Musee, N. 2011. Nanowastes and the environment: Potential new waste management paradigm. Environ. Int. 37: 112–128.

[12] Oza, G., A. Reyes-Calderón, A. Mewada, L.G. Arriaga, G.B. Cabrera, D.E. Luna, H. Iqbal, M. Sharon and A. Sharma. 2019. Plant-based metal and metal alloy nanoparticle synthesis: a comprehensive mechanistic approach. J. Mater. Sci. 55: 1309–1330.

[13] Kulkarni, N. and U. Muddapur. 2014. Biosynthesis of metal nanoparticles: a review. J. Nanotechnol 2014. Article ID 510246.

[14] Kumar, P.S., K.G. Pavithra and M. Naushad. 2019. Characterization techniques for nanomaterials. pp. 97–124. In Nanomaterials for Solar Cell Applications, Elsevier.

[15] Kumar, J.A., T. Krithiga, S. Manigandan, S. Sathish, A.A. Renita, P. Prakash, B.N. Prasad, T.P. Kumar, M. Rajasimman, A. Hosseini-Bandegharaei and D. Prabu. 2021. A focus to green synthesis of metal/metal based oxide nanoparticles: Various mechanisms and applications towards ecological approach. J. Clean. Prod. 324: 129198.

[16] Elemike, E.E., A.C. Ekennia, D.C. Onwudiwe and R.O. Ezeani. 2022. Agro-waste materials: Sustainable substrates in nanotechnology. pp. 187–214. In Agri-Waste and Microbes for Production of Sustainable Nanomaterials. Elsevier.

[17] Chen, Y., R. Guo, Y.C. Li, H. Liu and T.L. Zhan. 2016. A degradation model for high kitchen waste content municipal solid waste. Waste Manage. 58: 376–385.

[18] Mahanthesh, A.B., S. Haldar and S. Banerjee. 2022. Biotechnology for Zero Waste: Emerging Waste Management Techniques. John Wiley, 361–368.

[19] Bhardwaj, A.K., R. Naraian, S. Sundaram and R. Kaur. 2022. Biogenic and non-biogenic waste for the synthesis of nanoparticles and their applications. pp. 207–218. In Bioremediation: Green Approaches for a Clean and Sustainable Environment Bioremediation. CRC Press.

[20] Pal, G., P. Rai and A. Pandey. 2019. Green synthesis of nanoparticles: A greener approach for a cleaner future. pp. 1–26. In Green Synthesis, Characterization and Applications of Nanoparticles. Elsevier.

[21] Jha, S.K. and A. Jha. 2021. Plant extract mediated synthesis of metal nanoparticles, their characterization and applications: A green approach. Curr. Green Chem. 8: 185–202.

[22] Taran, M., M. Safaei, N. Karimi and A. Almasi. 2021. Benefits and application of nanotechnology in environmental science: an overview. Biointerface Res. Appl. Chem. 11: 7860–7870.

[23] Rao, M., A.K. Jha and K. Prasad. 2018. Nanomaterials: An upcoming fortune to waste recycling. pp. 241–271. In Exploring the Realms of Nature for Nanosynthesis. Cham: Springer International Publishing.

[24] Hoseinzadeh, E., P. Makhdoumi, P. Taha, H. Hossini, J. Stelling, M. Amjad Kamal and G. Md Ashraf. 2017. A review on nano-antimicrobials: metal nanoparticles, methods and mechanisms. Curr. Drug Metab. 18: 120–128.

[25] Virkutyte, J. and R.S. Varma. 2013. Green synthesis of nanomaterials: environmental aspects. In Sustainable nanotechnology and the environment: advances and achievements ACS Symp. Series 1124: 11–39.

[26] Iqbal, P., J.A. Preece and P.M. Mendes. 2012. Nanotechnology: the "Top-Down" and "Bottom-Up" Approaches. Supramolecular Chemistry: From Molecules to Nanomaterials. Wiley.

[27] Devatha, C.P. and A.K. Thalla. 2018. Green synthesis of nanomaterials. pp. 169–184. In Synthesis of Inorganic Nanomaterials. Woodhead Publishing.

[28] Pareek, V., A. Bhargava, R. Gupta, N. Jain and J. Panwar. 2017. Synthesis and applications of noble metal nanoparticles: a review. ASEM 9: 527–544.

[29] Tan, K.B., D. Sun, J. Huang, T. Odoom-Wubah and Q. Li. 2021. State of arts on the bio-synthesis of noble metal nanoparticles and their biological application. Chin. J. Chem. Eng. 30: 272–290.

[30] Ali, S., X. Chen, M.A. Shah, M. Ali, M. Zareef, M. Arslan, S. Ahmad, T. Jiao, H. Li and Q. Chen. 2021. The avenue of fruit wastes to worth for synthesis of silver and gold nanoparticles and their antimicrobial application against foodborne pathogens: A review. Food Chem. 359: 129912.

[31] Sharma, D., S.S. Gulati, N. Sharma and A. Chaudhary. 2022. Sustainable synthesis of silver nanoparticles using various biological sources and waste materials: A review. Emergent Mater. 5: 1649–1678.

[32] Saratale, R.G., G.D. Saratale, S. Ahn and H.S. Shin. 2021. Grape pomace extracted tannin for green synthesis of silver nanoparticles: Assessment of their antidiabetic, antioxidant potential and antimicrobial activity. Polymers 13: 4355.

[33] Saad, A.M., M.T. El-Saadony, A.M. El-Tahan, S. Sayed, M.A. Moustafa, A.E. Taha, T.F. Taha and M.M. Ramadan. 2021. Polyphenolic extracts from pomegranate and watermelon wastes as substrate to fabricate sustainable silver nanoparticles with larvicidal effect against Spodoptera littoralis. Saudi J. Biol. Sci. 28: 5674–5683.

[34] Sengupta, A. and A. Sarkar. 2022. Synthesis and characterization of nanoparticles from neem leaves and banana peels: a green prospect for dye degradation in wastewater. Ecotoxicology 31: 537–548.
[35] Ibrahim, H.M. 2015. Green synthesis and characterization of silver nanoparticles using banana peel extract and their antimicrobial activity against representative microorganisms. J. Radiat. Res. Appl. Sci. 8: 265–275.
[36] Cheng, J., X. Lin, X. Wu, Q. Liu, S. Wan and Y. Zhang. 2021. Preparation of a multifunctional silver nanoparticles polylactic acid food packaging film using mango peel extract. Int. J. Biol. Macromol. 188: 678–688.
[37] Pirathiba, S. and B.S. Dayananda. 2021. Potato peel waste as reductant for the biogenesis of gold and silver ultrafine particles. Mater. Today: Proc. 42: 1084–1090.
[38] Das, G., J.K. Patra, C.N.V. Nagaraj Basavegowda and H.S. Shin. 2019. Comparative study on antidiabetic, cytotoxicity, antioxidant and antibacterial properties of biosynthesized silver nanoparticles using outer peels of two varieties of *Ipomoea batatas* (L.) Lam. Int. J. Nanomed. 14: 4741.
[39] Edison, T.J.I. and M.G. Sethuraman. 2012. Instant green synthesis of silver nanoparticles using Terminalia chebula fruit extract and evaluation of their catalytic activity on reduction of methylene blue. Process Biochem. 47: 1351–1357.
[40] Kumar, K.M., B.K. Mandal, M. Sinha and V. Krishnakumar. 2012. Terminalia chebula mediated green and rapid synthesis of gold nanoparticles. Spectrochim. Acta A Mol. Biomol. Spectros. 86: 490–494.
[41] Agnihotri, S., D. Sillu, G. Sharma and R.K. Arya. 2018. Photocatalytic and antibacterial potential of silver nanoparticles derived from pineapple waste: process optimization and modeling kinetics for dye removal. Appl. Nanosci. 8: 2077–2092.
[42] Kadam, J., P. Dhawal, S. Barve and S. Kakodkar. 2020. Green synthesis of silver nanoparticles using cauliflower waste and their multifaceted applications in photocatalytic degradation of methylene blue dye and Hg^{2+} biosensing. SN Appl. Sci. 2: 1–16.
[43] Rajput, D., S. Paul and A. Gupta. 2020. Green synthesis of silver nanoparticles using waste tea leaves. Advanced Nano Research, Adv. Nano Res. 3: 1–14.
[44] Verma, A.K., N. Kumari and A.K. Jha. 2022. Biosynthesis of Silver Nanoparticles using Milk Whey and its Applications. IOSR J. Appl. Chem. 15: 60–66.
[45] Von White, G., P. Kerscher, R.M. Brown, J.D. Morella, W. McAllister, D. Dean and C.L. Kitchens. 2012. Green synthesis of robust, biocompatible silver nanoparticles using garlic extract. J. Nanomater. 2012: 55.
[46] Patra, J.K., Y. Kwon and K.H. Baek. 2016. Green biosynthesis of gold nanoparticles by onion peel extract: Synthesis, characterization and biological activities. Adv. Powder Technol. 27: 2204–2213.
[47] González-Ballesteros, N., J. Vidal-González and M.C. Rodríguez-Argüelles. 2021. Wealth from by-products: an attempt to synthesize valuable gold nanoparticles from *Brassica oleracea* var. acephala cv. Galega stems. J. Nanostruct. Chem. 11: 635–644.
[48] Teimouri, M., F. Khosravi-Nejad, F. Attar, A.A. Saboury, I. Kostova, G. Benelli and M. Falahati. 2018. Gold nanoparticles fabrication by plant extracts: synthesis, characterization, degradation of 4-nitrophenol from industrial wastewater, and insecticidal activity—a review. J. Clean. Prod. 184: 740–753.
[49] Carofiglio, M., S. Barui, V. Cauda and M. Laurenti. 2020. Doped zinc oxide nanoparticles: synthesis, characterization and potential use in nanomedicine. Appl. Sci. 10: 5194.
[50] Espitia, P.J.P., N.D.F.F. Soares, J.S.D.R. Coimbra, N.J. de Andrade, R.S. Cruz and E.A.A. Medeiros. 2012. Zinc oxide nanoparticles: synthesis, antimicrobial activity and food packaging applications. Food Bioprocess Technol. 5: 1447–1464.
[51] Ağbulut, Ü., M. Karagöz, S. Sarıdemir and A. Öztürk. 2020. Impact of various metal-oxide based nanoparticles and biodiesel blends on the combustion, performance, emission, vibration and noise characteristics of a CI engine. Fuel 270: 117521.
[52] Mahmood, T., S. ul Haq, A. Ahsan and W.A. Syed. 2019. Using cobalt and nickel oxide nanoparticles for the conversion of solid kitchen waste into biofuel. Curr. Anal. Energ. Environ. 1: 26–29.
[53] Chauhan, M., S. Yadav, R. Pasricha and P. Malhotra. 2021. Water chestnut peel facilitated biogenic synthesis of zinc oxide nanoparticles and their catalytic efficacy in the ring opening reaction of styrene oxide. Chem. Select 6: 8315–8322.

[54] Majumder, A., L. Ramrakhiani, D. Mukherjee, U. Mishra, A. Halder, A.K. Mandal and S. Ghosh. 2019. Green synthesis of iron oxide nanoparticles for arsenic remediation in water and sludge utilization. Clean Technol. Environ. Policy 21: 795–813.

[55] Rezania, S., M.A. Kamboh, S.S. Arian, N.A. Al-Dhabi, M.V. Arasu, G.A. Esmail and K.K. Yadav. 2021. Conversion of waste frying oil into biodiesel using recoverable nanocatalyst based on magnetic graphene oxide supported ternary mixed metal oxide nanoparticles. Bioresour. Technol. 323: 124561.

[56] Yorseng, K., S. Siengchin, B. Ashok and A.V. Rajulu. 2020. Nanocomposite egg shell powder with in situ generated silver nanoparticles using inherent collagen as reducing agent. J. Bioresour. Bioprod. 5: 101–107.

[57] Kashale, A.A., K.P. Gattu, K. Ghule, V.H. Ingole, S. Dhanayat, R. Sharma, J.Y. Chang and A.V. Ghule. 2016. Biomediated green synthesis of TiO_2 nanoparticles for lithium ion battery application. Compos. B: Eng. 99: 297–304.

[58] Rueda, D., V. Arias, Y. Zhang, A. Cabot, A.C. Agudelo and D. Cadavid. 2020. Low-cost tangerine peel waste mediated production of titanium dioxide nanocrystals: synthesis and characterization. Environmental Nanotechnology, Monitoring & Management 13: 100285.

[59] Permadani, R.L. 2019. Development of nanofluid detergent based on methyl ester sulfonates surfactant from waste cooking oil and titanium dioxide nanoparticles. IOP Conf. Series: Mater. Sci. Eng. 509: 012120.

[60] Rajeswari, V.D., E.M. Eed, A. Elfasakhany, I.A. Badruddin, S. Kamangar and K. Brindhadevi. 2021. Green synthesis of titanium dioxide nanoparticles using *Laurus nobilis* (bay leaf): Antioxidant and antimicrobial activities. Appl. Nanosci. 13: 1477–1484.

[61] Verma, V., M. Al-Dossari, J. Singh, M. Rawat, M.G. Kordy and M. Shaban. 2022. A review on green synthesis of TiO_2 NPs: Photocatalysis and antimicrobial applications. Polymer 14: 1444.

[62] Peng, Y., M. Azeem, R. Li, L. Xing, Y. Li, Y. Zhang, Z. Guo, Q. Wang, H.H. Ngo, G. Qu and Z. Zhang. 2022. Zirconium hydroxide nanoparticle encapsulated magnetic biochar composite derived from rice residue: Application for As (III) and As (V) polluted water purification. J. Hazard. Mater. 423: 127081.

[63] Iravani, S. and R.S. Varma. 2020. Green synthesis, biomedical and biotechnological applications of carbon and graphene quantum dots. A review. Environ. Chem. Lett. 18: 703–727.

[64] Shahraki, H.S., A. Ahmad and R. Bushra. 2022. Green carbon dots with multifaceted applications– Waste to wealth strategy. Flat. Chem. 31: 100310.

[65] Boruah, A., M. Saikia, T. Das, R.L. Goswamee and B.K. Saikia. 2020. Blue-emitting fluorescent carbon quantum dots from waste biomass sources and their application in fluoride ion detection in water. J. Photochem. Photobiol. B: Biol. 209: 111940.

[66] Fan, H., M. Zhang, B. Bhandari and C.H. Yang. 2020. Food waste as a carbon source in carbon quantum dots technology and their applications in food safety detection. Trends Food Sci. Technol. 95: 86–96.

[67] Hu, Y., J. Yang, J. Tian, L. Jia and J.S. Yu. 2014. Waste frying oil as a precursor for one-step synthesis of sulfur-doped carbon dots with pH-sensitive photoluminescence. Carbon 77: 775–782.

[68] Liu, H., L. Ding, L. Chen, Y. Chen, Y.T. Zhou, H. Li, Y. Xu, L. Zhao and N. Huang. 2019. A facile, green synthesis of biomass carbon dots coupled with molecularly imprinted polymers for highly selective detection of oxytetracycline. J. Ind. Eng. Chem. 69: 455–463.

[69] Himaja, A.L., P.S. Karthik, B. Sreedhar and S.P. Singh. 2014. Synthesis of carbon dots from kitchen waste: conversion of waste to value added product. J. Fluoresc. 24: 1767–1773.

[70] Min, S., P. Ezati and J.W. Rhim. 2022. Gelatin-based packaging material incorporated with potato skins carbon dots as functional filler. Ind. Crops Prod. 181: 114820.

[71] Kuldeep, A.R., R.D. Waghmare and K.M. Garadkar. 2022. Green synthesis of TiO_2/CDs nanohybrid composite as an active photocatalyst for the photodegradation of methyl orange. J. Mater. Sci.: Mater. Electron. 33: 7933–7944.

[72] Shivalkar, S., P.K. Gautam, A. Verma, K. Maurya, Md Palashuddin, S.K. Samanta and A.K. Sahoo. 2021. Autonomous magnetic microbots for environmental remediation developed by organic waste derived carbon dots. J. Environ. Manag. 297: 113322.

[73] Khalafallah, D., X. Quan, C. Ouyang, M. Zhi and Z. Hong. 2021. Heteroatoms doped porous carbon derived from waste potato peel for supercapacitors. Renew. Energy 170: 60–71.

[74] Prabakaran, E. and K. Pillay. 2020. Synthesis and characterization of fluorescent N-CDs/ZnONPs nanocomposite for latent fingerprint detection by using powder brushing method. Arab. J. Chem. 13: 3817–3835.

[75] Hu, Y., L. Zhang, X. Li, R. Liu, L. Lin and S. Zhao. 2017. Green preparation of S and N Co-doped carbon dots from water chestnut and onion as well as their use as an off–on fluorescent probe for the quantification and imaging of coenzyme A. ACS Sustain. Chem. Eng. 5: 4992–5000.

[76] Sun, C., Y. Zhang, P. Wang, Y. Yang, Y. Wang, J. Xu, Y. Wang and W.W. Yu. 2016. Synthesis of nitrogen and sulfur co-doped carbon dots from garlic for selective detection of Fe^{3+}. Nanoscale Res. Lett. 11: 1–9.

[77] Gattu, K.P., K. Ghule, A.A. Kashale, V.B Patil, D.M. Phase, R.S. Mane, S.H. Han, R. Sharma and A.V. Ghule. 2015. Bio-green synthesis of Ni-doped tin oxide nanoparticles and its influence on gas sensing properties. RSC Adv. 5: 72849–72856.

[78] Xu, J., T. Lai, Z. Feng, X. Weng and C. Huang. 2015. Formation of fluorescent carbon nanodots from kitchen wastes and their application for detection of Fe^{3+}. Luminescence. 30: 420–424.

[79] Supriya, S., G.S. Ananthnag, T. Maiyalagan and G. Hegde. 2022. Kitchen waste derived porous nanocarbon spheres for metal free degradation of azo dyes: An environmental friendly, cost effective method. J. Clust. Sci. 34: 243–254.

[80] Xu, C., M. Nasrollahzadeh, M. Selva, Z. Issaabadi and R. Luque. 2019. Waste-to-wealth: Biowaste valorization into valuable bio (nano) materials. Chem. Soc. Rev. 48: 4791–4822.

[81] Raul, P.K., P. Santra, D. Goswami, V. Tyagi, C. Yellappa, V. Mauka, R.R. Devi, P. Chattopadhyay, R.V. Jayaram and S.K. Dwivedi. 2021. Green synthesis of carbon dot silver nanohybrids from fruits and vegetable's peel waste: Applications as potent mosquito larvicide. Curr. Res. Green Sustain. Chem. 4: 100158.

[82] Saleh, A.K., H. El-Gendi, J.B. Ray and T.H. Taha. 2021. A low-cost effective media from starch kitchen waste for bacterial cellulose production and its application as simultaneous absorbance for methylene blue dye removal. Biomass Conv. Bioref. 13: 12437–12449.

[83] Ahmed, S.F., M. Mofijur, N. Rafa, A.T. Chowdhury, S. Chowdhury, M. Nahrin, A.S. Islam and H.C. Ong. 2022. Green approaches in synthesising nanomaterials for environmental nanobioremediation: Technological advancements, applications, benefits and challenges. Environ. Res. 204: 111967.

[84] Romanovs, A., I. Pichkalov, E. Sabanovic and J. Skirelis. 2019. Industry 4.0: methodologies, tools and applications. Proc. Open Conf. Elect., Electron. Info. Sci. (eStream), IEEE. 1–4.

[85] Moore, J.A. and J.C. Chow. 2021. Recent progress and applications of gold nanotechnology in medical biophysics using artificial intelligence and mathematical modeling. Nano Express. 2: 022001.

5

Nanofabrication Using Physical Methods

G.V.S. Subbaroy Sarma,[1] *Payal B. Joshi*[2] and *Murthy Chavali*[3],*

1. Introduction

Nanotechnology is the creation and use of functioning entities on atom and molecule level that has one unique size in the nm range [1]. Due to their tiny dimensions, these substances and structures may be deliberately constructed to display unique and considerably better fundamental characteristics, behaviours, and procedures. Materials are classified as nanomaterials when only any of their dimensions are between 1 and 100 nanometres. Asbestos nanofibers were used to strengthen ceramic compositions around 4500 years ago [2]. PbS nanomaterials were known by early Egyptians over 4000 years back, so they have been utilised through a primitive hair-dyeing method [3, 4]. The other noteworthy instance from earlier days would be the Lycurgus Cup. It was a diffracted bowl made mostly during the 4th century A.D. first by Romans. With illumination, it has a jade-like appearance, yet in transmittance, it has a transparent ruby appearance. Picture variability is visible based mostly on incident beam.

The existence of silver as well as gold nanoparticles causes such colour changes [5]. Richard Adolf Zsigmondy came up with the term "nanometer" in 1914. In his lecture at the American Physical Society's yearly conference, British scientist and Nobel Laureate Richard Feynman presented the first unique notion

[1] Department of Physics, Malla Reddy Engineering College (A), Maisammaguda, Dhulapally, Medchal, Malkajgiri. Secundrabad-500100 Telangana State, India.

[2] Shefali Research Laboratories, 203/454, Sai Section, Ambernath (East)-421501, Mumbai, Maharashtra, India.

[3] Office of the Dean Research & Development), # CK 106-P, Chanakya Bldg, Dr. Vishwanath Karad MITWPU, Pune 411038 Maharashtra, India.

* Corresponding author: ChavaliM@gmail.com, ChavaliM@outlook.com

of nanotechnology [6]. He gave a speech named "There's Plenty of Room at the Bottom." Feynman demonstrated during his presentation, he explained how the rules of matter need not restrict human capacity to operate only at atomic and molecular scales, but instead an absence of proper technology and approaches [7]. Regularly, the science of nanotechnology advances and today, sophisticated characterisation and fabrication methods are available for generating nanocomposites. Nanoparticles have developed into a fascinating category of materials in great interest with a variety of commercial uses. Nanomaterials are being used commercially in water-resistant paint, surface properties, electronic parts, beauty products, ecological clean-up, sensor systems, and energy storage devices [8]. The precise production, as well as assembly of nanoparticles and nanostructures, is going to be a key enabler in science and technology.

2. Classification of Nanomaterials

Nanomaterials have an extremely small size and have at least one dimension of 100 nm or less. As per Siegel, nanomaterials are categorized into 0-Dm, 1-Dm, 2-Dm, and 3-Dm nanostructures, as illustrated in Fig. 1.

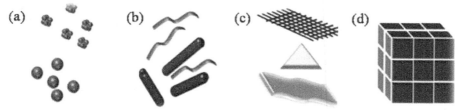

Fig. 1. (a) 0D spheres and clusters, (b) 1D nanofibers, wires, and rods, (c) 2D films, plates, and networks, (d) 3D nanomaterials.

3. Properties of Nanomaterials

Nanomaterials possess physical parameters that are midway among atoms as well as composite materials. The characteristics of nanometer-sized substances vary markedly from those in atom and composite substances. Nanomaterials have an extraordinarily wide surface-to-volume ratio because of their short widths, leading to high vast interfacial, creating enhanced interface-dependent material characteristics. The surface characteristics of nanoparticles may influence the overall substance, particularly whenever the dimensions of nanoparticles are equivalent to magnitude. As a result, the core substances' qualities might be enhanced or modified. Metallic nanomaterials, in particular, may be utilised in highly effective catalysts.

3.1 Optical Properties

The optical characteristics of nanoparticles are probably among the more exciting and relevant features. Nanomaterials' optical capabilities are influenced by factors like smaller dimensions, form, and surface morphology, including additional factors like adding impurities and making contact with the surroundings as well as similar nanoscale. Similarly, the form of metallic nanoparticles also has a significant impact on their optical characteristics. The optical characteristics of metallic nanoparticles vary as they become larger. Once anisotropy was introduced onto a nanoparticle, especially during its formation of nanostructures, the optical characteristics of the nanoparticles drastically altered. Whenever the size of the nanoparticles was lowered to less than 10 nm, dimension impacts upon optical characteristics were found [9].

3.2 Mechanical Properties

Mechanical properties of nanomaterials generally consist strength, brittleness, hardness, toughness, fatigue strength, plasticity, elasticity, ductility, rigidity, and yield stress. Having a better knowledge of the mechanical characteristics of such substances, model computations and molecular mechanics investigations is critical.

3.3 Electronic Transport in Nanostructures

Nanomaterials feature novel characteristics, which are typically not found in bulk materials related to their distinct electrical configuration and charge concentration. By making use of the nanostructure's unique features, modern electrical and optoelectronic components may be made. The 2D quantum theory field design is indeed the simplest to make of various nanomaterials. This is because, at the nanometer scale, it remains simply a single limited feature that might be the width of a thin layer that would be accurately modulated using advanced thin-film depositing methods like chemical vapour depositing. A quantum well design may be readily constructed by layering nm size tighter bandgap semiconductor among larger bandgap semiconductor materials. The movement of electrons across layered quantum well devices is governed by a tunnelling process.

3.4 Magnetic Properties

Although gold and platinum were quasi in bulk, both were magnetic at the nanoscale. Boundary atoms vary from bulk atoms as these could be transformed by interactions using various chemical species, i.e., by coating nanoparticles. Such a process allows for the modification of nanoparticle characteristics by encapsulating those using suitable compounds. Whenever quasi substances were synthesized at the nanoscale, they may display ferromagnetic-like properties. Non-magnetic substances may be used to make magnetic nanoparticles of Pd, platinum, and, more surprisingly, gold.

Mostly in sense of Pt and Pd, ferromagnetism is caused by compositional modifications due to size impacts. Whenever nanocomposites were coated using exactly suitable molecules, they turned ferromagnetic: the charge concentrated at the nanoscale interface causes magnetic properties. Highly concentrated carriers in the 5d band are found in molecules with diameters less than 2 nanometers. Bulk gold, like bare gold nps, exhibits an amazingly small concentration of regions and this will be diamagnetic. It is revealed how chemical bonding would create ferromagnetic properties in metallic groups by altering its d group configuration.

4. Nanomaterial Fabrication Techniques

Typically speaking, there are 2 methods of nanostructured materials' fabrication (Fig. 2):

1. Bottom-up approach
2. Top-down approach

Bottom-up procedures comprise continuous downsizing of material constituents, followed by a self-assembly mechanism that results in nanostructured synthesis. Mechanical influences occurring at the nanometer were employed to merge units forming bigger, structural shapes throughout self-assembly. With top-down techniques, bulkier starting configurations are used, that could be manipulated directly during nanostructured production [10]. The bigger molecule is chopped down into tiny components, which are subsequently transformed into a nanoparticle. Top-down fabrication techniques include crushing or milling, physical vapour deposition, as well as various damaging techniques [11].

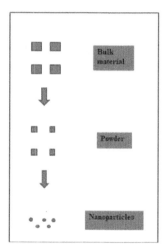 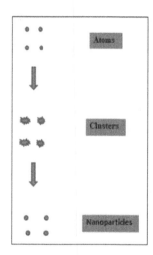

Fig. 2. (a) Top-down approach. (b) Bottom-up approach.

4.1 Mechanical Method

This represents a very low-cost approach for making nanoparticles in bulk. Ball milling is the easiest mechanical technique for transferring kinetic energy through the grinding material into any substance being reduced.

4.1.1 Mechanical/High Ball Milling Method

Milling is a consistently solid procedure for the fabrication of nanomaterials. Due to structural constraints, generating amazing nanoparticles with this approach is extremely tough as well as time-consuming. Mechanical milling, on the other hand, has several merits, including ease to use, relatively inexpensive nanomaterials' manufacturing, as well as the ability to increase up to huge proportions. The form of grinder, crushing rate, containers, duration, humidity, environment, width and width variation of the processing material, processing regulating agency, as well as the amount of filling its vial were some key aspects determining this finalized.

This was one of the quickest methods to synthesise nanoparticles from certain materials including composites. Milling comes in a variety of shapes and sizes, including planetary, vibratory, rod, and tumbling mills. After all addition, the width of the vessel is determined by the number of interests. The very first substance might have any dimension or form. Tight lids are used to lock the vessel. A 2:1 mass proportion of balls with the substance was generally recommended. Its grinding capacity is diminished whenever this vessel is higher over halfway full. When massive grinding balls collide, the impacting intensity is increased. Grinding with heavier pellets results in reduced particulate diameter yet higher flaws inside those nanoparticles.

Furthermore, certain pollutants inside these spheres might be introduced during this procedure. Non-crystalline particle production is enhanced by decreasing temperature. To discharge this energy created, cryo-cooling was occasionally utilized. Fluids may similarly be employed throughout its grinding. These vessels were revolved along their respective axis at a considerable rate. For synthesizing nanomaterials with their desired form, grinding rate and time are important [12, 13].

The substance was driven towards its boundaries, squeezed along the boundaries once its vessels rotate by about core direction as well as its inner axes, as observed in Fig. 3. It was essential that grind the substance into a small particle for which size can be relatively homogeneous. Simply by adjusting the rotational motion between the central axis and vessel, relatively homogeneous particles can be obtained. With the revolution of a singular vessel, the substance was forced toward the wall, with dark spots representing the powder form and vacant portions Fig. 4. The grinding device is used to make nanocrystalline substances such as cobalt, chromium, nickel-titanium, aluminium-iron and silver-iron nanoparticles in a matter of minutes to hours, ranging from a few milligrams to many kilograms.

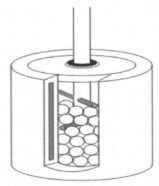

Fig. 3. A schematic diagram of a ball mill vessel.

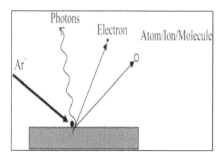

Fig. 7. Interaction of an ion with target.

to target atoms, and electron beams due to their own energy. The diagram depicts a schematic representation of numerous options (Fig. 7).

Direct Current (DC) sputtering, Radio Frequency (RF) sputtering, and magnetron sputtering are all possibilities for sputtering. In all the foregoing situations, discharges or plasma comprising compressed gases, ions or reacting gases are employed. Its deposits take place within a highly vacuum or extremely higher pressure pump comprising electrodes, each being a sputtering target as well as a substrate, often a gaseous injection capability among various components. While this mechanism would be under maximum gaseous compression while deposition which enables to get required purity.

4.2.5.1 DC Sputtering

It was an extremely simple depositing process where the sputtering targets were kept at a higher negative polarity while the substrates would remain near a positive, grounding, or floating voltage as shown in Figs. 8 and 9. According to that substance that is mounted, surfaces could be either warm or chilled around that same time. After this vacuum pump reached its desired basis level, argon gases were normally supplied under the stress of less than 10 Pa. Its commencement of depositing is indicated by a perceptible flame with power flow between both the cathode and anode. This glowing discharge was formed whenever a comparatively elevated potential is supplied across the anode and cathode having a gas particle, comprising various sections like cathode glow, Crooke's dark space, and negative light up, Faraday darkness space, positive column, anode dark area, and anode brightening.

Plasma, which contains a combination of particles, charges, and neutral atoms, with photons generated during numerous interactions, creates such zones. This compressed gas determines the overall quantity among distinct nanoparticles as well as the range through which these are spread. Gas ionisation is caused by intense particle collisions Fig. 7. The ion/neutral ratio is typically 10^{-4}. As a result, under a few more Pa pressure, a very big enough number of particles can be generated.

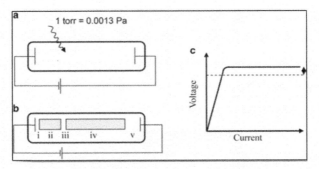

Fig. 8. (a) Plasma Generation (b) various regions of plasma and (c) i–v characteristic.

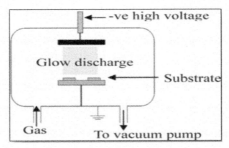

Fig. 9. Typical DC sputtering unit schematic layout.

4.2.5.2 RF Sputtering

Maintaining discharges among these terminals might demand their application at extremely strong voltages. Sputtering at 100–3,000 V was frequent among DC discharges. When a large intensity power is increased, its cathode and anode alternately modify polarizability, and its oscillatory particles induce enough ionisation. Frequencies of 5–30 MHz could be employed, while its terminals could become insulated. Nevertheless, while each frequency was allocated internationally for such purposes while various frequencies were accessible, 13.56 MHz was most often utilized in a deposition. Once this setup described in Fig. 10 is adopted, this targeting is inherently biased towards the negative electrode, turning negative.

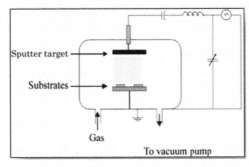

Fig. 10. RF sputtering set up with matching network.

4.2.5.3 Magnetron sputtering

The use of magnetism would boost RF/DC sputtered speeds even more. Lorentz force describes a force that a charging particle experiences whenever either electrical or magnetical fields operate at the same time.

$$\mathbf{F} = q\,(\mathbf{E} + \mathbf{v} \times \mathbf{B})$$

If E and B are parallel to one another, as shown in Fig. 11, single-particle leaves its terminal with an inclination of $0°$. While $v \times B = 0$, merely an applied potential operates mostly upon particles. Any particle creating an inclination θ, on the other hand, might be affected by all electromagnetic fields. $qv \cos \theta$ has been the amplitude of this particle acceleration within directions of an applied force. Considering the strength of $q\,v\,B \sin \theta$, this component owing to magnetic force might be transverse towards each v and B. The length of a particle orbiting all across the magnetic fields axis was r. Then $m\,(v \sin \theta)^2/r$ was their centrifugal force around there.

$$m\,(v \sin \theta)^2/r = q\,v\,B \sin \theta$$

$$\text{Thus} \quad r = \frac{mv\sin\theta}{qB}$$

Each electron can ionise additional particles inside the gas by moving in a helix pattern. In reality, magnetic fields that were simultaneously parallel and perpendicular to its axis of the applied field were applied to enhance the ionizing of the gas and hence, It's sputtering effectiveness. Metal oxides such as Al_2O_3, nitrides such as TiN, and carbides such as WC could be produced by sputtering metallic substrates with gases such as O_2, N_2, NH_3, CH_4, and H_2S. It was described as 'reactive sputtering'.

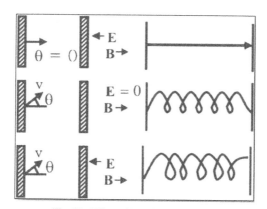

Fig. 11. Effect of E and B on electron.

4.2.5.4 Electron Cyclotron Resonance (ECR) Plasma Deposition

Utilizing microwaves' frequencies as well as associating the resonant frequencies of particles within a magnetic field, its plasma concentration could be increased even more.

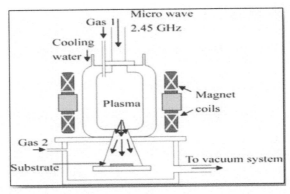

Fig. 12. Electron Cyclotron Resonance schematic diagram for deposition.

$$\omega = \frac{eB}{m}$$

Here ω is the microwave frequency, which was usually 2.45 GHz, e represents the charge of the electron, m is the mass of the electron, and B is the magnetic field. ECR plasma ionisation density is around 2–3 times of scale higher than prior approaches. With such a method, thin films and nanomaterials of SiO_2, SiN, and GaN were produced. Figure 12 depicts a diagram illustrating such a strategy.

5. Other Physical Methods

5.1 Electric Arc Deposition

It was among the most basic and effective processes for bulk fullerenes, carbon nanotubes, and other materials. This arrangement was depicted in Fig. 13, consisting mostly of a liquid vacuum with electrodes that form an arc among themselves. This positive electrode alone serves as a substance resource. Whenever catalysts were employed, an extra heating supply of evaporation could be required. Inert gas is required based on the targeted outcomes. An extremely strong current of 50–100 A was transmitted through a lower voltage source across a 1 mm separation across its terminals. Inside the vacuum pump, an inert atmosphere pressure is sustained. Anode substance disappears if the arc was formed. Once these electrodes are burned while their separation is widening, this gets increasingly necessary to regulate this electrode spacing before destroying a continuous vacuum. Such an approach involved creating an arc between two graphene sheets to obtain vast quantities of fullerenes. Under lower helium pressure, fullerenes develop, while nanotubes establish with increased pressure. Fullerenes can be made through purifying dust gathered near its vacuum chamber's internal side, but nanotubes can exclusively be generated with higher He gas pressures and even inside its cathode's mid-section. There were almost no carbon nanotubes just on the inner wall.

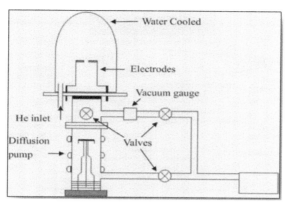

Fig. 13. Arc deposition set up.

Carbon nanoparticles have been frequently observed just at sites in which nanotubes were generated. When an arc discharge occurs, the temperatures might exceed 3,500 degree Celsius. Different nanoparticles might potentially be feasible to acquire using a similar process. Furthermore, it has been discovered that such an approach was best suited for the production of fullerenes or carbon nanotubes.

5.2 Ion Beam Technique

There exist many instances where lower or higher energetic ions were employed for creating nanoparticles. Ion gun typically generate metallic ions that is specifically supposed to generate metallic ions that have been pushed to lower or higher energies and directed towards such a surface warmed up to only a few thousand °C. Different mechanisms such as sputtering and electromagnetic radiation may occur in combination during sputtering depositing, based on the overall strength of such impacting ions. For such cases, heating was employed to enhance the crystalline nature of certain substances. Ion implantation was also used to synthesize doped nanoparticles in certain instances. Manufacturing nanoparticles with rapid ion beams and highly energetic ion accelerators may potentially be a feasible prospect.

5.3 Plasma

A further approach for producing nanoparticles includes the plasma technique. Radiofrequency heating circuits create this plasma. The first material was placed inside a pestle, which was then placed inside a fully isolated tube. Relatively high coils looped over that evacuation tube subsequently warmed solid material beyond its vaporization limit. Helium seems to be the gas employed mostly during the process, but upon entering into the device produces higher plasma within this vicinity of such coils. Such metals form vapourised nuclei mostly on helium atoms that disperse up to just a cool collecting rod, in which nanoparticles are then gathered but also properly sanitized with gaseous oxygen. Thermal plasma procedures, as well as plasma spray syntheses, are different sorts of plasma procedures. Plasma spray synthesizing seems to be a process for making nanoparticles which could be done out in free air. The

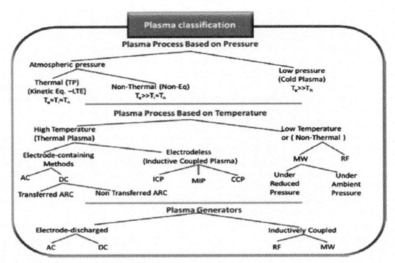

Fig. 14. Different plasma classification.

gathering of such created nanoparticles becomes challenging due to the fast flow speed with those nanoparticles. Nanoparticles bearing electrical charges emerge from the plasma region within the thermal plasma procedure. Thus, as a consequence of such advantages of using energetic ions, aggregation, as well as coagulation, could significantly be decreased [22, 23].

Different reaction rates could generally reach over vapour deposition since the reactants were ionised and then separated; however, their electrostatic interactions of the particles stay. Massive manufacturing prices, a thin grain size, as well as the capacity to make unagglomerated particles have all been major benefits of its technique [24]. This technique's benefits include its flexibility, low price, and capacity to attain larger yields. This technique's scope is restricted by the need for safe and reliable particulate gathering [25]. Plasma processes are classified depending upon the substances supplied into the reactors as well as the thermal mechanism Fig. 14.

5.4 Microwave Irradiation

By their well-known merits beyond chemically synthesized approaches, microwave irradiation was already frequently utilized in the preparation of biological, and chemical, including artificial nanocomposites [26]. The rapid and efficient oxidizing of chemical molecules during microwave conditions was studied using a new stage transmission-oxidizing agent called CTAMABC. CTAMABC initially dissolved in acetonitrile, and then alcohol was applied rapidly around room temperature with synthesized solution forcefully mixed. After microwave irradiation, this liquid remained homogenous over a brief period until the black-brown reducing chemical was collected. These interactions were monitored using paper chromatography as well as ultra-violet spectroscopy [27]. Some other researchers used hexamine as a reductant and bio-based pectin as a stabiliser for the synthesis of Ag NPs through an aqueous solution with a quick, effective, and cost-effective microwave-assisted synthesis method. These nanoparticles are discovered to have an overall circular form with a diameter of 18.84 nm. Its activated strength was estimated to be 47.3 kJ mol^{-1} [28], and its reactants increased upon its rise in temperatures.

5.5 Pulsed Laser Method

A pulsed laser approach is typically utilised for the manufacture of nanoparticles with a fast speed of around 3 gm/min. Inside a blender-like appliance, silver nitrate solutions with some reduction reaction were injected. Its mechanism includes a hard disk, which spins in with these solutions. To generate warm spots upon that disc's surfaces, it was subjected to pulse using laser light. Its silver nitrate interacts only with reduction solution to generate silver nanoparticles that may be extracted using centrifugation near hot regions. Their average particle diameter is determined mostly by the laser's intensity and its disc's rotational speed shown in Fig. 15.

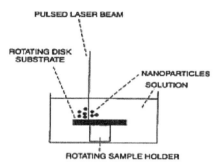

Fig. 15. Pulsed laser setup.

5.6 Gamma Radiation

Gamma radiation would be the best route for the fabrication of metallic nanoparticles since this is repeatable, can regulate the structure of the particulate. Mainly produces narrow sized nanoparticles, which are simple, inexpensive, as well as requires minimal toxins' precursors: through the water as well as a solvent like ethanol, this has used a fewest reaction mixture, this utilises a reaction condition nearer to room temperature and reduces its portions as by-products and waste [29]. Radiolytic reductions were seen to be very effective methods for producing monosized and widely scattered metallic clusters [30]. The stimulation and ionizing of its liquid were the principal consequences of elevated gamma radiation interacting with aqueous solutions containing ions [31]. Water could be produced, for example, by irradiating a sequence of reduction and oxidation substances, as illustrated in the expression below.

$$H_2O \Rightarrow e^-_{aq}, H_3O +, H \cdot, OH \cdot, H_2, H_2O_2$$

The compounds e$^-$ aq and H• seem to be the core components for this way of producing nanoparticles using metallic dissolved salts. However, some specific hydroxyl scavengers were applied, and this formation of hydroxyl OH• hinders its effectiveness. Isopropanol [32] would be a popular choice with them. One such method had been frequently employed to develop nanoparticle fluids, especially silver and gold, in the past. Gamma Ray has been employed to capture nanoparticles within polymeric structures including mesoporous [33–35].

5.7 Lithographic Methods

Lithographic techniques were top-down approaches capable of creating micron-sized features for most parts, although they are power complex and expensive apparatus. For centuries, lithography has been employed to create printable circuits and computers. Nanoimprint lithography would be a more specific variety of lithography than traditional lithography. It was a pretty lot similar pattern creation. Templates are created initially; subsequently, some softer polymer substance is pressed that makes a final design. Stamping materials were formed via the top-down process. Nanospheres lithography uses latex spheres to create functionalized matrices. Photolithography, e$^-$ beam lithography, soft lithography, focussed ion lithography, microlithography, and dipped pinning lithography are some of the patterning processes.

5.8 Sputtering

Sputtering would be a phenomenon in which nanoparticles are deposited by ejecting particles from that [36]. The heat treatment process is just a great way to build a thin sheet of nanomaterials. Both dimensions and shapes of nanoparticles are governed by the parameters mentioned: (i) temperatures (ii) layers' width (iii) thermal treatment time (iv) surface, etc. [37].

6. Application of Nanoparticles

6.1 Food Packaging

Carbon nanotubes, which are cylindrical structures having nanoscale level width, represent an advancement in nanotechnologies for packaged foods. Nanosensors include detectors that are embedded in packing materials that identify gases that escape into defective foods, thus minimising gas penetration and condensation. Silica nanoparticles reduce losses of humidity out from substance while also preventing oxygen entry within the container [38]. Nanotechnology has yet to be used to monitor food. Nanosensors, which are small microchips implanted inside foods and create an electronic signal, will be used in the monitoring systems to help to follow quality ingredients through the field via factories to major retailers. Bacterial deterioration is, however, detected when the product is encased in a smart package.

6.2 Food Processing

In the categories of efficient nutrition delivery, and biological isolation of proteins, including nanoencapsulation of nutritional supplements, the possible influence of nanotechnologies in food manufacturing is a fast-growing trend. Nutrients, antibacterial agents, and antioxidants, including food ingredients like colourants, and preservatives have all been essential constituents of food products. Food qualities such as colour, tasting, texture, and storage stability were suitable with all of those ingredients. Nano encapsulating, nano emulsified, and other methods of preservation may be used.

6.3 Medicine

Nanoscience and technology are now being explored in the domain of medicine towards timely identification of diseases like cancers and atherosclerotic, as well as drug targeting to a specific biological cell. Timing of medication distribution and the speciality of sick cells were two essential characteristics of nanotechnology in drug delivery applications that enhance effective accessibility. Vast interfacial proportion enhances orthopaedic performance and reduces patient satisfaction by increasing bone interconnections [39].

6.4 Antimicrobial Activity

The bacteriostatic impact of metal nanoparticles has been related to their tiny dimensions and surface area to volume ratio, which allows interaction carefully with microorganism's membranes, allowing metal nanoparticles to penetrate quickly into cells excluding the intrinsic parts of the cell, effectively inactivating the microorganisms.

6.5 Agriculture

Agriculture is the main source of livelihood for several nations, such as India and China, which draw almost a percentage of their national wealth from this. However, mostly because of climatic change, ecological issues such as pesticide and fertiliser deposition, and urbanisation, such industry is currently facing multiple difficulties. Mostly in areas of nutrition absorption, identification of diseases, infection management, and intelligent supply networks, nanotechnology is revolutionising farming [40]. Nanocatalyst will improve accessible with pesticides and fertilisers within upcoming to improve energy effectiveness with reduced dose rates, and environmental protection against elevated pesticides.

6.6 Textile

Nanotechnology's application within garment industries has been receiving attention as potential technology for various applications [41]. Water repellence, wrinkling resistance, anti-bacterial, anti-static, and UV protection are just a few features.

7. Conclusion

This paper provided a comprehensive summary of nanoparticles, including their categorization, production, characterization, and uses. Around a minimum of 1 nm, groupings of elements are worked within nanotechnologies. Nanoparticles were frequently classified as things with large sizes. Nanotechnology involves the scientific knowledge of substances, which display extraordinary qualities, functions, and processes because of their small size. Nanoparticles had sparked a lot of attention because of their unusual physical and chemical characteristics, and they can be used in a variety of applications. Nanotechnology nowadays takes advantage of the latest advances in material science, biotechnology, and electronics that produce innovative substances with special characteristics due to their nanometric structures.

Several of these substances, including sunscreens and stain-resistant plants, have indeed made their way inside consumer items. Some were being studied in-depth seeking remedies for humankind's most pressing issues, such as sickness, clean technology, and freshwater. Future nanotechnology goods, which would be accessible within the next generations, promise much more transformative uses than the present and relatively close nanotechnologies. Nanoparticles can be used in a variety of fields, including medical, agro-food, electronics, and energy generation. Nanoparticles, in a nutshell, have rendered our lives easier and more comfortable. Nanotechnology has a promising future because of its applications in numerous disciplines of research. Several nanoparticle-manufacturing processes were created, and they are appropriate for the synthesis of nanomaterials in a variety of applications.

Acknowledgement

We thank previous and current lab members for their valuable contributions.

Author Contributions

All authors read and equally contributed to this manuscript.

References

[1] Satya Narayana, T., M.V. Ramana Reddy and J. Siva Kumar. 2016. Synthesis and characterization of pure and indium doped SnO_2 nanoparticles by sol-gel methods. International Journal of Scientific & Engineering Research 7(12). December-2016. ISSN 2229-5518.

[2] Heiligtag, F.J. and M. Niederberger. 2013. The fascinating world of nanoparticle research. Research Review, Mat. Today 16: 262–271.

[3] Walter, P., E. Welcomme, P. Hallegot, N.J. Zaluzec, C. Deeb, J. Castaing, P. Veyssiere, R. Breniaux, J. Leveque and G. Tsoucaris. 2006. Early use of PbS nanotechnology for an ancient hair dyeing formula. Nano Lett. 6: 2215–2219.

[4] Jeevanandam, J., A. Barhoum, Y.S. Chan, A. Dufresne and M.K. Danquah. 2018. Review on nanoparticles and nanostructured materials: history, sources, toxicity and regulations. Beilstein J. Nanotech. 9: 1050–1074.

[5] Freestone, I., N. Meeks, M. Sax and C. Higgitt. 2007. The Lycurgus Cup—A Roman Nanotechnology. Gold Bull. 40: 270–277.

[6] Santamaria, A. 2012. Nanotoxicity, Historical Overview of Nanotechnology and Nanotoxicology. Humana Press, Totowa, chap-1: 1–12.

[7] Nasrollahzadeh, M., M. Sajadi, M. Atarod, M. Sajjadi and Z. Issaabadi. 2019. An Introduction to Green Nanotechnology. Interface Science and Technology, Elsevier, 28: 1–27.

[8] Sharifi, S., S. Behzadi, S. Laurent, M. Laird Forrest, P. Stroeve and M. Mahmoudi. 2012. Toxicity of nanomaterials. Chem. Soc. Rev. 41: 2323–2343.

[9] Karak, N. 2019. Fundamentals of nanomaterials and polymer nanocomposites. pp. 1–45. *In*: Nanomaterials and Polymer Nanocomposites.

[10] Namita, R. 2015. Methods of preparation of nanoparticles—a review. International Journal of Advances in Engineering & Technology Jan. 2015. ISSN: 22311963.

[11] Iravani, S. 2011. Green synthesis of metal nanoparticles using plants. Green Chem. 13: 2638–2650.

[12] Konrad, A., U. Herr, R. Tidecks, F. Kummer and K. Samwer. 2001. Luminescence of bulk and nanocrystalline cubic yttria. J. App. Physics 90: 3516–23.

[13] Andrievskii, R.A. 1994. The synthesis and properties of nanocrystalline refractory compounds. Russian Chem. Rev. 63: 411–427.

[14] Rastogi, A. 2017. A mini-review practice of formulations of nanoparticles. Int. J. Chem. Synthesis Chem. Reactions 3: 1–7.

[15] Dikusar, A.I., P.G. Globa, S.S. Belevskii and S.P. Sidel nikova. 2009. On limiting rate of dimensional electrodeposition at meso and nanomaterial manufacturing by template synthesis. Surface Eng. Appl. Electrochem. 45: 171–9.

[16] Karthikeyan, B. and B. Loganathan. 2013. A close look of Au/Pt/Ag nanocomposites using SERS assisted with optical, electrochemical, spectral and theoretical methods. Phys E 49: 105–10.

[17] Amendola, V. and M. Meneghetti. 2009. Laser Ablation synthesis in solution and size manipulation of noble metal nanoparticles. Phys. Chem. Chem. Phys. 11: 3805–3821.

[18] Dudoitis, V. et al. 2011. Lith. J. Phys. 51: 03.

[19] Skandan, G. and A. Singhal. 2006. *In*: Y. Gogotsi (ed.). Nanomaterials Handbook. Taylor and Francis Group, Florida.

[20] Sudarsanam, P. and B.M. Reddy. 2013. *In*: T. Tsuzuki (ed.). Nanotechnology Commercialization. Pan Stanford Publishing, Singapore.

[21] Behera, S. and P.L. Nayak. 2013. *In vitro* antibacterial activity of green synthesized silver nanoparticles using Jamun extract against multiple drug-resistant bacteria. World J. Nano Sci. Technol. 2: 62–65.

[22] Vollath, D. and K.E. Sickafus. 1992. Synthesis of nanosized ceramic oxide powders by microwave plasma reactions. Nano Struct. Mat. 1: 427–437.

[23] Vollath, D. 1994. Mater. Res. Soc. Symp. Proc. 347: 629.

[24] Vollath, D. 2008. Nanomaterials: An Introduction to Synthesis, Properties and Applications. Wiley-VCH, Weinheim 7: 865–870.

[25] Luther, W. 2004. In Industrial application of nanomaterials-chances and risks. W. Luther (ed.). Future Technologies Division, Dusseldorf.

[26] Horikoshi, S. and N. Serpone. 2013. Introduction to Nanoparticles, Microwaves in Nanoparticle Synthesis. 1st ed: Wiley-VCH Verlag GmbH and Co. KGaA.

[27] Riaz, U., S.M. Ashraf and A. Madan. 2014. Effect of microwave irradiation time and temperature on the spectroscopic and morphological properties of nanostructured poly (carbazole) synthesized within bentonite clay galleries. New Journal of Chemistry 38: 4219–4228.

[28] Tiwary, K.P., S.K. Choubey and K. Sharma. 2013. Structural and optical properties of ZnS nanoparticles synthesized by microwave irradiation method. Chalcogenide Letters 10: 319–323.

[29] Rao, Y.N., D. Banerjee, A. Datta, S.K. Das, R. Guin and A. Saha. 2010. Gamma irradiation route to the synthesis of highly re-dispersible natural polymer capped silver nanoparticles. Radiation Physics and Chemistry 79: 1240–1246.

[30] Marignier, J., J. Belloni, M. Delcourt and J. Chevalier. 1985. New micro aggregates of non-noble metals and alloys prepared by radiation-induced reduction. Nature 317: 344–345.

[31] Abidi, W. and H. Remita. 2010. Gold-based nanoparticles generated by radiolytic and photolytic methods. Recent Patents on Engineering 4(3): 170–188.

[32] Temgire, M.K., J. Bellare and S.S. Joshi. 2011. Gamma radiolytic formation of alloyed Ag-Pt nanocolloids. Advances in Physical Chemistry 9 p. Article ID: 249097.

[33] Krklješ, A. 2011. Radiolytic synthesis of nanocomposites based on noble metal nanoparticles and natural polymer, and their application as biomaterial (IAEA-RC--12071). International Atomic Energy Agency (IAEA).

[34] Chen, Q., J. Shi, R. Zhao and X. Shen. 2010. Radiolytic syntheses of nanoparticles and inorganic-polymer hybrid microgels (IAEA-RC--11242). International Atomic Energy Agency (IAEA).

[35] Hornebecq, V., M. Antonietti, T. Cardinal and M. Treguer-Delapierre. 2003. Stable silver nanoparticles immobilized in mesoporous silica. Chemistry of Materials 15(10): 1993–1999.

[36] Shah, P. and A. Gavrin. 2006. Synthesis of nanoparticles using high-pressure sputtering for magnetic domain imaging. J. Magn. Magn. Mater. 301(1): 118–123.

[37] Lugscheider, E. et al. 1998. Magnetron-sputtered hard material coatings on thermoplastic polymers for clean room applications. Surf. Coat. Technol. 108: 398–402.

[38] Sozer, N. and J.L. Kokini. 2009. Trends in Biotechnology 27(2): 82–89.

[39] Sahoo, S.K., S. Parveen and J. Panda. 2007. Nanomedicine: Nanotechnology, Biology and Medicine 3: 20–31.

[40] Rai, M. and A. Ingle. 2012. Applied Microbiology and Biotechnology 94: 287–293.

[41] Wong, Y.W.H., C.W.M. Yuen, M.Y.S. Leung, S.K.A. Ku and H.L.I Lam. 2006. Autex Research Journal 6: 1–8.

6

Zno Nanostructured Materials for Surface and Biological Applications

Mohamed S. Selim,[1] *Shimaa A. Higazy,*[1] *Sherif A. El-Safty,*[2,]*
Ahmed A. Azzam,[2,3] *Notaila M. Nasser*[2] and
Mohamed A. Shenashen[1,2,]*

1. Introduction

Nanomaterials' research play an important role in solving problems and improving our lives in every aspect of technology. In this context, a lot of research endeavors have been devoted to providing several promising strategies to manufacturing surfaces and coatings based on nanostructured materials to enhance structural properties of surfaces as well as physical and chemical properties [1–4]. As is notable, the design of nanostructured thin-layer films, surfaces and coatings occupies a privileged position in numerous applications associated with the environmental, energy, and biological applications [5–10].

Interest in polymer composite systems research has been rapidly expanding in recent years due to their numerous potential applications [11–13], dielectrics [14], biological field [15–17], food packaging [18], bioplastics [19], extraction and water treatment [20–22], and coatings [23–26]. Adding inorganic nanofillers to polymers increases polymer properties that are radically different from standard polymer

[1] Petroleum Application Department, Egyptian Petroleum Research Institute (EPRI), Nasr City 11727, Cairo (Egypt).
[2] Research Center for Macromolecules and Biomaterials, National Institute for Materials Science (NIMS), 1-2-1 Sengen, Tsukuba-shi, Ibaraki-ken 305-0047, Japan.
[3] Environmental Research Department, Theodor Bilharz Research Institute, 12411, Cairo, Egypt.
* Corresponding authors: sherif.elsafty@nims.go.jp; shenashen.mohameda@nims.go.jp

properties, according to the researchers [27–32]. Nanoparticles (NPs) have been found to have a significant impact on the characteristics of basic polymers when used to produce nanocomposite [33–35]. A multicomponent structure having microscopic fillers (less than 100 nm in at least one dimension) is referred to as a polymeric nanocomposite [33, 36, 37]. Because of their high aspect ratio and enormous surface area, nanofillers behave as intelligent improver in the polymeric resins. As a hot spot at the moment, nanofillers with controlled size and morphology are desirable reinforcing materials for polymers [38]. Moreover, various organic-inorganic hybrid nanocomposite materials have been designed for various applications [39–42]. In this regards, diverse nano-inorganic dopants including SiO_2, Al_2O_3, TiO_2, SiO_2, ZnO, and other nano-metal oxide are commonly utilized as nano-dopants in the polymeric resins [43–46]. In this context, this study will focus on studying the features of ZnO nanofillers to develop new structural surfaces with advanced properties. ZnO can adopt various nanomaterials including NPs, nanowires (NWs), and nanorods (NRs). ZnO has a broad-band gap (3.4 eV) and is an n-type (II–V) semiconductor with several functions.

Even in the presence of sunlight, water, and air, it possesses excellent chemical stability, UV absorbance, and binding energy (60 meV) [47]. ZnO can be used in biomedical applications because it is non-toxic and safe for the environment [48]. ZnO NPs have unique features that allow them to exist in both an anti-electrostatic and conductive form, as well as having excellent chemical, optical, magnetic, and electrical features. Polymer coatings, semiconductors, photochemical, UV-shielding materials, piezoelectric devices, optical waveguides, antibacterial agents, UV-laser emitters, cosmetics, solar cells, self-purification, and gas sensors materials (Fig. 1) [49–52] have a lot of potential. ZnO exhibits bactericidal activity in the absence of light and at pH 7–8 [53]. Additionally, visible fluorescence is detected in ZnO NPs, especially when synthesized by sol-gel, but hydrothermal synthesis renders them ideal for usage in UV emitters. Traditional metal oxides, such as ZnO, are combined with polymers in certain structural layouts to achieve the desired performance [13], which is a commonly utilized major method for producing ZnO/polymer nanocomposite.

The components' characteristics, the filler's large surface area, polymer-nanofiller interfacial bindings and nanofiller's well-distribution within the resins are all thought to contribute to the improvement in attributes. This can be fulfilled by tailoring the characteristics of nanofillers, polymers, and the hybrid nanocomposite to achieve outstanding features. In the required application, selecting an appropriate polymeric resin is crucial. Chemical and heat resistance, mechanical durability, biological activity, and friction coefficient can all be improved by incorporating ZnO into a polymer matrix [54]. The benefits of ZnO NPs are shown in Fig. 2.

In general, controlling the structure of the ZnO/polymer composite well contributes to the improvement of the desired properties of the final structure, so many efforts have emerged regarding the adaptability and management of the filler particle interactions with the polymer matrix. Studying the ZnO nanofillers' structure-property relationship is inevitable to develop newly structured surfaces

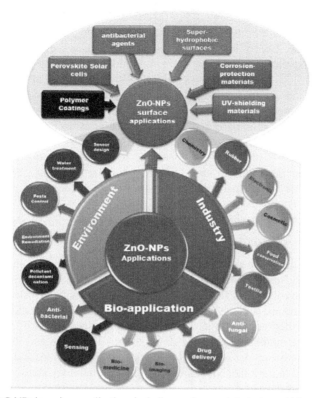

Fig. 1. ZnO NPs in various applications including environment, industry and bioapplications.

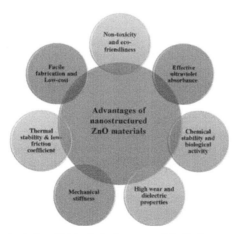

Fig. 2. Chemical, physical, and biological advantages of the ZnO nanostructured materials.

with advanced properties. It takes into account the impacts of functionalization, surface area to volume ratio of nanofillers, the antifouling effect, sustainability, and multifunctionality. Controlled ZnO nanostructures aid in the creation of a rough morphology and the generation of extra functionalities for the superhydrophobic surface. The influences of dispersing nano-ZnO within different polymeric resins is investigated in depth in this chapter, which covers production, processing, characterization methods, and a wide range of applications. Our research focuses on ZnO effects on modulating polymer nanocomposites' surface, mechanical, photo-induced, antifouling, and antibacterial characteristics. Incorporation of nano-ZnO structure within various polymeric resins is an excellent technique for generating better performance even at low nanofillers loading percentages, thus producing feasible and applied nanocomposite surface materials.

2. Synthesis Methodologies of Nanostructured ZnO Particles and Polymer Composites

A variety of methods are used to synthesize ZnO NPs with different morphologies from distinct precursor materials. The most widely used methods are solid-state reactions [55], pyrolysis via flame spray [56], chemical, sonochemical, microwave, sol-gel, hydrothermal, and solvothermal methodologies [57–61]. ZnO NPs are made via the co-precipitation technique. Two important concerns in all of these synthesis processes are the homogeneity of the ZnO particle dispersion and the low reaction temperature. Nanostructures, on the other hand, contain impurities and metal ions that need be removed to optimize NP formation. Some of the many nano-ZnO shapes are NPs, NRs, nanorings, nanotubes, flower-like, and nanobelts. These nanostructures can be dispersed in a wide range of liquids and polymeric resins. ZnO NPs cluster like other NPs, compromising their uniform distribution in the polymer medium. Inorganic particles or polymers can be grafted onto the ZnO surface to alleviate this problem [62].

This would improve the distribution and interfacial bonding of nano-ZnO within the polymeric resin to produce improved nanocomposite materials. Such desired composite performance is influenced by the size of the nanofillers as well as the polymer matrix's properties. This is often accomplished by selecting appropriate chemical and physical mixing procedures to reinforce the polymeric resin. Chemical reactions create chemical connections between polymers and fillers, unlike physical procedures that involve polymer/nanofillers mixing within a suitable solvent. Chemical synthesis yields composites that are multi-structured and stable, with stronger polymer/nanofiller connections. On the other hand, physical methods create polymer/nanofillers static connections, such as Lewis acid/base and/or van der Waals force interactions. Chemical-grafting of polymers onto ZnO surfaces yields homogenous, clear products that are easily removed from the system of reaction [63]. The breakdown temperatures of such composites are usually higher than those of ordinary polymers, and there is no significant phase separation. This assures that the system's polymer-ZnO linkages are strong, and that the stronger the contact, the more stable the nanocomposites will be and can be applied for various industrial applications.

3. Surface and Biological Applications of ZnO Nanostructures

In every field of technology, ZnO nanomaterials help to solve problems and make our lives easier. There is an urgent need to develop innovative nanomaterials with improved properties to meet the demand for improvement [64, 65]. If new structured nanomaterials with enhanced properties are to be produced, the investigation of the structure-property relationship is a necessity. Engineering applications for ZnO-based surfaces include self-cleaning, anti-biofouling, anti-icing, anticorrosion, and textiles. To make superhydrophobic nano-surfaces, researchers employed a straightforward method of NP's distribution within the polymer resin and then coating water-repellent polymeric nanocomposite film on a suitable substrate [66]. Controlled NP structures help create a rough morphology and provide additional characteristics for a superhydrophobic surface.

3.1 Self-cleaning Surfaces

Superhydrophobic nanostructured surfaces have piqued attention in a variety of industrial applications around the globe. Biomimetic [67] is an engineering architecture with a hierarchy, tectonics of materials, nano-surfaces, and machineries model based on the function and structure of biological systems. Biological systems could develop superhydrophobic coating materials. The development of biomimetic surfaces with micro and nanostructures is used to reduce fouling in the maritime environment. As a result, it is vital to clarify the process and precision for constructing bio-replicated multiscale structures [68]. Many natural surfaces are superhydrophobic and self-cleaning, such as butterfly wings as well as cabbage leaves [69]. The term "*Lotus Effect*" was named after the Lotus plant leaves (*Nelumbo nucifera*) [70], representing a well-known water-repellent example. Electron microscopy revealed projecting nubs 20–40 μm apart on the surface of lotus leaves that were covered by a waxy-rough crystalloid surface. WCAs $\geq 150°$ and low contact angle hysteresis are all characteristics of so-called superhydrophobic surfaces. Micro/nano binary roughness in combination with a low surface free energy (SFE) can facilitate such operations [71].

Since the initial synthetic ultra-hydrophobic coating was conducted in 1996 [72], there have been a slew of new ways to create surface roughness that displays superhydrophobicity. Superhydrophobicity is a technique for ensuring important surface qualities are protected. Creating a hierarchical, rough morphology with low energy molecules is required for the fabrication of superhydrophobicity surfaces [73]. A simple method of dispersing NPs in a hydrophobic polymer matrix followed by surface coating the hydrophobic polymer/NP composite dispersion on a suitable substrate [74] was used to fabricate superhydrophobic nano-surfaces in addition to etching, lithography, biomimetic, and stamping processes. Controlled NP structures contribute in the formation of a rough morphology and the establishment of extra superhydrophobic surface capabilities [75].

Surface roughness and hydrophobicity can be increased not only by increasing the solid–liquid contact, but also by trapping air between the surface and the liquid droplet on a rough surface. The surface water-repellency will be enhanced by trapping of air as it has a WCA of 180° [76]. A hierarchical micro-nano structured surface with a low SFE is responsible for superhydrophobicity [77]. ZnO nanostructures in zero dimensional (0D), 1-dimensional (1D), 2-dimensional (2D), as well as 3-dimensional (3D) dimensions have been described in the literature. Zero-dimension NPs are virtually spherical NPs. Using ZnO particles manufactured by a hydrothermal process, Gao et al. [78] constructed ultrahydrophobicity on a hierarchical nano-surface by dropping on glass substrates for a thorough experimental technique. To minimize surface energy and roughness, this method used a functional fluoroethylene-vinylether polymer with inorganic ZnO particles. The WCA can range from 135° ± 4° to 145° ± 3° and even 152° ± 2° depending on the reaction medium composition, and the ZnO particles can be formed in various shapes by adjusting reaction medium composition.

Furthermore, "chestnut" ZnO particles were more flexible than 1D nano-ZnO rods that proved useful in large-area grounding. The most prevalent 1D structures include NRs, nano-needles, nanotubes, NWs, and nanocombs. Lotus leaves have extremely hydrophobic surfaces and micro/nano-structured topology that have the potential to self-clean. Chakradhar et al. [79] used a 155° WCA to make ultrahydrophobic PDMS/nano-ZnO composite surfaces. To produce ZnO nanowires over tin oxide substrate doped with fluorine, Pauporte et al. [80] used a one-step electrochemical technique. The temperature at which ZnO NWs are deposited has been discovered to be a key factor in defining their morphology and structure. The surface non-wettability of a surface treated with stearic acid was changed from hydrophilicity to hydrophobicity (WCA of 168.3°). An *in-situ* photo-reduction approach can prepare rGO/ZnO nanocomposite for self-cleaning, and pollution-removal characteristics were also studied [81–83] (Fig. 3A). Kumbhakar et al. [82] reported a green fabrication method to produce 2D rGO-ZnO nanocomposites using zinc acetate and apple juice for self-cleaning and photocatalytic applications (Fig. 3B). The results show the photo-degradation of methylene blue dye (~ 91%) within 1 h.

The 2D architectures of ZnO include nanosheets, nanoplates, and nanopellets [84]. Li and co-workers [85] created nano-ZnO sheets on the bamboo-like substrate after utilizing chemical vapour deposition to alter the surface with fluoroalkyl silane. In the acidic rains, pH = 3. UV radiation for this newly formed structure displayed good water repellency and superhydrophobicity stability.

Examples of three-dimensional morphologies of ZnO include Snowflakes, coniferous urchin, flower, dandelion, etc. formations and other 3D morphologies of ZnO have been discovered [86, 87]. Dai et al. [88] developed a 3D hierarchical ZnO film with variable wettability and lotus leaf-like micro/nano patterns. This superhydrophobic surface was created using ZnO micro pillars with a homogenous ZnO coating, which was then followed by the formation of ZnO NRs on the micropillars structure. The highest contact angle after 24 hours of growth is 160°. Developing ZnO hierarchical micro/nano structures with customizable morphology and surface topologies, as well as programmable wettability, remains a major challenge, despite

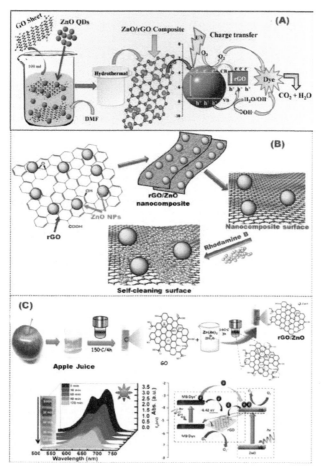

Fig. 3. Self-assembly and photocatalytic production of rGO/ZnO hybrid nanocomposite for dye removal. (A) photocatalytic ZnO/rGO nanocomposite for toxic dyes degradation [81]; Copyright © 2018 Elsevier B.V. All rights reserved, (B) photocatalytic degradation of Rhodamine B [82]; Copyright 2012, with ACS permission, and (C) rGO/ZnO hybrid photocatalyst nanocomposite synthesized from zinc acetate and apple juice for self-cleaning and photo-degradation of methylene blue dye [83]; Copyright © 2018 Elsevier B.V. All rights reserved.

the fact that there are multiple approaches for creating diverse morphologies of ZnO. The mean length and diameter size of nano-ZnO pillars can be changed in a hydrothermal reaction system by altering the solution concentration, growth time, and reaction temperature, according to Hao et al. [89]. Anchored graphene materials are well-defined photo-catalysts that can be used to make outstanding superhydrophobic, self-cleaning, and photocatalytic surface materials. He [90] developed a low-cost photocatalytic self-cleaning rGO/ZnO nanocomposite film. A trendy and environmentally sustainable trend is to use graphenic nanocomposite as strong fouling-release (FR) surface (Fig. 4).

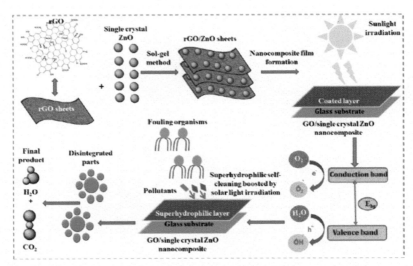

Fig. 4. A single-phase method was employed to develop rGO/ZnO hybrid composite coated on a glassy surface and subjected to UV-Vis irradiation for photocatalytic self-cleaning application. It produced a pollutant-repellant and FR nanosurface. Solar light may fragment soil, which can then be transformed to CO_2 and H_2O [90]. In 2015, the copyright was granted by Elsevier Ltd.

3.2 Antifouling Coating Surface

In the maritime industry, biofouling is a fast-moving and complex problem [91]. Shipping is responsible for over 90% of all global trade. When the friction drag caused by fouling layers rises, the ship's velocity drops. As a result, significant feasting of fuel is required for attaining the desired velocity, resulting in increased travel costs as well as the release of destructive substances into the environment [92]. Biofouling has typically been avoided by using leachant anti-fouling coatings, which release toxicants into the maritime environment, killing non-target creatures such as fish and dolphins. As global embargoes and constraints have grown, the usage of biocidal antifouling technologies has spurred the development of environmentally benign alternatives, such as FR technology. Silicone FR paints employ a method that prevents fouling attachments which decrease coating-fouling adhesion strength and improve the fouling-resistance.

PDMS has many advantages over tin-free antifouling paints including non-stick, eco-friendly, non-leaching and a CH_3 group, including ultra-smooth topology, extremely mobile surface, and reduced surface tension [93]. Thermally stable, anti-oxidant, anti-ozone, and UV resistant, PDMS is a great choice for a variety of applications. Although silicone paints already have good FR capabilities, inorganic boosting nano-additives are now required for better mechanical and FR performance. Inorganic–organic interactions can boost FR surface self-cleaning capabilities and performance by developing ultra-water-repellent surfaces with

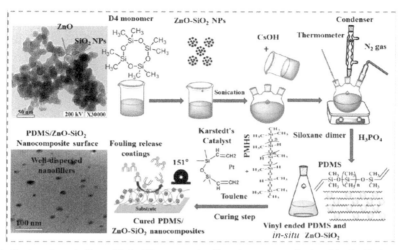

Fig. 6. Engineering of silicone/ZnO-SiO₂ composite film via *in-situ* method and hydrosilation curing technique. The TEM image of ZnO-SiO₂ nanofiller and SEM of silicone resin enriched with this nanofiller were illustrated [101]. Copyright 2017; reprinted with Elsevier's permission.

corrosion inhibitor by restricting the flow of external current between the anodes and cathodes [106].

Surface stability is a problem with most thin organic corrosion prevention coatings [107]. Corrosion-resistance and water-repellent surfaces can be developed using organic–inorganic nanocomposite [108]. It is advantageous to build corrosion-resistant coatings using nano-ZnO fillers. Coatings with exceptional barrier qualities can be made using a graphene nanosheet-like structure [109]. To avoid closely packed GO structures, GO nanosheets can be decorated with nano-metal oxide particles [110, 111]. 1D metal oxide NPs, notably NRs, have been used to anchor graphene materials by researchers [108]. Water-repellency of PDMS/GO-TiO₂-diatomaceous Earth hybrid nanocomposite surface achieved surface durability and 96.7% corrosion inhibition [112]. NRs of ZnO exhibit large surface area as well as water-repellent characteristics [113]. A ternary composite of silicone resin filled with GO-ZnO exhibited corrosion-protection and ultrahydrophobic surface [114] (Fig. 7). To create GO nanosheets with a thickness of 2 nm, a modified Hummers' method was employed.

Nano-ZnO rods with 40 nm mean diameter and a prominently exposed crystal facet of [0001] were manufactured using a controlled hydrothermal methodology. A chemical bath deposition process was used to make a GO-ZnO hybrid nanofiller with precise size and morphology. To analyze such nanocomposites' corrosion barrier characteristics, they were exposed to a 3.5% NaCl solution on the surface. According to Tafel polarization and EIS investigations, the addition of the nanofiller improved the coating's corrosion protection. The maximum impedance value is found in the ternary nanocomposite coating of silicone resin enriched with 1 wt.% of GO-ZnO fillers. The PDMS coating system has been improved by 1 wt.%. The anticorrosion of GO-ZnO hybrid fillers were also demonstrated. The exceptional corrosion resistance was attributed to the efficient dispersion of the graphene-based nanocomposite.

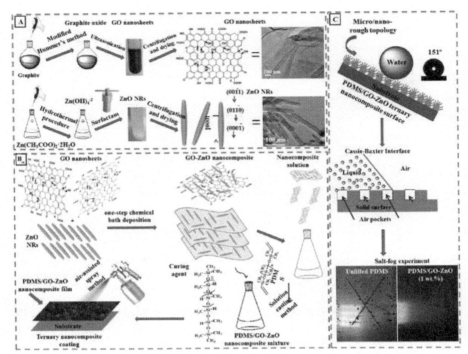

Fig. 7. (A) A modified Hummers' procedure and a surfactant-assisted hydrothermal method are used to synthesize GO nanosheets and ZnO NRs. (B) Chemical bath deposition methodology to prepare GO-ZnO nanofillers which were dispersed in the silicone matrix to produce ternary surface which is explained by the Cassie-Baxter approach for water-repellency [114]. Copyright 2021, reprinted with Elsevier's permission.

3.4 Perovskite Solar Cells (PSCs)

PSCs research has advanced significantly in the previous decade [115, 116]. PSCs can be divided into two classes, namely mesoporous PSCs and planar perovskite thin film solar cells, depending on whether a mesoporous layer is included in their structure or not [117]. TCO/hole transport layer/perovskite absorber/PC61BM/ cathode inverted structure revealed great commercialization prospects for planar PSCs [118]. This is due to the low-temperature processing, ease of use, high PCE, and large-scale manufacturing capacity. Their electrical properties are greatly influenced by charge injection and extraction at the cathode contact [119]. When a barrier remains between the interfacial contact between the Fermi level of certain electrode metals and the lowest unoccupied molecular orbital of organic material (PCBM) in organic optoelectronic devices, electron injection and extraction are poorer [120]. The interfacial contact between PCBM layer and metal electrode can reduce electronic extraction and injection.

PSCs can be made more efficient using interfacial materials. The interfacial engineering of PSCs has received more attention as a result of this paradigm. PSC interfacial engineering has gotten a lot more attention as a result of this methodology. Because of its wide band gap semiconductor and high electron mobility, ZnO is widely used as a hole blocking layer and electron transport in modern photovoltaics [121]. Nano-ZnO is a suitable option for interfacial engineering as a CBL [122] because of its exceptional material stability and charge carrier extraction efficiency.

In terms of nanostructures, shape, modification of surface, and composite hybrid, the performance of ZnO (employed as CBLs in polymeric resin and organic solar cells) has been investigated [123]. The influences of ZnO geometric structures on the solar cells' photovoltaic efficiency has been investigated. The NR shape of ZnO is an excellent morphology for making photovoltaic instrument because it increases the active area of the solar cell while lowering electrical losses. Nano-ZnO seed layer serves as a hole barrier, preventing recombination at the cathode, while ZnO-NRs facilitate electron collection and transmission [124]. Changes in the crystallinity of the seed layer have no effect on ZnO-NR growth since it happens exclusively in the [002] plane. The NR shape, [002] orientation, reduced size, and enhanced solar cell hole blocking layer are all benefits of the NR form.

Jia et al. [125] reported a ZnO-based solar cell surface device using (poly[(9,9-bis(3'-(N,N-dimethylamion)propyl)-2,7-fluorene)-alt-2,7-(9,9-dioctyl)-fluorene)-alt-2,7-(9,9-diocty). The device's efficiency was considerably increased as a result of more selective electron extraction. Between the PCBM layer and Ag electrode, Zhu et al. [126] employed a ZnO/TIPD film to improve inverted PSCs. In the ambient atmosphere, PCBM/ZnO/TIPD PSCs have a PCE and stability of 13.7%, which is greater than ZnO:TIPD or bare PCBM-based PSCs. For inverted PSCs with excellent power conversion efficiency (PCE), advanced cathode buffer layers (CBLs) based on ZnO [127] were developed (Fig. 8). After combining with bathocuproine (BCP), a controlled hydrothermal technique can be used to produce nano-ZnO rods with a mean diameter of 40 nm. Planar PSCs (p-i-n) with a device structure of (indium tin oxide/PEDOT:PSS/$CH_3NH_3PbI_3$xClx/$PC_{61}BM$/CBLs/Ag) were fabricated using the produced composite ZnO-NRs/BCP as a basis. The produced PSC composite exhibited 18.13% PCE and longer-term stability as compared with single-layer BCP (15.17%) or NRs of ZnO (16.55%) devices. The Narayanan group [128] created ZnO-NRs on microslide glass substrates with 150–450 nm mean size.

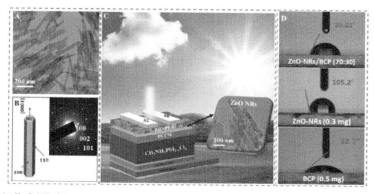

Fig. 8. (A) ZnO NRs' TEM capture; (B) schematic illustration as well as SAED results for ZnO-NRs; (C) schematic illustration of ITO/PEDOT:PSS/$CH_3NH_3PbI_3$xClx/$PC_{61}BM$/CBLs/Ag surface. (D) represents WCAs of ZnO NRs/BCP, ZnO NRs as well as BCP thin films [127]. Copyright 2020, with permission from the ACS.

3.5 Antibacterial Active Agents

Controlled NPs hold a lot of promise in biological and health-related domains because of their non-toxicity and biocompatibility [129–134]. NPs of ZnO, in particular, are antimicrobial and can deform and destroy bacterial cell membranes, causing intracellular material leaks and, eventually, bacterial cell passing. ZnO NPs could be used to preserve crops and food, according to these studies [135]. The antibacterial effectiveness of ZnO NPs in controlling *Rothia secludes* in biofilm formation was established in biofilm growth experiments on polystyrene plates [136]. The ciprofloxacin's bacterial resistance could be improved by enriching with ZnO NPs against *S. aureus E. coli.* The notion that the particles interfere with NorA protein pumping could explain the enhanced activity of *S. aureus* in the presence of ZnO NPs [137]. ZnO's antibacterial mobility may be influenced by the size and closeness of regular white light. Preliminary research found that the smaller the molecule size, the more effective it is at preventing microbial growth. Furthermore, the author speculated that ZnO surface coatings exhibit high antibacterial activity against different microorganisms [138]. ZnO sensitivity was higher in gram-positive bacteria than in gram-negative bacteria. Manufactured ZnO was also tested for antibacterial action against a variety of pathogens, including foodborne illnesses. The antibacterial activity against Salmonella typhimurium and *S. aureus* was checked and the synthesized ZnO showed good performance suggesting its conceivable application in the sustenance safeguarding field [139].

ZnO NPs can also be used in antibacterial coating materials to prevent microorganisms from forming biofilms by connecting, colonizing, diffusing, and shaping them. A comparable study between the antibacterial actions of ZnO NRs and SiC NWs with varied diameter sizes, crystal orientation, and topological surface was investigated by Askar et al. [140]. Both materials have high aspect ratio, surface area, and active centres to microbes. ZnO NRs had better antibacterial performance than SiC NWs based on MIC, immunomodulatory effect, and inhibitory zone. ZnO NRs outperformed SiC NWs in killing pathogenic bacteria, morphological disorder, and cellular membrane damage, as revealed by scanning microscopic and confocal laser captures. Electrostatic interaction between the negative bacterial surfaces and positive Zn^{+2} ions causes ZnO NRs to have a strong bacterial-resistance capability (Fig. 9). Gram-positive bacterial strains are more susceptible to ZnO NRs-induced microbial suppression than Gram-negative organisms because of their outer membrane proteins which protect them from cytotoxicity. ZnO NRs-based fabrics were also used to demonstrate wearable detection and antibacterial control without the use of an antiperspirant [134].

3.5.1 ZnO with Other Metals

Bacterial-resistant inorganic nanomaterials are widely used against various microbial strains for various biological applications. When ZnO is coupled with other metals, it has antibacterial properties (Table 1). Inorganic antibiotic NPs are useful for a variety of antibacterial industrial fields. Mg/ZnO and Sb/ZnO nanocrystals have

studies reported that the majority of research on metal oxide-based polymeric nanostructured composites exhibited various surface and biological applications. ZnO NPs' dispersion in the polymer resin improve the chemical, physical, and antibacterial properties. ZnO added to a variety of polymer matrices would boost modulus and strength considerably. ZnO has emerged as a new green broad-spectrum antibacterial agent with low bacterial resistance and sustained release properties. The fundamental functions of size- and shape-controlled hybrid nanocomposites have been introduced for various ZnO applications. In addition, ZnO's chemical variety provides the polymer with distinct characteristics. Surface, electrical, physico-mechanical, thermal, sensing, energy storage, and fuel cell features of ZnO/polymer composites are improved by well-distribution of ZnO nanofillers. Nanotechnology will be transformed by these prospective nanocomposites, which will have uses in electrical, mechanical, and chemical fields. Each example also contains remedies/proposals for overcoming hurdles and suturing extremely efficient ZnO nanocomposites. The final features are strongly influenced by the polymer/ZnO interfacial contact which can improve the mechanical, physical, and biological characteristics. ZnO nanofillers' distribution is controlled during the manufacturing process, which affects reinforcing and, as a result, material properties. The cytotoxic effect on mammalian cells has also been investigated in recent years. Electrostatic interaction with the bacterial cells, oxidative stress, and cell entrapment are all well-known mechanisms for ZnO bacterial resistance. The necessary processes must be followed when using the appropriate reaction media, dissolution medium, polymer molecular weight, ZnO architecture, and desired output. The effect of structurally folded ZnO nanoagents tectonics, polymer nanocomposites, and building blocks on the production of exceptional antibacterial surface coatings is discussed in this chapter. Because of the functional groups in ZnO, the surface charge can be decreased even at low concentrations. This improves filler-polymer compatibility, resulting in composites with outstanding dielectric properties. The surface and biological percolation concentration displays efficient distribution of ZnO NPs with non-toxic and light-weight structure in various industry. As a result, many additional studies must be conducted in order to industrialize ZnO/polymer nanocomposites for human applications. This chapter will provide inspiration to the researchers in the field of material science, chemistry, physics, biology, and engineering. It will promote both academic and industrial research on various ZnO applications.

References

[1] Idumah, C.I., C.M. Obele, E.O. Emmanuel and A. Hassan. 2020. Recently emerging nanotechnological advancements in polymer nanocomposite coatings for anti-corrosion, anti-fouling and self-healing, surfaces interfaces. Surf. Interfaces 21: 100734.

[2] Xavier, J.R. 2020. Electrochemical, mechanical and adhesive properties of surface modified NiO-epoxy nanocomposite coatings on mild steel. Mater. Sci. Eng. B 260: 114639.

[3] Arukalam, I.O., E.O. Oguzie and Y. Li. 2016. Fabrication of FDTS-modified PDMS-ZnO nanocomposite hydrophobic coating with anti-fouling capability for corrosion protection of Q235 steel. J. Colloid Interface Sci. 484: 220–228.

[4] Hu, Y., S. Li, W. Kang, H. Lin and Y. Hu. 2021. Surface modification of Ti6Al4V alloy by polydopamine grafted GO/ZnO nanocomposite coating. Surf. Coat. Tech. 422: 127534.

[5] Panwar, V., G. Anoop, S.S. Gaur and S. Park. 2022. Enhanced sensing and electrical performance of hierarchical porous ionic polymer-metal nanocomposite via minimizing cracks in electrode. J. Colloid Interface Sci. 606: 837–847.

[6] Behera, R. and K. Elanseralathan. 2022. A review on polyvinylidene fluoride polymer based nanocomposites for energy storage applications. J. Energy Storage 48: 103788.

[7] Idumah, C.I. 2021. Novel advancements in green and sustainable polymeric nanocomposites coatings. Current Res. in Green Sustain. Chem. 4: 100173.

[8] Karki, S., M.B. Gohain, D. Yadav and P.G. Ingole. 2021. Nanocomposite and bio-nanocomposite polymeric materials/membranes development in energy and medical sector: A review. Inter. J. Biological Macromol. 193: 2121–2139.

[9] El-Safty, S.A. and M.A. Shenashen. 2020. Advanced nanoscale build-up sensors for daily life monitoring of diabetics. Adv. Mater. Interfaces 7(15): 2000153.

[10] El-Safty, S.A. and M.A. Shenashen. 2020. Nanoscale dynamic chemical, biological sensor material designs for control monitoring and early detection of advanced diseases. Mater. Today Bio. 5(15): 2000153.

[11] Ponnamma, D., K.T. Varughese, M.A.A. Al-Maadeed and S. Thomas. 2017. Curing enhancement and network effects in multi-walled carbon nanotube-filled vulcanized natural rubber: evidence for solvent sensing. Polym. Int. 66: 931–938.

[12] Goutham, S., S. Kaur, K.K. Sadasivuni, J.K. Bal, N. Jayarambabu, D.S. Kumar and K.V. Rao. 2017. Nanostructured ZnO gas sensors obtained by green method and combustion technique. Mater. Sci. Semicond. Process. 57: 110–115.

[13] Goutham, S., D.S. Kumar, K.K. Sadasivuni, J.J. Cabibihan and K.V. Rao. 2017. Nanostructure ZnFe$_2$O$_4$ with *Bacillus subtilis* for detection of LPG at low temperature. J. Electron. Mater. 46: 2334–2339.

[14] Deshmukh, K., M.B. Ahamed, K.K. Sadasivuni, D. Ponnamma, M.A. AlMaadeed, S.K. Pasha and K. Chidambaram. 2017. Graphene oxide reinforced poly (4-styrenesulfonic acid)/polyvinyl alcohol blend composites with enhanced dielectric properties for portable and flexible electronics. Mater. Chem. Phys. 186: 188–201.

[15] Stodolak, E., C. Paluszkiewicz, M. Bogun and M. Blazewicz. 2009. Nanocomposite fibres for medical applications. J. Mol. Struct. 924–926: 208–213.

[16] Reda, A., S.A. El-Safty, M.M. Selim and M.A. Shenashen. 2021. Optical glucose biosensor built-in disposable strips and wearable electronic devices. Biosens. Bioelectronics 185: 113237.

[17] Shenashen, M.A., M.Y. Emran, A. El Sabagh, M.M. Selim, A. Elmarakbi and S.A. El-Safty. 2022. Progress in sensory devices of pesticides, pathogens, coronavirus, and chemical additives and hazards in food assessment: Food safety concerns. Prog. Mater. Sci. 124: 100866.

[18] Maizurah, M., A. Fazilah, M.H. Norzia and A.A. Karim. 2007. Antibacterial activity and mechanical properties of partially hydrolyzed sago starch-alginate edible film containing lemongrass oil. J. Food Sci. 72: C324–C330.

[19] Domenek, S., P. Feuilloley, J. Gratraud, M.H. Morel and S. Guilbert. 2004. Biodegradability of wheat gluten based bioplastics. Chemosphere 54: 551–559.

[20] Gomaa, H., S.A. El-Safty, M.A. Shenashen, S. Kawada, H. Yamaguchi, M. Abdelmottaleb and M.F. Cheira. 2018. Three-dimensional, vertical platelets of ZnO carriers for selective extraction of cobalt Ions from waste printed circuit boards. ACS Sustainable Chem. Eng. 6(11): 13813–13825.

[21] Gomaa, H., M.A. Shenashen, A. Elbaz, S. Kawada, T.A. Seaf El-Nasr, M.F. Cheira, A.I. Eid and S.A. El-Safty. 2021. Inorganic-organic mesoporous hybrid segregators for selective and sensitive extraction of precious elements from urban mining. J. Colloid Interface Sci. 604: 61–79.

[22] Awual, M.R., M.A. Shenashen, A. Jyo, H. Shiwaku and T. Yaitaa. 2014. Preparing of novel fibrous ligand exchange adsorbent for rapid column-mode trace phosphate removal from water. J. Ind. Engin. Chem. 20(5): 2840–2847.

[23] Selim, M.S., S.A. El-Safty, A.M. Azzam, M.A. Shenashen, M.A. El-Sockary and O.M. Abo Elenien. 2019. Superhydrophobic silicone/TiO$_2$–SiO$_2$ nanorod-like composites for marine fouling release coatings. ChemistrySelect 4: 3395.

[24] Selim, M.S., S.A. El-Safty, M.A. El-Sockary, A.I. Hashem, O.M. Abo Elenien, A.M. EL-Saeed and N.A. Fatthallah. 2015. Tailored design of Cu$_2$O nanocube/silicone composites as efficient foul-release coatings. RSC Adv. 5(26): 19933–19943.

[25] Selim, M.S., M.A. Shenashen, S.A. El-Safty, M. Sakai, S.A. Higazy, M.M. Selim, H. Isago and A. Elmarakbi. 2017. Recent progress in marine foul-release polymeric nanocomposite coatings. Prog. Mater. Sci. 87: 1–32.

[26] Selim, M.S., S.A. El-Safty, M.A. El-Sockary, A.I. Hashem, O.M. Abo Elenien, A.M. EL-Saeed and N.A, Fatthallah. 2015. Modeling of spherical silver nanoparticles in silicone-based nanocomposites for marine antifouling. RSC Adv. 5(78): 63175–63185.

[27] Nagaraj, A., D. Govindaraj and M. Rajan. 2018. Magnesium oxide entrapped Polypyrrole hybrid nanocomposite as an efficient selective scavenger for fluoride ion in drinking water. Emerg. Mater. 1: 25–33.

[28] Selim, M.S., Z. Hao, P. Mo, J. Yi and H. Ou. 2020. Biobased alkyd/graphene oxide decorated with β–MnO_2 nanorods as a robust ternary nanocomposite for surface coating. Colloid Surf. A: Physicochem. Engin. Asp. 601: 125057.

[29] Selim, M.S., M.A. Shenashen, A.I. Hashem and S.A. El-Safty. 2018. Linseed oil-based alkyd/Cu_2O nanocomposite coatings for surface applications. New J. Chem. 42: 10048–10058.

[30] Selim, M.S., F.Q. Wang, H. Yang, Y. Huang and S. Kuga. 2017. Hyperbranched alkyd/magnetite-silica nanocomposite as a coating material. Mater. Des. 135: 173–183.

[31] Selim, M.S., H. Yang, Y. Li, F.Q. Wang, X. Li and Y. Huang. 2018. Ceramic hyperbranched alkyd/γ-Al_2O_3 nanorods composite as a surface coating. Prog. Org. Coat. 120: 217–227.

[32] Sadasivuni, K.K., A. Saiter, N. Gautier, S. Thomas and Y. Grohens. 2013. Effect of molecular interactions on the performance of poly (isobutylene-co-isoprene)/graphene and clay nanocomposites. Colloid Polym. Sci. 291: 1729–1740.

[33] Selim, M.S., S.A. El-Safty and M.A. Shenashen. 2019. Chapter 8 - Superhydrophobic foul resistant and self-cleaning polymer coating. pp. 181–203. *In*: Samal, S.K., S. Mohanty and S.K. Nayak (eds.). Superhydrophobic Polymer Coatings. Elsevier.

[34] Mazrouaa, A.M., N.A. Mansour, M.Y. Abed, M.A. Youssif, M.A. Shenashen and M.R. Awual. 2019. Nano-composite multi-wall carbon nanotubes using poly (p-phenylene terephthalamide) for enhanced electric conductivity. J. Environ. Chem. Eng. 7(2): 103002.

[35] Ponnamma, D., K.K. Sadasivuni, Y. Grohens, Q. Guo and S. Thomas. 2014. Carbon nanotube based elastomer composites–an approach towards multifunctional materials. J. Mater. Chem. 2: 8446–8485.

[36] Selim, M.S., M.A. Shenashen, N.A. Fatthallah, A. Elmarakbi and S.A. El-Safty. 2017. *In situ* fabrication of onedimensional-based lotus-like silicone/γ-Al_2O_3 nanocomposites for marine fouling release coatings. ChemistrySelect 2(30): 9691–9700.

[37] Kafy, A., K.K. Sadasivuni, A. Akther, S.K. Min and J. Kim. 2015. Cellulose/graphene nanocomposite as multifunctional electronic and solvent sensor material. Mater. Lett. 159: 20–23.

[38] Selim, M.S., N.A. Fatthallah, S.A. Higazy, Z. Hao and P.J. Mo. 2022. A comparative study between two novel silicone/graphene-based nanostructured surfaces for maritime antifouling. J. Colloid Interface Sci. 606: Part 1, 367–383.

[39] Khairy, M., S.A. El-Safty, M.A. Shenashen and E.A. Elshehy. 2013. Hierarchical inorganic–organic multi-shell nanospheres for intervention and treatment of lead-contaminated blood. Nanoscale 5(17): 7920–7927.

[40] Azzam, A.M., M.A. Shenashen, M.M. Selim, H. Yamaguchi, I.M. El-Sewify, S. Kawada, A.A. Alhamid and S.A. El-Safty. 2017. Nanospherical inorganic α-Fe core-organic shell necklaces for the removal of arsenic (V) and chromium (VI) from aqueous solution. J. Phys. Chem. Solids 109: 78–88.

[41] Soliman, A.E., M.A. Shenashen, I.M. El-Sewify, G.M. Taha, M. El-Taher, H. Yamaguchi, A.S. Alamoudi, M.M. Selim and S.A. El-Safty. 2017. Mesoporous organic–inorganic core–shell necklace cages for potentially capturing Cd^{2+} ions from water sources. ChemistrySelect 2(21): 6135–6142.

[42] El-Sewify, I.M., M.A. Shenashen, A. Shahat, H. Yamaguchi, M.M. Selim, M.M.H. Khalil and S.A. El-Safty. 2017. Ratiometric fluorescent chemosensor for Zn^{2+} ions in environmental samples using supermicroporous organic-inorganic structures as potential platforms. ChemistrySelect 2(34): 11083–11090.

[43] Wang, Z.S., C.H. Huang, Y.Y. Huang, Y.J. Hou, P.H. Xie, B.W. Zhang and H.M. Cheng. 2001. A highly efficient solar cell made from a dye-modified ZnO-covered TiO_2 nanoporous electrode. Chem. Mater. 13: 678–682.

[44] Khalifa, H., S.A. El-Safty, A. Reda, M.A. Shenashen and A.I. Eid. 2020. Anisotropic alignments of hierarchical Li_2SiO_3/TiO_2@nano-C anode//$LiMnPO_4$@nano-C cathode architectures for full-cell lithium-ion battery. Nation. Sci. Rev. 7(5): 863–880.

[45] Selim, M.S., S.A. El-Safty, M.A. Shenashen, S.A. Higazy and A. Elmarakbi. 2020. Progress in biomimetic leverages for marine antifouling using nanocomposite coatings. J. Mater. Chem., B 8: 3701.

[46] Hirvikorpi, T., M. Vähä-Nissi, J. Nikkola, A. Harlin and M. Karppinen. 2011. Thin Al_2O_3 barrier coatings onto temperature-sensitive packaging materials by atomic layer deposition. Surf. Coat. Technol. 205: 5088–5092.

[47] Janotti, A. and C.G. Van de Walle. 2009. Fundamentals of zinc oxide as a semiconductor. Rep. Prog. Phys. 2: 126501.

[48] Hezam, A., K. Namratha, Q.A. Drmosh, D. Ponnamma, A.M. Saeed, V. Ganesh, B. Neppolian and K. Byrappa. 2018. Direct Z-scheme $Cs_2O–Bi_2O_3–ZnO$ heterostructures for photocatalytic overall water splitting. J. Mater. Chem. A 6: 21379–21388.

[49] Parangusan, H., D. Ponnamma, M.A.A. Al-Maadeed and A. Marimuthu. 2018. Nanoflowerlike yttrium-doped ZnO photocatalyst for the degradation of methylene blue dye. Photochem. Photobiol. 94: 237–246.

[50] Seo, M., Y. Jung, D. Lim, D. Cho and Y. Jeong. 2013. Piezoelectric and field emitted properties of controlled ZnO nanorods on CNT yarns. Mater. Lett. 92: 177–180.

[51] Yi, G.C., C. Wang and W.I. Park. 2005. ZnO nanorods: synthesis, characterization and applications. Semicond. Sci. Technol. 20: 22–34.

[52] Li, R., S. Yabe, M. Yamashita, S. Momose, S. Yoshida, S. Yin and T. Sato. 2002. Synthesis and UV-shielding properties of ZnO- and CaO-doped CeO_2 via soft solution chemical process. Solid State Ionics 151: 235–241.

[53] Tam, K.H., A.B. Djurišić, C.M.N. Chan, Y.Y. Xi, C.W. Tse, Y.H. Leung and D.W.T. Au. 2008. Antibacterial activity of ZnO nanorods prepared by a hydrothermal method. Thin Solid Films 516: 6167–6174.

[54] Thangamani, G.J., K. Deshmukh, K.K. Sadasivuni, K. Chidambaram, M.B. Ahamed, D. Ponnamma, M.A.A. AlMaadeed and S.K.K. Pasha. 2017. Recent advances in electrochemical biosensor and gas sensors based on graphene and carbon nanotubes (CNT)—a review. Adv. Mater. Lett. 3: 196–205.

[55] Suwanboon, S., P. Amornpitoksuk, A. Sukolrat, and N. Muensit. 2013. Optical and photocatalytic properties of La-doped ZnO nanoparticles prepared via precipitation and mechanical milling method. Ceram. Int. 39: 2811–2819.

[56] Lee, S.D., S.H. Nam, M.H. Kim and J.H. Boo. 2012. Synthesis and photocatalytic property of ZnO nanoparticles prepared by spray-pyrolysis method. Phys. Procedia 32: 320–326.

[57] Stanković, A., L. Veselinović, S.D. Škapin, S. Marković and D. Uskoković. 2011. Controlled mechanochemically assisted synthesis of ZnO nanopowders in the presence of oxalic acid. J. Mater. Sci. 46: 3716–3724.

[58] Sharma, D., S. Sharma, B.S. Kaith, J. Rajput and M. Kaur. 2011. Synthesis of ZnO nanoparticles using surfactant free in-air and microwave method. Appl. Surf. Sci. 257: 9661–9672.

[59] Kazeminezhad, I., A. Sadollahkhani and M. Farbod. 2013. Synthesis of ZnO nanoparticles and flower-like nanostructures using nonsono- and sono-electrooxidation methods. Mater. Lett. 92: 29–32.

[60] Ba-Abbad, M.M., A.A.H. Kadhum, A.B. Mohamad, M.S. Takriff and K. Sopian. 2013. The effect of process parameters on the size of ZnO nanoparticles synthesized via the sol–gel technique. J. Alloys Compd. 550: 63–70.

[61] Aneesh, P.M., K.A. Vanaja and M.K. Jayaraj. 2007. Synthesis of ZnO nanoparticles by hydrothermal method. Proc. SPIE 6639: 66390J-1–66390J-9.

[62] Wang, D., Y. Feng, L. Han and Y. Tian. 2008. Effect of wet surface treated nano-SiO_2 on mechanical properties of polypropylene composite. J. Wuhan Univ. Technol. Mater. Sci. Ed. 23: 354–357.

[63] Xiong, H.M., D.P. Xie, X.Y. Guan, Y.J. Tan and Y.Y. Xia. 2007. Water-stable blue-emitting ZnO@ polymer core–shell microspheres. J. Mater. Chem. 17: 2490.

[64] Shenashen, M.A., S.A. El-Safty and E.A. Elshehy. 2014. Synthesis, morphological control, and properties of silver nanoparticles in potential applications. Part. Part. Syst. Charact. 31(3): 293–316.

[65] Shenashen, M.A., A. Derbalah, A. Hamza, A. Mohamed and S.A. El-Safty. 2017. Antifungal activity of fabricated mesoporous alumina nanoparticles against root rot disease of tomato caused by *Fusarium oxysporium*. Pest Manag. Sci. 73(6): 1121–1126.

[66] Dong, C., Y. Gu, M. Zhong, L. Li, K. Sezer, M. Ma and W. Liu. 2011. Fabrication of superhydrophobic Cu surfaces with tunable regular micro and random nano-scale structures by hybrid laser texture and chemical etching. J. Mater. Process. Technol. 211(7): 1234–1240.

[67] Salta, M., J.A. Wharton, P. Stoodley, S.P. Dennington, L.R. Goodes, S. Werwinski, U. Mart, R.J.K. Wood and K.R. Stokes. 2010. Designing biomimetic antifouling surfaces. Philos. Trans. R. Soc., A 368: 4729–4754.

[68] Sharma, B., P. Malik and P. Jain. 2018. Biopolymer reinforced nanocomposites: A comprehensive review. Mater. Today Commun. 16: 353–363.

[69] Barthlott, W. and C. Neinhuis. 1997. Purity of the sacred lotus, or escape from contamination in biological surfaces. Planta 202(1): 1–8.

[70] Mohamed, A.M.A., A.M. Abdullah and N.A. Younan. 2015. Corrosion behavior of superhydrophobic surfaces: A review. Arab. J. Chem. 8: 749–765.

[71] Martines, E., K. Seunarine, H. Morgan, N. Gadegaard, C.D.W. Wilkinson and M.O. Riehle. 2005. Superhydrophobicity and superhydrophilicity of regular nanopatterns. Nano Lett. 5: 2097–103.

[72] Onda, T., S. Shibuichi, N. Satoh and K. Tsujii. 1996. Super-water-repellent fractal surfaces. Langmuir 12: 2125–2127.

[73] Selim, M.S., M.A. Shenashen, S.A. El-Safty, M. Sakai, S.A. Higazy, M.M. Selim, H. Isago and A. Elmarakbi. 2017. Recent progress in marine foul-release polymeric nanocomposite coatings. Prog. Mater. Sci. 87: 1–32.

[74] Ding, Y., Y. Chen and J. Zheng. 2018. Dispersion of nanoparticles in polymer matrices with well-designed ligands as dispersant/emulsifier/comonomer. Compos. Sci. Technol. 156: 215–222.

[75] Gao, X. and Z. Guo. 2017. Biomimetic superhydrophobic surfaces with transition metals and their oxides: A review. J. Bionic Engin. 14: 401–439.

[76] Ma, M., Y. Mao, M. Gupta, K.K. Gleason and G.C. Rutledge. 2005. Superhydrophobic fabrics produced by electrospinning and chemical vapor deposition. Macromolecules 38(23): 9742–9748.

[77] Yang, F. and Z. Guo. 2015. Characterization of micro-morphology and wettability of lotus leaf, waterlily leaf and biomimetic ZnO surface. J. Bionic Engin. 12: 88–97.

[78] Gao, D. and M. Jia. 2015. Hierarchical ZnO particles grafting by fluorocarbon polymer derivative: Preparation and superhydrophobic behavior. Appl. Surf. Sci. 343: 172–180.

[79] Chakradhar, R.P.S., V.D. Kumar, J.L. Rao and B.J. Basu. 2011. Fabrication of superhydrophobic surfaces based on ZnO–PDMS nanocomposite coatings and study of its wetting behaviour. Appl. Surf. Sci. 257(20): 8569–8575.

[80] Pauporté, Th., G. Bataille, L. Joulaud and F.J. Vermersch. 2011. Well-aligned ZnO nanowire arrays prepared by seed-layer-free electrodeposition and their Cassie−Wenzel transition after hydrophobization. J. Phys. Chem. C 114: 194–202.

[81] Mandal, S.K., K. Dutta, S. Pal, S. Mandal, A. Naskar, P.K. Pal, T.S. Bhattacharya, A. Singha, R. Saikh, S. De, and D. Jana. 2019. Engineering of ZnO/rGO nanocomposite photocatalyst towards rapid degradation of toxic dyes. Mater. Chem. Phys. 223: 456–465.

[82] Wang, J., T. Tsuzuki, B. Tang, X. Hou, L. Sun and X. Wang. 2012. *In-situ* synthesis of rGO-ZnO nanocomposite for demonstration of sunlight driven enhanced photocatalytic and self-cleaning of organic dyes and tea stains of cotton fabrics. ACS Appl. Mater. Interfaces 4(6): 3084–3090.

[83] Kumbhakar, P., A. Pramanik, S. Biswas, A.K. Kole, R. Sarkar and P. Kumbhakar. 2018. Reduced Graphene oxide/ZnO composite: Reusable adsorbent for pollutant management. J. Hazardous Mater. 360: 193–203.

[84] Chiu, W.S., P.S. Khiew, M. Cloke, D. Isa, T.K. Tan, S. Radiman, R. Abd-Shukor, M.A. Hamid, N.W. Huang, H.N. Lim and C.H. Chia. 2010. Photocatalytic study of two-dimensional ZnO nanopellets in the decomposition of methylene blue. Chem. Engin. J. 158: 345–352.

[85] Li, J., Q. Sun, Q. Yao, J. Wang, S. Han and C. Jin. 2015. Fabrication of robust superhydrophobic bamboo based on ZnO nanosheet networks with improved water-, UV-, and fire-resistant properties. J. Nanomater. 2015: 431426.

[86] Polshettiwar, V., B. Baruwati and R.S. Varma. 2009. Self-assembly of metal oxides into three-dimensional nanostructures: Synthesis and application in catalysis. ACS Nano 3: 728–736.

[87] Bitenc, M. and Z.C. Orel. 2009. Synthesis and characterization of crystalline hexagonal bipods of zinc oxide. Mater. Res. Bullet. 44: 381–387.

[88] Dai, S., D. Zhang, Q. Shi, X. Han, S. Wang and Z. Du. 2013. Biomimetic fabrication and tunable wetting properties of three-dimensional hierarchical ZnO structures by combining soft lithography templated with lotus leaf and hydrothermal treatments. Crystengcomm 15: 5417–5424.

[89] Hao, X., G. Wu, L. Wang, D. Lv, Y. Luo, L. Li and N. He. 2015. Superhydrophobic surfaces based on ZnO constructed hierarchical architectures. Microelectron. Engin. 141: 44–50.

[90] He, H-Y. 2015. Photoinduced superhydrophilicity and high photocatalytic activity of ZnO–reduced graphene oxide nanocomposite films for self-cleaning applications. Mater. Sci. Semicon. Proc. 31: 200–208.

[91] Grant, T.M., D. Rennison and G. Cervin. 2022. Towards eco-friendly marine antifouling biocides – Nature inspired tetrasubstituted 2,5-diketopiperazines. Sci. Total Environ. 812: 152487.

[92] Jin, H., L. Tian, W. Bing, J. Zhao and L. Ren. 2022. Bioinspired marine antifouling coatings: Status, prospects, and future. Prog. Mater. Sci. 124: 100889.

[93] Selim, M.S., S.A. El-Safty, N.A. Fatthallah and M.A. Shenashen. 2018. Silicone/graphene oxide sheet-alumina nanorod ternary super hydrophobic antifouling coating. Prog. Org Coat. 121: 160–172.

[94] Selim, M.S., A. Elmarakbi, A.M. Azzam, M.A. Shenashen, A.M. EL-Saeed and S.A. El-Safty. 2018. Ecofriendly design of superhydrophobic nano-magnetite/silicone composites for marine foul-release paints. Prog. Org. Coat. 116: 21–34.

[95] Selim, M.S., H. Yang, F.Q. Wang, X. Li, Y. Huang and N.A. Fatthallah. 2018. Silicone/Ag@SiO$_2$ core–shell nanocomposite as a self-cleaning antifouling coating material. RSC Adv. 8: 9910–9921.

[96] Bressy, C., J.-F. Briand, S. Lafond, R. Davy, F. Mazeas, B. Tanguy, C. Martin, L. Horatius, C. Anton, F. Quiniou and C. Compère. 2022. What governs marine fouling assemblages on chemically-active antifouling coatings? Prog. Org. Coat. 164: 106701.

[97] Barthwal, S., W. Barthlott, B. Singh and N.B. Singh. 2020. Multifunctional and fluorine-free superhydrophobic composite coating based on PDMS modified MWCNTs/ZnO with self-cleaning, oil-water separation, and flame retardant properties. Colloids Surf. A: Physicochem. Eng. Asp. 597: 124776.

[98] Padmavathi, A.R., P.S. Murthy, A. Das, P. Veeramani and T.S. Rao. 2021. Inorganic nanoparticle embedded Polydimethyl siloxane nanocomposites for biofouling mitigation. Surf. Interf. 25: 101171.

[99] Selim, M.S., S.A. El-Safty, M.A. Shenashen, M.A. El-Sockary, O.M. Abo Elenien and A.M. EL-Saeed. 2019. Robust alkyd/exfoliated graphene oxide nanocomposite as a surface coating. Prog. Org. Coat. 126: 106–118.

[100] Selim, M.S., H. Yang, F.Q. Wang, N.A. Fatthallah, Y. Huang and S. Kuga. 2019. Silicone/ZnO nanorod composite coating as a marine antifouling surface. Appl. Surf. Sci. 466: 40–50.

[101] Selim, M.S., M.A. Shenashen, S. Hasegawa, N.A. Fatthallah, A. Elmarakbi and S.A. El-Safty. 2017. Synthesis of ultrahydrophobic and thermally stable inorganic–organic nanocomposites for self-cleaning foul release coatings. Chem. Eng. J. 320: 653–666.

[102] Ammar, S., K. Ramesh, I.A.W. Ma, Z. Farah, B. Vengadaesvaran, S. Ramesh and A.K. Arof. 2017. Studies on SiO$_2$-hybrid polymeric nanocomposite coatings with superior corrosion protection and hydrophobicity. Surf. Coat. Technol. 324: 536–545.

[103] Shaban, S.M., E.A. Badr, M.A. Shenashen and A.A. Farag. 2021. Fabrication and characterization of encapsulated Gemini cationic surfactant as anticorrosion material for carbon steel protection in down-hole pipelines. Environ. Tech. Innov. 23: 101603.

[104] Qing, Y., C. Yang, Y. Sun, Y. Zheng, X. Wang, Y. Shang, L. Wang and C. Liua. 2015. Facile fabrication of superhydrophobic surfaces with corrosion resistance by nanocomposite coating of TiO$_2$ and polydimethylsiloxane. Colloids Surf. A: Physicochem. Eng. Asp. 484: 471–477.

[105] Arukalam, I.O., E.E. Oguzie and Y. Li. 2018. Nanostructured superhydrophobicpolysiloxane coating for high barrier and anticorrosion applications in marine environment. J. Colloid Interface Sci. 512: 674–685.

[106] Yilgör, E. and I. Yilgör. 2014. Silicone containing copolymers: Synthesis, properties and applications. Prog. Polym. Sci. 39(6): 1165–1195.

[107] Ejenstam, L., A. Swerin, J. Pan and P.M. Claesson. 2015. Corrosion protection by hydrophobic silica particle-polydimethylsiloxane composite coatings. Corros. Sci. 99: 89–97.

[108] Selim, M.S., S.A. El-Safty, M.A. Shenashena, M.A. El-Sockary, O.M. Abo Elenien and A.M. EL-Saeed. 2019. Robust alkyd/exfoliated graphene oxide nanocomposite as a surface coating. Prog. Org. Coat. 126: 106–118.

[109] Othman, N.H., M.C. Ismail, M. Mustapha, N. Sallih, K.E. Kee and R.A. Jaal. 2019. Graphene-based polymer nanocomposites as barrier coatings for corrosion protection. Prog. Org. Coat. 135: 82–99.

[110] McAllister, M.J., J.-L. Li, D.H. Adamson, H.C. Schniepp, A.A. Abdala, J. Liu, M. Herrera-Alonso, D.L. Milius, R. Car, R.K. Prud'homme and I.A. Aksay. 2007. Single sheet functionalized graphene by oxidation and thermal expansion of graphite. Chem. Mater. 19: 4396.

[111] Gutierrez-Gonzalez, C.F., A. Smirnov, A. Centeno, A. Fern´andez, B. Alonso, V.G. Rocha, R. Torrecillas, A. Zurutuza and J.F. Bartolome. 2015. Wear behavior of graphene/alumina composite. Ceram. Inter. 41(6): 7434–7438.

[112] Nine, M.J., M.A. Cole, L. Johnson, D.N.H. Tran and D. Losic. 2015. Robust superhydrophobic graphene-based composite coatings with self-cleaning and corrosion barrier properties. ACS Appl. Mater. Interfaces 7: 28482–28493.

[113] Wang, T., Y. Yun, M. Wang, C. Li, G. Liu and W. Yang. 2019. Superhydrophobic ceramic hollow fiber membrane planted by ZnO nanorod-array for high-salinity water desalination. J. Taiwan. Inst. Chem. Eng. 105: 17–27.

[114] Selim, M.S., S.A. El-Safty, M.A. Abbas and M.A. Shenashen. 2021. Facile design of graphene oxide-ZnO nanorod-based ternary nanocomposite as a superhydrophobic and corrosion-barrier coating. Colloid. Surf. A: Physicochem. Engin. Asp. 611: 125793.

[115] Green, M.A., A. Ho-Baillie and H.J. Snaith. 2014. The Emergence of Perovskite solar cells. Nat. Photonics 8: 506–514.

[116] Nogay, G., F. Sahli, J. Werner, R. Monnard, M. Boccard, M. Despeisse, F. Haug, Q. Jeangros, A. Ingenito and C. Ballif. 2019. 25.1%-efficient monolithic Perovskite/silicon tandem solar cell based on A p-type monocrystalline textured silicon wafer and high-temperature passivating contacts. ACS Energy Lett. 4: 844–845.

[117] Ball, J.M., M.M. Lee, A. Hey and H.J. Snaith. 2013. Low-temperature processed meso-superstructured to thin-film Perovskite solar cells. Energy Environ. Sci. 6: 1739–1743.

[118] You, J., Z. Hong, Y. Yang, Q. Chen, M. Cai, T.B. Song, C.C. Chen, S. Lu, Y. Liu, H. Zhou and Y. Yang. 2014. Low-temperature solution-processed Perovskite solar cells with high efficiency and flexibility. ACS Nano 8: 1674–1680.

[119] Elseman, A.M., L. Luo and Q.L. Song. 2020. Self-doping synthesis of trivalent Ni_2O_3 as a hole transport layer for high fill factor and efficient inverted Perovskite solar cells. Dalton Trans. 49: 14243–14250.

[120] Yip, H.L., S.K. Hau, N.S. Baek, H. Ma and A.K.Y. Jen. 2008. Polymer solar cells that use self-assembled-monolayer-modified Zno/metals as cathodes. Adv. Mater. 20: 2376–2382.

[121] Wang, K., V. Körstgens, D. Yang, N. Hohn, S.V. Roth and P. Müller-Buschbaum. 2018. Morphology control of low temperature fabricated ZnO nanostructures for transparent active layers in all solid-state dye-sensitized solar cells. J. Mater. Chem. A 6: 4405–4415.

[122] Liang, Z., Q. Zhang, O. Wiranwetchayan, J. Xi, Z. Yang, K. Park, C. Li and G. Cao. 2012. Effects of the morphology of a ZnO buffer layer on the photovoltaic performance of inverted polymer solar cells. Adv. Funct. Mater. 22: 2194–2201.

[123] Liang, Z., R. Gao, J.L. Lan, O. Wiranwetchayan, Q. Zhang, C. Li and G. Cao. 2013. Growth of vertically aligned ZnO nanowalls for inverted polymer solar cells. Sol. Energy Mater. Sol. Cells 117: 34–40.

[124] Wang, J.C., W.T. Weng, M.Y. Tsai, M.K. Lee, S.F. Horng, T.P. Perng, C.C. Kei, C.C. Yu and H.F. Meng. 2010. Highly efficient flexible inverted organic solar cells using atomic layer deposited ZnO as electron selective layer. J. Mater. Chem. 20: 862–866.

[125] Jia, X., L. Zhang, Q. Luo, H. Lu, X. Li, Z. Xie, Y. Yang, Y.Q. Li, X. Liu and C.Q. Ma. 2016. Power conversion efficiency and device stability improvement of inverted Perovskite solar cells by using a ZnO:PFN composite cathode buffer layer. ACS Appl. Mater. Interfaces 8: 18410–18417.

[126] Zhu, L., C. Chen, Y. Weng, F. Li and Q. Lou. 2019. Enhancing the performance of inverted Perovskite solar cells by inserting a ZnO:TIPD film between PCBM layer and Ag electrode. Sol. Energy Mater. Sol. Cells 198: 11–18.

[127] Selim, M.S., A.M. Elseman and Z. Hao. 2020. ZnO nanorods: An advanced cathode buffer layer for inverted Perovskite solar cells. ACS Appl. Energy Mater. 3(12): 11781–11791.

[128] Narayanan, G.N. and K. Annamalai. 2016. Role of hexamethylenetetramine concentration on structural, morphological, optical and electrical properties of hydrothermally grown zinc oxide nanorods. J. Mater. Sci.: Mater. Electron. 27: 12209–12215.

[129] Selim, M.S., A.M. Azzam, M.A. Shenashen, S.A. Higazy, B.B. Mostafa and S.A. El-Safty. 2024. Comparative study between three carbonaceous nanoblades and nanodarts for antimicrobial applications. J. Environ. Sci. 136: 594–605.

[130] Azzam, A.M., M.A. Shenashen, B.B. Mostafa, W.A. Kandeel and S.A. El-Safty. 2019. Antibacterial activity of magnesium oxide nano-hexagonal sheets for wastewater remediation. Environ. Prog. Sustainable Energy 38: S260–S266.

[131] Emran, M.Y., M.A. Shenashen, AI Eid, M.M. Selim and S.A. El-Safty. 2022. Portable sensitive and selective biosensing assay of dopamine in live cells using dual phosphorus and nitrogen doped carbon urchin-like structure. Chem. Eng. J. 430: 132818.

[132] Azzam, A.M., M.A. Shenashen, M.M. Selim, A.S. Alamoudi and S.A. El-Safty. 2017. Hexagonal Mg(OH)$_2$ nanosheets as antibacterial agent for treating contaminated water sources. ChemistrySelect 2(35): 11431–11437.

[133] Azzam, A.M., M.A. Shenashen, A. Tawfik, N.A. Safwat, B.B. Mostafa and S.A. El-Safty. 2022. Antimicrobial activity of mesoporous organic functionalized hexagon Fe$_3$O$_4$ nanosheets for wastewater treatment. Environ. Nanotech. Monit. Manag. 18: 100739.

[134] Hatamie, A., A. Khan, M. Golabi, A.P. Turner, V. Beni, W.C. Mak, A. Sadollahkhani, H. Alnoor, B. Zargar, S. Bano and O. Nur. 2015. Zinc oxide nanostructure-modified textile and its application to biosensing, photocatalysis, and as antibacterial material. Langmuir 31: 10913–10921.

[135] Liu, Y., L. He, A. Mustapha, H. Li, Z.Q. Hu and M. Lin. 2009. Antibacterial activities of zinc oxide nanoparticles against *Escherichia coli* O157:H7. J. Appl. Microbiol. 107: 1193–1201.

[136] Khan, S.T., M. Ahamed, J. Musarrat and A.A. Al-Khedhairy. 2014. Anti-biofilm and antibacterial activities of zinc oxide nanoparticles against the oral opportunistic pathogens, *Rothia dentocariosa* and *Rothia mucilaginosa*. Eur. J. Oral Sci. 122: 397–403.

[137] Banoee, M., S. Seif, Z.E. Nazari, P. Jafari-Fesharaki, H.R. Shahverdi, A. Moballegh, K.M. Moghaddam and A.R. Shahverdi. 2010. ZnO nanoparticles enhanced antibacterial activity of ciprofloxacin against *Staphylococcus aureus* and *Escherichia coli*. J. Biomed. Mater. Res. B Appl. Biomater. 93: 557–561.

[138] Jones, N., B. Ray, K.T. Ranjit and A.C. Manna. 2008. Antibacterial activity of ZnO nanoparticle suspensions on a broad spectrum of microorganisms. FEMS Microbiol. Lett. 279: 71–76.

[139] Tayel, A.A., W.F. El-Tras, S. Moussa, A.F. El-Baz, H. Mahrous, M.F. Salem and L. Brimer. 2011. Antibacterial action of zinc oxide nanoparticles against food borne pathogens. J. Food Saf. 31: 211–218.

[140] Askar, A.A., M.S. Selim, S.A. El-Safty, A.I. Hashem, M.M. Selim and M.A. Shenashen. 2021. Antimicrobial and immunomodulatory potential of nanoscale hierarchical one-dimensional zinc oxide and silicon carbide materials. Mater. Chem. Phys. 263: 124376.

[141] Zhang, X., R. Zhou, P. Liu, L. Fu, X. Lan and G. Gong. 2011. Improvement of the antibacterial activity of nanocrystalline zinc oxide by doping Mg (II) or Sb (III). Int. J. Appl. Ceram. Technol. 8: 1087–10981.

[142] Ravichandran, K., K. Karthika, B. Sakthivel, N.J. Begum, S. Snega, S. Swaminathan and V. Senthamilselvi. 2014. Tuning the combined magnetic and antibacterial properties of ZnO nanopowders through Mn doping for biomedical applications. J. Magn. Magn. Mater. 358: 50–55.

2. Experimental Methods

The process of electrochemical exfoliation was used to create graphene. $FeSO_4$ (AR grade) in the concentration of 0.1 M was dissolved in 40 ml of distilled water to create the electrolyte for the exfoliation. The bath was then loaded with two high quality natural graphite rods. Throughout the experiment, the spacing between the two high quality electrodes was maintained at around 2 cm. The two electrodes were subjected to static potential of 15 V. After 30 minutes, the anode graphite electrode started to corrode, and after that, at the bottom of the reaction chamber, a black precipitate began to develop gradually. The electrolyte was finally created in a homogeneous solution. After six hours, the precipitate was removed from the reaction chamber. The precipitate underwent a thorough cleaning with ethanol and distilled water before being dried for two hours at 60°C. For additional characterization, the finished product was acquired. With a scan rate of 3°/minute, the XRD of graphene and graphite was carried out on the Rigaku MiniFlex 600 apparatus from 20 to 90° of 2θ. Graphene's morphology was examined with the Jeol JSM-6390LV at a 20 kV accelerating voltage with EDS detector. A laser beam with an agitation wavelength of 514 nm was used to record the Raman spectra using a Renishaw Plo Micro Raman spectrometer. Using Shimadzu Corp. IR - Prestige 21, FTIR spectrum of graphene was obtained. Graphene exfoliation absorption spectra were examined using spectrophotometer type-117.

3. Results and Discussion

3.1 Structural Analysis

X-ray diffraction has been used to examine the crystal structures of exfoliated graphene and natural graphite. Figure 2 displays a photograph of natural graphite and graphene. Peeled-off graphene and graphite exhibit reflection peaks at 2θ = 26.4°, as shown in the picture. For all graphene generated using various electrolytes, the (002) and (004) planes, comparable to those in graphite, were generally represented by the peaks at 2θ = 26° and 2θ = 54° [27]. On the other hand, the peak at 2θ = 26° widened. This might be caused by its corrugated structure and the increase in inter-lameller spacing inside the graphitic structure, which indicated the presence of graphene. Exfoliated graphene (002) has a significantly lower intensity than graphite (002). The intensity of exfoliated graphene (002) significantly decreases due to the break of the interplanar carbon inside the graphitic structure during the electrochemical process, and the thickness of the graphite also decreases as a result [25]. The availability of the sample and energetic intercalation of SO_4^{2-} ions may be to blame for the generation of oxygen gas, other side reactions, and the formation of CO_2 and CO between the stratified layers of graphite electrode, which promoted hydroxylation to the surface and edge of exfoliated graphene. Therefore, the inter-lamellar distance will grow as a result of surface functionalization [28]. Additionally, the graph demonstrates that no extra crystal plane diffraction peak was seen in graphene, excluding the possibility of oxidation. Graphite (002) has a higher intensity than graphene, which suggests

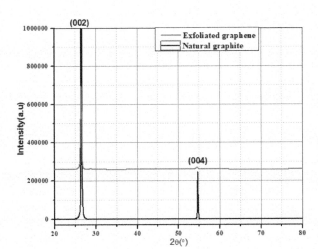

Fig. 2. XRD spectra of exfoliated graphene (EG) and natural graphite. Reprinted from Reference 42 with permission. Copyright (2022), Elsevier.

Table 2. Structural parameters of natural graphite and exfoliated graphene (EG) obtained through XRD.

Samples	Peak ° (2θ)	$d_{(002)}$ (Å)	β (radian)	D (nm)
Graphite	26.4	3.36	0.00243	58.60
Exfoliated graphene (EG)	26.4	3.37	0.00521	27.32

that it has more crystallinity. Graphene (002) has a larger full width at half maxima (FWHM) than graphite (002). The Scherrer formula,

$$D = \frac{0.9\lambda}{\beta \cos \theta} \tag{1}$$

was employed to determine the crystallite size of exfoliated graphene and graphite, where θ is the diffracted angle, β is the full width at half maximum of the (002) peak in radians and λ is the wavelength of the incident X-ray (= 0.154 nm) [29]. Table 2 displays the FWHM, interplanar spacing, and crystallite size of exfoliated graphene and graphite.

The size of the crystallites of graphene formed by electrochemical exfoliation is reduced because inter-lamellar spacing ($d_{(002)}$) rises due to cavitation energy generation during the exfoliation process [26]. This leads to the conclusion that an electrochemical method is used to exfoliate graphite.

3.2 Surface Morphology and Energy Dispersive Spectroscopy (EDS) Analysis

The exfoliated graphene's surface morphology has been depicted using a scanning electron microscope (SEM). The SEM was used to view the powered samples at a 20 kV accelerating voltage in a high vacuum environment. The SEM image of exfoliated graphene is exhibited in Fig. 3. The image supports the formation of

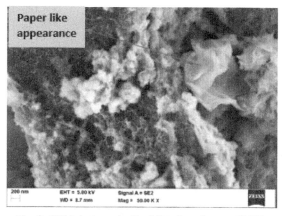

Fig. 3. SEM photograph of exfoliated graphene at 50 KX.

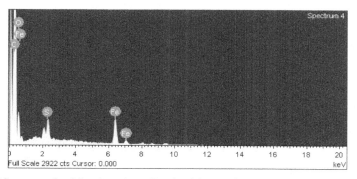

Fig. 4. EDS spectra of exfoliated graphene. Reprinted from Reference 42 with permission. Copyright (2022), Elsevier.

Table 3. Atomic percentage of exfoliated graphene.

S.No.	Elements	Atomic %
1.	C	81.81
2.	O	1.25
3.	Fe	0.43
4.	S	16.50

graphene, which exhibits roughened surface, out of plane deformation, and a crumpled or wrinkled appearance similar to paper [30]. Surfaces become roughened as a result of distortion during exfoliation and restacking. All of these features of graphene support the idea that it forms in aqueous media through an electrochemical exfoliation process.

The compositional analysis of exfoliated graphene is shown in Fig. 4. Using EDS, the compositional analysis was done. The presence of C, O, S, and Fe with proportions close to unity is confirmed by the EDS spectra. Table 3 displays the atomic proportion of exfoliated graphene.

3.3 FTIR Analysis

Figure 5 displays the FTIR spectra of graphene powders that have been exfoliated electrochemically. To ascertain the bonding of the chemical, the frequency range of the FTIR spectra was 4000 cm^{-1} to 400 cm^{-1} (mid-infrared range). It is evident from the entire spectrum that the specimen is free of any non-bonded SO^{4-} ions. Peaks linked with OH (3466 cm^{-1}) and the C=C (1634 cm^{-1}) are visible in the spectra in Fig. 5. Due to the adsorbed water molecules, the stretching vibrations of the O-H functional group emerged, producing a powerful and broad peak at 3466 cm^{-1}. Infrared (IR) absorption at 1634 cm^{-1} provides evidence for the stretching of the C=C bond in the aromatic ring of the carbon sheet [31]. The presence of a C=C linkage in an aqueous solution shows that graphene dispersion is present [32]. The Sp^2 character is also visible on the C=C bond [33]. The hydrocarbon group's C-H stretching vibrations, which are inherited from graphite are visible in the peak at 2927 cm^{-1} [32]. The peaks that occurred at 1022 cm^{-1} and 1400 cm^{-1}, respectively, demonstrate C-O stretching, alkoxide, and COO-H/CO-H stretching [31, 34]. The aromatic signal was linked to the sharp band at 800 cm^{-1}. The various functional groups found in exfoliated graphene are listed in Table 4. The findings are in line with the study by Htwe et al. [27].

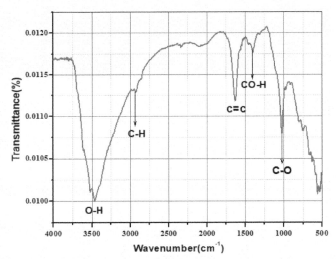

Fig. 5. FTIR spectra of exfoliated graphene. Reprinted from Reference 42 with permission. Copyright (2022), Elsevier.

Table 4. Different functional groups appeared in exfoliated graphene.

S.No.	Functional groups	Wavenumber(cm^{-1})
1.	C=C	~ 1634
2.	-OH	~ 3466
3.	C-O	~ 1022
4.	COO-H/CO-H	~ 1400
5.	C-H	~ 2927

3.4 UV-Visible Spectra of Exfoliated Graphene (EG)

The UV-visible spectra of graphene in aqueous media are demonstrated in Fig. 6. A UV-Visible spectrometer spanning wavelengths between 200 and 800 nm is used to record data. To see the absorption peak, the UV-visible spectrum was recorded. This approach is based on the notion that the colour of the material being characterized is directly proportional to the absorption in a specific wavelength range. According to the UV-Visible spectrum, the highest absorption is found at a specific wavelength [35]. Due to the π-π* transition of aromatic CAC bonds, the absorbance peak of exfoliated graphene was noticed at 267 nm [35, 36]. Graphene oxide (GO), on the other hand, displays π-π* transition of aromatic C-C rings. Due to the electronic configuration of graphene during the reduction of graphene oxide, this shift, which is a red shift, occurred [26].

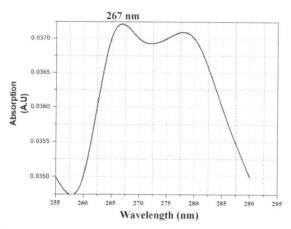

Fig. 6. UV-Visible spectra of exfoliated graphene. Reprinted from Reference 42 with permission, Copyright (2022), Elsevier.

3.5 Raman Analysis

For research on graphene, Raman spectroscopy is regarded as the most significant analysis. The number and orientation of layers, the quality and types of edges, strain, disorderly crystallinity, and functional groups are all determined by it. Additionally, it provides important details about the existence of Sp^2 and Sp^3 hybridization. Raman spectroscopy is a rapid, non-destructive technology that may be used on a variety of materials that have undergone various modifications. Raman spectroscopy, which analyses samples chemically by utilizing light to induce molecular vibration and then deciphering this interaction, falls under the genre of vibrational spectroscopy. The exfoliated graphene's Raman spectra are illustrated in Fig. 7. With an exposure time of 0.5 seconds and 15 mW of power, the Raman spectra are acquired at a wavelength of 514 nm. As can be seen from the figure, the graphene specimen exhibits three different peaks that are labelled D band, G band, and 2D band, respectively. The structural disorder of graphene, which is mostly linked to surface dislocations, is what causes the D band to appear at 1343 cm^{-1} [37]. The two-fold degenerate E$_{2g}$ mode at the zone centre corresponds to the G band's emergence at 1570 cm^{-1} [37]. All Sp^2 hybridized carbons exhibit this peak, which results from the stretching of C-C bonds [37, 38]. The third and final one occurs at 2706 cm^{-1} and is frequently referred to as the 2D band; however, it is also known as the G1 band because the G1 band is an overtone of the D band [39, 40]. The graphene signature is shown by the 2D band. The origin of the 2D or G1 band, which is explained by double-resonant, is sometimes referred to as the second order Raman spectrum [40]. Additionally, the I$_{2D}$/I$_G$ intensity ratio reveals the number of graphene layers. According to the intensity ratios I$_{2D}$/I$_G$ of > 2, 1–2 and < 1, respectively, graphene is made up of a single layer, two layers, and several layers [38]. In this instance, the I$_{2D}$/I$_G$ intensity ratio is 0.5, which is consistent with multilayer graphene. Using the formula provided here, we also determine the average diameter La of the graphene planes making up the domain here [41].

$$L_a = \frac{4.4}{R} \tag{2}$$

where R is the intensity ratio of D to G band. L$_a$ was determined to be 4.7 nm in this instance. By adjusting the process parameter, the number of graphene layers and average graphene plane diameter will be increased.

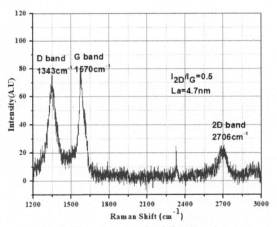

Fig. 7. Raman spectra of exfoliated graphene.

4. Conclusion

Electrochemical exfoliation was used to create graphene in an aqueous media. The electrochemical exfoliation process is becoming a crucial method for obtaining different types of graphene compounds. The production of graphene by electrochemical exfoliation has various benefits, including a one-step process, environmental friendliness, a straightforward experimental setup, and a lack of the use of harsh chemicals. SEM, XRD, and Raman studies have all confirmed the production of graphene. Out of plane deformation, rough surfaces, and a wrinkled paper appearance are all characteristics of exfoliated graphene. The hexagonal configuration of graphene at (002) is also confirmed by the XRD. As a result of the breakage of the interplanar carbon atom inside the graphitic structure, the intensity of exfoliated graphene is significantly reduced when compared to graphite. Exfoliated graphene exhibits an absorption peak at 267 nm, which is comparable to graphene's typical values. At around 2706 cm^{-1}, the Raman analysis reveals the distinctive peak of graphene. All of this data points to the notion that graphene exfoliates in aqueous medium. This work also shows that a variety of parameters, including the use of graphite electrodes, electrolytes, applied potential, and others, affect the properties of graphene materials formed via electrochemical exfoliation. Low voltage, cathodic exfoliation, and thin graphite electrodes are advantageous.

Acknowledgements

For all characterizations, the author thanks CIF, BIT Mesra, CRF, IISc Bengaluru, and SMITA Research Lab, IIT Delhi.

References

[1] Stoller, M.D., S. Park, Y. Zhu, J. An and R.S. Ruoff. 2008. Graphene-Based Ultracapacitors, Nano Lett. 8(10): 3498–3502.

[2] Liang, M. and L. Zhi. 2009. Graphene-based electrode materials for rechargeable lithium batteries. J. Mater. Chem. 19: 5871–5878.

[3] Han, M.Y., B. Özyilmaz, Y. Zhang and P. Kim. 2007. Energy band-gap engineering of graphene nanoribbons. Phys. Rev. Lett. 98: 206805.

[4] Ponomarenko, L.A., F. Schedin, M.I. Katsnelson, R. Yang, E.W. Hill, K.S. Novoselov and A.K. Geim. 2008. Chaotic dirac billiard in graphene quantum dots. Science 320(5874): 356–358.

[5] Hong, W., Y. Xu, G. Lu, C. Li and G. Shi. 2008. Transparent graphene/PEDOT–PSS composite films as counter electrodes of dye-sensitized solar cells. Electrochem. Commun. 10(10): 1555–1558.

[6] Liu, Q., X. Liu, X. Zhong, L. Yang, N. Zhang, G. Pan, S. Yin, Y. Chen and J. Wei. 2009. Photovoltaic cells based on solution-processable graphene and P3HT. Adv. Funct. Mater. 894–904.

[7] Liu, Y., X. Dong and P. Chen. 2012. Biological and chemical sensors based on graphene materials. Chem. Soc. Rev. 41(6): 2283–2307.

[8] Wang, Y., K. Huang, A. Derre, P. Puech, S. Rouziere, P. Launois, C. Castro, M. Monthioux and A. Penicaud. 2017. Conductive graphene coatings synthesized from graphenide solutions. Carbon 121: 217–225.

[9] Kim, H., Y. Miura and C.W. Macosko. 2010. Nanocomposites for improved gas barrier and electrical conductivity, Chem. Mater. 22: 3441–3450.

[10] Balandin, A.A., S. Ghosh, W. Bao, I. Calizo, D. Teweldebrhan, F. Miao and C.N. Lau. 2008. Superior thermal conductivity of single-layer graphene. Nano Lett. 8(3): 902–907.

[11] Kuilla, T., S. Bhadra, D. Yao, N.H. Kim, S. Bose and J.H. Lee. 2010. Recent advances in graphene based polymer composites. Prog. Polym. Sci. 35(11): 1350–1375.

[12] Li, X. and L. Zhi. 2018. Graphene hybridization for energy storage applications. Chem. Soc. Rev. 47: 3189–3216.

[13] Yi, M. and Z. Shen. 2015. A review on mechanical exfoliation for the scalable production of graphene. J. Mater. Chem. A 3(22): 11700–11715.

[14] Novoselov, K.S., V.I. Fal'Ko, L. Colombo, P.R. Gellert, M.G. Schwab and K. Kim. 2012. A roadmap for graphene. Nature 490: 192–200.

[15] Dong, L., J. Yang, M. Chhowalla and K.P. Loh. 2017. Synthesis and reduction of large sized graphene oxide sheets. Chem. Soc. Rev. 46: 7306–7316.

[16] Dreyer, D.R., R.S. Ruoff and C.W. Bielawski. 2010. From conception to realization: an historial account of graphene and some perspectives for its future. Angew. Chem. Int. Ed. 49(49): 9336–9344.

[17] Xu, Y., H. Cao, Y. Xue, B. Li and W. Cai. 2018. Liquid-phase exfoliation of graphene: an overview on exfoliation media, techniques, and challenges. Nanomaterials 8(11): 942.

[18] Cooper, D.R., B. D'Anjou, N. Ghattamaneni, B. Harack, M. Hilke, A. Horth, N. Majlis, M. Massicotte, L. Vandsburger, E. Whiteway and V. Yu. 2012. Experimental review of graphene. ISRN, Condens. Matter Phys. 2012: 1–56.

[19] Yin, P.T., S. Shah, M. Chhowalla and K.-B. Lee. 2015. Design, synthesis, and characterization of graphene–nanoparticle hybrid materials for bioapplications. Chem. Rev. 115: 2483–2531.

[20] Novoselov, K.S., V. Fal, L. Colombo, P. Gellert, M. Schwab and K. Kim. 2012. A roadmap for graphene. Nature 490: 192–200.

[21] Randviir, E.P., D.A.C. Brownson and C.E. Banks. 2014. A decade of graphene research: Production, applications and outlook. Mater. Today 17: 426–432.

[22] Kuila, T., S. Bose and A.K. Mishra. 2012. Chemical functionalization of graphene. J. Process Mater. Sci. 57: 1061–1105.

[23] Yi, M. and Z. Shen. 2016. Fluid dynamics: An emerging route for the scalable production of graphene in the last five years. RSC Adv. 6: 72525–72536.

[24] Amiri, A., M.N.M. Zubir, A.M. Dimiev, K.H. Teng, M. Shanbedi, S.N. Kazi and S. Bin Rozali. 2017. Facile, environmentally friendly, cost effective and scalable production of few-layered graphene. Chem. Eng. J. 326: 1105–1115.

[25] Saiful Badri, M.A., M.M. Salleh, N.F. Md Noor, M.Y.A. Rahman and A.A. Umar. 2017. Green synthesis of few-layered graphene from aqueous processed graphite exfoliation for graphene thin film preparation. Mater. Chem. Phys. 193: 212–219.

[26] Thema, F.T., M.J. Moloto, E.W. Dikio, N.N. Nyangiwe, L. Kotsedi, M. Maaza and M. Khenfouch. 2012. Synthesis and characterization of graphene thin films by chemical reduction of exfoliated and intercalated graphite oxide. J. Chem.

[27] Htwe, Y.Z.N., W.S. Chow, Y. Suda, A.A. Thant and M. Mariatti. 2019. Effect of electrolytes and sonication times on the formation of graphene using an electrochemical exfoliation process. Appl. Surf. Sci. 469: 951–961.

[28] Sahoo, S. and A. Mallik. 2015. Simple, Fast and cost–effective electrochemical synthesis of few layer graphene nanosheets. Nano 10(02): 1550019.

[29] Cullity, B.D. 1978. Elements of X-ray Diffraction, Addison Wesley Reading, M.A., USA, 197.

[30] Nishijo, J., Ch. Okabe, O. Oishi and N. Nishi. 2006. Synthesis, structures and magnetic properties of carbon-encapsulated nanoparticles via thermal decomposition of metal acetylide. Carbon 44: 2943–2949.

[31] Boehm, H. 2002. Surface oxides on carbon and their analysis: a critical assessment. Carbon 40: 145–149.

[32] Ahmad, A.F., F.H. Moin Abd, H.M. Mohd Kabir, I.A. Rahman, F. Mohamed, C.C. Hua, S. Ramli and S. Radiman. 2013. Graphene Colloidal dispersion in various organic solvents. Malaysian J. Anal. Sci. 17(3): 475–480.

[33] Dato, A., Z. Lee, K.J. Jeon, T.R. Erni, V. Radmilovic, T.J. Richardson and M. Frenklach. 2009. Clean and highly ordered graphene synthesized in the gas phase. Chem. Commun. 40: 6095–6097.

[34] Liu, J., H. Yang, S.G. Zhen, C.K. Poh, A. Chaurasia, J. Luo et al. 2013. A green approach to the synthesis of high-quality graphene oxide flakes via electrochemical exfoliation of pencil core. RSC Adv. 3: 11745–11750.

[35] Singh, R. and C.C. Tripathi. 2016. Flexible supercapacitors using liquid phase exfoliated graphene with enhanced specific capacitance. Int. J. Electrochem. Sci. 11: 6336–6346.

[36] Kumar Anurag and S.R. Kumar. 2021. Synthesis of graphene through electrochemical exfoliation technique in aqueous medium. Materials Today: Proceedings 44: 2695–2699.

[37] Swapan Das, Chandan K. Ghosh, Chandan K. Sarkar and Sunipa Roy. 2018. Facile synthesis of multi-layer graphene by electrochemical exfoliation using organic solvent. Nanotechnol Rev. 7: 497–508.

which ultrasound applies such effects has been proposed as "acoustic cavitation", in which the ultrasonic wave passes through a solution while forming bubbles that consecutively grow and collapse in the solution (7). The laser ablation (LA) method, on the other hand, is a complicated process used to reduce the size of bulk materials while breaking down one part by using a laser pulse. Also, substances from the surface can be removed by the laser pulse. Melting and crushing large selenium particles in a liquid medium exposed to laser radiation produces high-quality nanoparticles (7). This method is an economical technique that is free of contaminations common with chemical agents, leading to highly-stable nanoparticles which can be collected rapidly after synthesis (8). Microwave-aided synthesis of SeNPs is another method that has recently attracted attention. Microwave irradiation is a regular heating technique in the laboratory, and in microwave-aided SeNP synthesis, selenium salts are used as the primary reagent in an aqueous solution without any surfactants. This method leads to the formation of SeNPs after 4 minutes of heating (9). Due to its unique advantages, including faster reaction rate and subsequent decrease in reaction time, quick heating procedures, high reaction selectivity, and energy-saving, microwave-aided synthesis has rapidly grown as a favored nanofabrication method.

2.2 Chemical Synthesis

Chemical synthesis of SeNPs is usually rapid and possible with a wide range of materials; however, this method is often considered energy-consuming and relies on toxic chemicals (10). Controlled decay of organometallic complexes and metal-surfactant compounds, electrochemical synthesis, reduction of metal salt precursors, and wet chemical method (which is based on solution-phase technique) are some examples of the chemical synthesis methods (10). Two types of agents, namely protective and reducing agents, are commonly employed in these methods. Surfactants are usually applied as protective agents, and sodium citrate, hydrazine hydrate, and borohydride are often used as reducing agents. Also, the carboxylic group of common organic acids, including ascorbic acid, folic acid, sialic acid, oxalic acid, benzoic acid, gallic acid, and acetic acid can cause a reduction in selenium salts, leading to the acid-induced synthesis of SeNPs (9). However, the most popular method of SeNPs chemical synthesis has been the reduction of selenium dioxide, selenate, or selenite via hydrazine, glycol, or sodium ascorbate as reducing agents. According to some reports, varied ratios of 100 mM sodium selenite and 50 mM ascorbic acid result in the production of SeNPs. Ascorbic acid possesses antioxidative features and has an important role in the reduction and transformation of SeNPs (11). In a study by Patil et al. in 2019, SeNPs were synthesized by the chemical reduction method at room temperature, using glutathione as a reducing agent. Glutathione acts as both a reducing agent and a stabilizer to prevent aggregation of SeNPs (12). This technique, which leads to the reduction of sodium selenite by glutathione, is one of the simplest chemical techniques for the synthesis of SeNPs. Mentioned chemical methods should be carried out in harsh experimental situations (13).

Wet chemical methods, or solution-phase techniques, which can be performed in aqueous or non-aqueous solutions, are considered an excellent method for SeNP synthesis. Different sizes of nanomaterials, ranging from 12–50 nm, can be produced by wet chemical methods. Chemical synthesis of SeNPs in aqueous solvent results in homogeneous, small, and stable particles, which are favorable for biomedical studies. In this method, sodium selenite and selenious acid (H_2SeO_3) are generally employed as primary agents, which are used along with reducing agents and stabilizers. Potassium/sodium borohydride and ascorbic acid are common reducing agents, with the former being considered more toxic. It is important to note that the concentration of primary substances and reducing agents affect the growth and nucleation of nanoparticles (14). Stabilizers are also used to prevent the potential aggregation of SeNPs in aqueous solvents, including polysaccharides, gallic and ascorbic acid, polyvinyl alcohol, and quercetin (7). This outlines the importance of sustaining the stability of SeNPs in aqueous solutions. For example, an increase in the size of nanoparticles leads to greater reactivity and a subsequent increase in the risk of particle interaction. A solution to avoid such interactions is to coat the particles with agents known as "capping agents". A single layer coating of any dense matrix, such as a surfactant or polymer, is the simplest method to stabilize the particles, which enhances the viscosity of the solution, causing less interaction between nanoparticles and preventing their growth (12). Moreover, polysaccharides can be used for the dispersion and stabilization of SeNPs, due to their hydrophilic groups which can react with nanosized materials and avoid their aggregation (15). Both natural and modified water-soluble polysaccharides can be used as stabilizers in SeNPs synthesis. Chitosan, carboxymethyl chitosan, konjac glucomannan (KGM), acacia gum, sulfated polysaccharides, and carboxymethyl cellulose are some examples. Also, the combination of SeNPs with polysaccharides may potentially lead to useful materials for the pharmaceutical and food industry.

Water-soluble, hyperbranched polysaccharide (HBP) is taken from sclerotia of *Pleurotus tuber-regium* and used as a stabilizer for the selenious acid-reducing system, leading to the successful synthesis of well-dispersed, spherical SeNPs. Chitosan (CTS) is another abundant natural polysaccharide and the N-deacetylated production of chitin. A great number of reports have indicated the non-toxic, non-allergic, biodegrading, and biocompatible features of chitosan. CTS decomposes into amino sugars, which are safe products and can be absorbed completely by the human body. Chitosan is known as a proper stabilizer for SeNPs synthesis, and, due to its intrinsic antioxidant activity, the *in vitro* antioxidative features of chitosan-loaded selenite increased significantly compared to selenite, as reported by Zeng et al. (15).

The sol-gel technique is another wet chemical method that causes the production of micro- and nano-crystalline powders, thin films, ceramics, metal oxide, and organic-inorganic hybrid NPs' powders (10). Sol-gel technology is an appropriate method to change material features and merge several functionalities in one material. This technique can be carried out in low-temperature conditions and without environment sensitivity, which eases the utilization of this technique for a range of materials.

2.3 Biological Synthesis

In contrast to chemical methods, living organisms including fungi, plants, yeast, and bacteria are involved in the biological synthesis of SeNPs. Thus, biological synthesis is known as an eco-friendly, non-toxic method that leads to nanomaterial with significant pharmacological properties.

As a result of the complexity inherent in chemical synthesis methods, biological-based synthesis, also known as "green synthesis", has gained enormous popularity, since it avoids costly and complicated chemical reagents required in chemical methods. Hence, the chemistry and properties of green synthesis have been thoroughly investigated by researchers to realize the interaction between living organisms and inorganic compounds. Various types of microorganisms, plant extracts, and fungi have been implemented in the production of SeNPs (2).

2.3.1 Plants

Selenium nanoparticles can be synthesized through a one-step process in the presence of biologically-active plant extracts, which include different metabolites such as alkaloids, phenols, saponins, and flavonoids. These phytoconstituents carry out the biosynthesis of SeNPs through acting as capping, reducing, and stabilizing agents, increasing the efficiency of synthesis as compared to chemical methods. Various plant organs, such as leaves, flowers, and buds can be used for the biosynthesis of SeNPs (2). Leaf extracts of Aloe vera, which are a rich source of polysaccharides, sterols, phenolic compounds, flavonoids, lignin, and proteins, are well-known reducing and stabilizing reagents for the synthesis of SeNPs (7). Moreover, biosynthesis of spherical and crystalline SeNPs with a stable pH has been reported with the aqueous extract of *Allium sativum*, as well as *Asteriscus graveolens*, which leads to spherical SeNPs in the size of 20.06 nm that have been applied as anticancer drug carriers (16, 17). *Catharanthus roseus* and *Peltophorum pterocarpum* extracts are also an attractive alternative for the physical/chemical synthesis of SeNPs, due to the production of biocompatible, hollow SeNPs (18). The extract of *Clausena dentata* has also been applied in SeNP biosynthesis (19). Moreover, crystalline SeNPs with a 65 nm size has been green synthesized by *Diospyros Montana* extract, in which flavonoids and phenols act as stabilizers and reducing agents (20). In addition, the combination of sodium selenite (Na_2SeO_3) with green tea extract as a reducing agent, and *Lycium barbarum* as a surface capping agent, leads to the production of spherical SeNPs with a size range of 83–160 nm, which have shown robust biological activities, including free radical scavenging and antioxidant activity (21). Further, lemon leaf extracts have been used in the synthesis of SeNPs with the size range of 50–80 nm, which have been reported to protect human lymphocytes from UV radiation-induced DNA damage (14). Altogether, various plant extracts have been employed in the synthesis of different types of SeNPs with various size ranges, which offer a promising, green alternative to the physical/chemical synthesis methods.

2.3.2 Microbes

The rhythmic connection between inorganic materials and living organisms has led to the maintenance of life on this planet. Over the last few years, researchers have under-investigated the relationship between inorganic molecules and biological organisms. Studies proved that some micro-organisms possess the ability to produce nanoparticles, which can be performed through intracellular or extracellular pathways. Microbial synthesis of selenium nanoparticles can be performed via bacterial, fungal, and yeast-mediated synthesis.

2.3.2.1 Bacteria

Since handling and expansion of prokaryotic micro-organisms are more feasible and facile, they are considered as a preferred source for SeNPs production. The biosynthesis of SeNPs can be carried out through intracellular, extracellular, and membrane-bound mechanisms. Of interest, selenium was observed on the cell wall and membrane of *Escherichia coli* for the first time in bacteria via electron microscopy (22). In the early studies, the gram-negative, obligate anaerobic, *Sulfurospirillum barnesii* SES-3 strain, which is a selenium respiring bacterium, was demonstrated to reduce selenate to elemental selenium, through which 3000-nm, uniform nanospheres were synthesized (23). Other examples of selenium-respiring bacteria include *Selenihalanaerobacter*, and *Bacillus selenitireducens* (24). The size of the resulting SeNPs produced by different bacterial strains is dependent on the concentration of sodium selenite (Na_2SeO_3) available to the bacteria, and biomass concentration. For instance, a low concentration of *Shewanella* sp. biomass synthesizes 1–20 nm SeNPs after 2 hours of incubation, while larger SeNPs, ranging from 51 to 60 nm, can be produced with a higher concentration of bacteria after 24–72 hours of incubation (25). Few studies have focused on the synthesis of SeNPs via aerobic microorganisms, including soil bacteria *Pseudomonas aeruginosa* and *Bacillus* sp. (26). However, these studies have elucidated limited characterization aspects of the selenium nanospheres produced. Probiotic bacteria, including *Lactobacillus* sp., *Streptococcus thermophilus*, and *Bifidobacteria* sp. can reduce sodium hydrogen selenite ($NaHSeO_3$) salt to elemental selenium. Of note, it has been demonstrated that lactic acid bacteria are able to merge selenium into intracellular proteins in the form of the amino acid selenocysteine (SeCys), which is the dominant form of selenium found in the lactobacillus species (27). Further, production of monoclinic SeNPs with 200-nm size and well dispersity via *Pseudomonas alcaliphila* has been reported, taking place at 28°C with ambient pressure. The transformation of SeNPs from nanospheres into nanorods takes place after 24 hours of the reaction; however, PVP (polyvinylpyrrolidone) is a capping agent and controls the size of produced SeNPs that causes an interruption in the mentioned transformation (28). Hence, according to the above examples, selenium respiring bacteria as well as many other strains can be used for the microbial synthesis of selenium nanoparticles.

2.3.2.2 Fungi

One of the most common methods for the production of metal nanoparticles is via fungi since they harbor metal accumulation activity. Almost all fungi are sensitive to selenium, meaning that selenium-containing compounds possess antifungal properties. It is now established that incubation of fungal bodies with a high concentration of selenium leads to the activation of detoxifying procedures and subsequent cell damage in fungal cells. However, according to the study by Wangeline et al., fungi exposed to environments that contain high amounts of selenium are more tolerant to selenium-containing compounds (29). Studies by Sarkar et al. and Zare et al. have reported the extracellular synthesis of SeNPs by *Alternaria alternate* and *Aspergillus terreus*, respectively (30, 31). *Aspergillus terreus* incubated with selenium ions produces spherical SeNPs with a size of 47 nm after an incubation time of 60 minutes (31). Also, stable and uniform SeNPs can be synthesized via the *Alternaria alternate* fungus, in which the presence of a protein matrix in the outer shell of SeNPs acts as a stabilizing agent, enhancing their dispersion in liquid suspension for a longer period.

2.3.2.3 Yeast

Yeast cells harbor the potential to bioaccumulate numerous trace elements, including selenium, through their growth period. *Saccharomyces cerevisiae* is able to produce SeNPs in the selenium-rich medium under variable fermentation conditions including duration of fermentation, pH value, temperature, and shaking speed (32). However, few studies have reported the production of SeNPs via yeast cells, and green synthesis of SeNPs with yeast cells has not been investigated in-depth to date. Thus, it is crucial for nanobiotechnology researchers to better elucidate the mechanism and potentialities of yeast-mediated green synthesis of selenium and other nanometal particles.

Although biological synthesis of SeNPs overcomes some serious issues associated with chemical and physical methods, it is not free of drawbacks. For instance, the complexity of the extraction step in case the nanoparticles are produced intracellularly by the microorganisms is one of the disadvantages of the biological method. Furthermore, sustaining appropriate growth conditions for microorganisms, as well as large-scale nanoparticle production with larger amounts of biomass are other important concerns that need to be addressed through further studies (10).

3. Biomedical Applications

Several nano-based pharmaceuticals have been approved for specific indications by the American Food and Drug Administration (FDA). Nanoparticles with the size range of 10–100 nm are ideal for therapeutic purposes since they are small enough to be protected from ingestion by the reticuloendothelial system (RES), and large enough not to pass through renal filtration (14). Importantly, when anti-tumor applications are intended, the pathologic vasculature conditions of the tumor microenvironment aids nanoparticle accumulation in tumor tissues. This effect is known as the Enhanced Permeability and Retention (EPR) effect, which allows macromolecules of specific size ranges to better accumulate and retain in tumors, rather than normal tissues (33). Among the available metal nanoparticles, SeNPs are one of the most useful in the biomedical industry. According to the properties of SeNPs discussed earlier, including the unique physiochemical features and low toxicity, they are constantly being studied for their potential pharmaceutical effects. Notable efficacy of SeNPs has been observed in various diseases, including anti-diabetic, anti-cancer, anti-inflammatory, and anti-microbial activity. Also,

SeNPs are gaining increasing attention as a suitable drug carrier in novel nano-based drug-delivery systems.

3.1 Anti-cancer Activity

The pathology of cancer is associated with uncontrolled cell division and migration, and it is considered a serious cause of mortality, morbidity, and low quality of life (QoL) in many societies. Approximately 19.3 million new cancer cases have been diagnosed in 2020, with the occurrence of almost 10 million cancer-related deaths in the same year (34). Radical surgery in early stages, as well as chemotherapy, radiotherapy, hormone therapy, and immunotherapy, are the most important cancer treatment modalities. Recently, nano-based drugs have drawn enormous attention as a game-changer in the treatment of cancer. In this regard, specific metal nanoparticles, including SeNPs, have demonstrated anti-cancer activities through several studies. The cytotoxic effects of SeNPs against various cancer cell lines, including human cervical carcinoma cells (HeLa, HeLa-S3, C-33A) (35), hepatic cancer cells (HepG2) (36), human lung adenocarcinoma cells (A549) (37), human breast adenocarcinoma cells (MCF-7) (38), and murine mammary carcinoma cells (4T1) (38) have been demonstrated. Of note, these nanoparticles have shown excellent safety and biocompatibility in normal epithelial, skeletal muscle, hepatic, and blood cells, especially when produced through "green synthesis" methods (39). Different mechanisms have been proposed through which SeNPs exert their anti-cancer effects, including activation of apoptosis pathways and cell cycle arrest, inducing mitochondrial dysfunction, production of reactive specious oxygen (ROS), disruption of cellular homeostasis, and DNA fragmentation. Triggering the apoptosis pathways by SeNPs starts with ROS accumulation associated with SeNP internalization in cancer, but not normal, cells. ROS starts a series of mitochondria-associated pathways which lead to endoplasmic reticulum stress and eventual activation of caspases. First, the mitochondrial membrane potential is affected, leading to cytochrome-c leakage into the cytosol, which leads to activation of several pathways, including MAPK-Erk, PI3K, NF-κB, and apoptosis pathways, leading to caspase-9 activation. Caspase-9 activation induces caspase-3 activity, which finally leads to DNA degradation and apoptosis. Moreover, the subsequent influx of modulated Ca^{2+} causes caspase activity and cell apoptosis. Thus, in cancer cells, ROS is known as a mediator for SeNP-induced anti-cancer activity (10). In a study by Vahidi et al., cancer cells treated with biologically-synthesized SeNPs have a notably higher caspase-3 activity than normal cells treated with biogenic SeNPs, outlining the exquisite safety of these nanoparticles in normal cells (39). Biologically synthesized SeNPs via *Bacillus* and *Lactobacillus* strains have been shown to stimulate anti-cancer immune responses in cancer-bearing mice and prevent tumor progression (40). Some of the immunostimulatory properties of biogenic SeNPs are assumed to occur due to the special functional groups located on the surface of SeNPs, which are absent on those synthesized chemically. *Lactobacillus* sp. possess immunomodulatory effects as the normal intestinal flora, and their antigen is thought to be expressed on the surface of biogenic SeNPs (41). Such immunostimulatory effects are important for cancer patients in whom the immune system is compromised, and might present a novel immunotherapeutic modality for these patients.

Several other compounds in combination with SeNPs have been investigated for their possible synergistic anti-cancer effects. Based on a study by El Batal et al., the combination of fermented wheat germ extract (FWGE) with SeNPs decreases tumor volume in an ascites carcinoma model in mice (42). FWGE inhibits oxidative damage in normal tissues, thereby leading to apoptosis in cancer cells, and is thus known as a nutritional supplement for cancer patients. This study revealed the superior anti-cancer efficacy of this supplement when combined with SeNPs. Moreover, the incorporation of selenium in the structure of hydroxyapatite (HA), which is the main inorganic mineral in hard tissues such as bones and teeth, reduces the recurrence of osteosarcoma in mice and is used as a supporting agent for bone regeneration in the bone graft (43).

3.2 Antimicrobial Activity

Selenium-containing compounds, including sodium selenite (Na_2SeO_3), sodium selenate (Na_2SeO_4), sodium selenide (Na_2Se), and selenium dioxide (SeO_2) have shown antibacterial effects against *E. coli* through inducing DNA damage (44). The same effect has been demonstrated with SeNPs, with the proposed mechanism being ROS generation and subsequent destruction of cell DNA and essential enzymes. Several anti-microbial potentials have been observed with SeNPs, including antibacterial (45), antifungal (46), and antialgal (47) properties. These properties can also be enhanced through modification with other agents. As an example, SeNPs were modified with the positively charged spider silk protein eADF4 (κ16), causing a surface positive charge that increases the bactericidal efficiency against gram-negative bacteria, including *E. coli* (2). The anti-bacterial properties of SeNPs have been shown to be strongly dependent on their size. Thus, the highest inhibition in the growth of methicillin-sensitive *Staphylococcus aureus* (MSSA) and methicillin-resistant *Staphylococcus aureus* (MRSA) have been observed with SeNPs with a concentration of 10 μg.mL^{-1} and a size of 81 nm (48).

Recently, the activity of metal nanoparticles against pathogenic fungi have attracted the attention of many researchers. *Candida albicans* is an opportunistic pathogenic yeast that can cause mild to severe fungal infections, especially in long-term antibiotic consumers and immunocompromised patients. Based on several studies, selenium nanoparticles-enriched *Lactobacillus* spp. co-cultured with *C. albicans* inhibited the growth of *C. albicans* colony in the culture. In addition to the antifungal properties of SeNPs against *C. albicans*, it is assumed that *Lactobacillus* release metabolites that prevent *C. albicans* colony growth (46). Moreover, other studies have shown the potential of silver and selenium nanoparticles to prevent biofilm formation in *C. albicans* (2). A large amount of SeNPs accumulates in the cell wall of *C. albicans* through chemisorption, and selenium causes sulfur displacement from methionine and cysteine, thus damaging the cell wall. In addition, biogenic SeNPs produced via *Klebsiella pneumonia* demonstrate anti-fungal characteristics, inhibiting the mycelial growth of *Alternaria solani* and *Colletotrichum capsica* (47).

3.3 Drug Delivery Applications

One of the most important potentials of nanoparticles is their gene and drug loading capacity. In the context of gene therapy, nanoparticles are classified as nonviral vectors, with the advantage of inducing minimal immunogenic responses compared to viral vectors, and the potential to transport larger nucleic acid molecules (1). SeNPs have also been studied as drug carriers, especially in the context of chemotherapeutic drugs, since SeNPs have been shown to reduce their systemic toxicity while improving their efficacy. The binding of the drug to SeNPs occurs through physical dispersion or chemical binding, and specific modifying agents, e.g., polymers, can increase the efficiency of the combination. Polymers are easy to modify and have high potentials for drug loading, condensation of nucleic acids, and targeting. Polymers can also act as a drug reservoir layer coating the nanoparticle, thus enhancing drug solubility and loading capacity, while protecting them from degradation (49). Cisplatin-, 5-flurouracil-, and doxorubicin-loaded SeNPs have indicated enhanced anti-cancer effects compared to their non-nano-based counterparts (14). Further, according to the study by Huang et al., a transferrin-conjugated SeNP delivery system increased the uptake of doxorubicin in the mammalian breast cancer cell line MCF-7. Based on the results of this study, this drug delivery system effectively caused apoptosis and inhibition of cancer cell growth compared to control (50). A delivery system based on irinotecan and SeNPs in mice model and *in vivo* study indicated enhanced cytotoxicity, compared with each of the components used solely, in the human ileocecal adenocarcinoma cell line HCT-8, causing a 62.1% reduction in tumor size. Collectively, based on the results discussed above and those of many other similar studies, SeNPs offer a promising nano-based drug carrier platform due to their unique properties, especially for chemotherapeutic drugs.

3.4 Anti-diabetic Activity

Diabetes mellitus (DM) is a metabolic disorder resulting from pancreas dysfunction. Pancreas secrets insulin, which is a hormone controlling the level of blood glucose. DM is classified into two major types, including type-I and type-II. Damage to many organs, including the eye, liver, heart, and kidneys are common complications in DM patients. Since the etiology of DM is in part associated with inflammation and oxidative response, selenium supplements and SeNPs might provide benefit in these patients from a theoretical point of view (2). A study by Ashrafizadeh et al. in 2020 showed the exceptional anti-diabetic potential of chitosan-stabilized selenium nanoparticles (CsS-SeNPs) in rat models of DM (51). Further studies concluded that modified SeNPs with peptide-conjugated chitosan (SCD) can activate VPAC-2, which is a receptor moderating glucose-dependent insulin secretion, eventually leading to reduction of blood glucose levels. SCD treatment *in vitro* indicated improved insulin sensitivity and lipid profile compared to control (52).

3.5 Anti-inflammatory Activity

Since the process of inflammation is involved in the pathology of many diseases, the potential anti-inflammatory activities of SeNPs have recently attracted enormous attention. In the process of inflammation, stimulants triggering cellular stress activate the NF-κB transcription factor, which is regulated by mitogen-activated protein kinase (MAP-K), thus triggering the expression of various pro-inflammatory genes. SeNPs have demonstrated inhibition of MAP-K, NF-κB, and reduction in TNF-α levels, which are important markers of inflammation (2). Moreover, a combination of SeNPs with silymarin in low concentration indicated a marked reduction in NF-κB activity, as well as reductions in the level of IL-1β, MPO, and TNF-α (53). Further studies showed SeNPs modified with polysaccharides to harbor anti-inflammatory properties by inhibiting the degradation of Iκ-B, which prevents the NF-κB pathway, and phosphorylation of JNK1/2 and p38 (5). Iκ-B is an inhibitory protein that can be phosphorylated by Iκ-B kinase, then ubiquitinated and degraded. Degradation of Iκ-B leads to the initiation of the NF-κB pathway. Taken together, it can be inferred that the anti-inflammatory activity of SeNPs is one of their vital properties which needs to be further evaluated for possible translation into the clinic.

4. Conclusion

Selenium is an essential micronutrient for a living organism that is taken through diet. Nanoparticle-based formulations for a variety of metal elements are available, one of which is SeNPs. SeNPs have indicated distinct properties, including antioxidant and pro-oxidant effects, by affecting the catalytic activity of various physiologic enzymes. In comparison to selenium-containing compounds, SeNPs harbor less toxicity for living organisms and thus can widely be applied in different industries, especially in biomedicine. In this chapter, various methods of SeNPs synthesis have been discussed, with a focus on biological synthesis. Biologic synthesis of SeNPs is cost-effective, safe, and with less contamination compared with chemical methods, which require hazardous chemicals, extreme pH conditions, and high temperature. Further, we have discussed the several applications of SeNPs, including anti-microbial, anti-diabetic, and anti-inflammatory activities. More importantly, SeNPs offer promising potentials for cancer treatment, since they have shown potent anti-cancer effects through several studies. Furthermore, SeNPs offer a unique platform for drug delivery, especially for chemotherapeutic drugs. Further investigation regarding their properties and detailed mechanisms of action are needed to enhance our knowledge and better harness the distinctive potentials of these nanoparticles.

References

[1] Tapiero, H., D.M. Townsend and K.D. Tew. 2003. The antioxidant role of selenium and seleno-compounds. Biomedicine & Pharmacotherapy 57(3): 134–44.

[2] Nayak, V., K.R.B. Singh, A.K. Singh and R.P. Singh. 2021. Potentialities of selenium nanoparticles in biomedical science. New Journal of Chemistry 45(6): 2849–78.

[3] Khanna, P.K., N. Bisht and P. Phalswal. 2022. Selenium nanoparticles: a review on synthesis and biomedical applications. Materials Advances.

[4] Forootanfar, H., M. Adeli-Sardou, M. Nikkhoo, M. Mehrabani, B. Amir-Heidari, A.R. Shahverdi et al. 2014. Antioxidant and cytotoxic effect of biologically synthesized selenium nanoparticles in comparison to selenium dioxide. Journal of Trace Elements in Medicine and Biology 28(1): 75–9.

[5] Khurana, A., S. Tekula, M.A. Saifi, P. Venkatesh and C. Godugu. 2019. Therapeutic applications of selenium nanoparticles. Biomedicine & pharmacotherapy = Biomedecine & pharmacotherapie. 111: 802–12.

[6] Kondaparthi, P., S.J.S. Flora and S. Naqvi. 2019. Selenium nanoparticles: An insight on its Pro-oxidant and antioxidant properties. Frontiers in Nanoscience and Nanotechnology 6.

[7] Varlamova, E.G., E.A. Turovsky and E.V. Blinova. 2021. Therapeutic potential and main methods of obtaining selenium nanoparticles. International Journal of Molecular Sciences 22(19): 10808.

[8] Menazea, A.A., A.M. Ismail, N.S. Awwad and H.A. Ibrahim. 2020. Physical characterization and antibacterial activity of PVA/Chitosan matrix doped by selenium nanoparticles prepared via one-pot laser ablation route. Journal of Materials Research and Technology 9(5): 9598–606.

[9] Skalickova, S., V. Milosavljevic, K. Cihalova, P. Horky, L. Richtera and V. Adam. 2017. Selenium nanoparticles as a nutritional supplement. Nutrition 33: 83–90.

[10] Yazdi, M., Z. Sepehrizadeh, M. Mahdavi, A.R. Shahverdi and M. Faramarzi. 2016. Metal, metalloid, and oxide nanoparticles for therapeutic and diagnostic oncology. Nano Biomedicine and Engineering 8.

[11] Sarkar, B., S. Bhattacharjee, A. Daware, P. Tribedi, K.K. Krishnani and P.S. Minhas. 2015. Selenium nanoparticles for stress-resilient fish and livestock. Nanoscale Research Letters 10(1): 371.

[12] Patil, D.P., M. Usharani, A.G. Reddy, B. Kalakumar, G.K. Sawale and K. Vanitha. 2019. Chemical synthesis and characterization of selenium nanoparticles. Chemical Science Review and Letters 8(32): 161–5.

[13] Langi, B., C. Shah, K. Singh, A. Chaskar, M. Kumar and P.N. Bajaj. 2010. Ionic liquid-induced synthesis of selenium nanoparticles. Materials Research Bulletin 45(6): 668–71.

[14] Maiyo, F. and M. Singh. 2017. Selenium nanoparticles: potential in cancer gene and drug delivery. Nanomedicine (London, England) 12(9): 1075–89.

[15] Zeng, S., Y. Ke, Y. Liu, Y. Shen, L. Zhang, C. Li et al. 2018. Synthesis and antidiabetic properties of chitosan-stabilized selenium nanoparticles. Colloids and surfaces B, Biointerfaces 170: 115–21.

[16] Anu, K., G. Singaravelu, K. Murugan and G. Benelli 2017. Green-synthesis of selenium nanoparticles using garlic cloves (Allium sativum): Biophysical characterization and cytotoxicity on vero cells. Journal of Cluster Science 28.

[17] Zeebaree, S.Y.S., A.Y.S. Zeebaree and O.I.H. Zebari. 2020. Diagnosis of the multiple effect of selenium nanoparticles decorated by Asteriscus graveolens components in inhibiting HepG2 cell proliferation. Sustainable Chemistry and Pharmacy 15: 100210.

[18] Deepa, B. and V. Ganesan. 2014. Bioinspiredsynthesis of selenium nanoparticles using flowers of Catharanthus roseus (L.) G. Don. and Peltophorum pterocarpum (DC.) Backer ex Heyne—A comparison. International Journal of ChemTech Research 77: 974–4290.

[19] Sowndarya, P., G. Ramkumar and M.S. Shivakumar. 2017. Green synthesis of selenium nanoparticles conjugated Clausena dentata plant leaf extract and their insecticidal potential against mosquito vectors. Artificial Cells, Nanomedicine, and Biotechnology 45(8): 1490–5.

[20] Kokila, K., N. Elavarasan and V. Sujatha. 2017. Diospyros montana leaf extract-mediated synthesis of selenium nanoparticles and their biological applications. New Journal of Chemistry 41(15): 7481–90.

[21] Zhang, W., J. Zhang, D. Ding, L. Zhang, L.A. Muehlmann, S.E. Deng et al. 2018..Synthesis and antioxidant properties of Lycium barbarum polysaccharides capped selenium nanoparticles using tea extract. Artificial Cells, Nanomedicine, and Biotechnology 46(7): 1463–70.

[22] Wadhwani, S.A., U.U. Shedbalkar, R. Singh and B.A. Chopade. 2016. Biogenic selenium nanoparticles: current status and future prospects. Applied Microbiology and Biotechnology 100(6): 2555–66.

[23] Oremland, R.S., J.S. Blum, C.W. Culbertson, P.T. Visscher, L.G. Miller, P. Dowdle et al. 1994. Isolation, growth, and metabolism of an obligately anaerobic, selenate-respiring bacterium, strain SES-3. Appl. Environ. Microbiol. 60(8): 3011–9.

[24] Bansal, V., A. Bharde, R. Ramanathan and S.K. Bhargava. 2012. Inorganic materials using 'unusual' microorganisms. Advances in Colloid and Interface Science 179-182: 150–68.

[25] Tam, K., C.T. Ho, J.H. Lee, M. Lai, C.H. Chang, Y. Rheem et al. 2010. Growth mechanism of amorphous selenium nanoparticles synthesized by Shewanella sp. HN-41. Bioscience, Biotechnology, and Biochemistry 74(4): 696–700.

[26] Torres, S.K., V.L. Campos, C.G. León, S.M. Rodríguez-Llamazares, S.M. Rojas, M. González et al. 2012. Biosynthesis of selenium nanoparticles by Pantoea agglomerans and their antioxidant activity. Journal of Nanoparticle Research 14(11): 1236.

[27] Eszenyi, P., A. Sztrik, B. Babka and P. Joe. 2011. Elemental, nano-sized (100–500 nm) selenium production by probiotic lactic acid bacteria. International Journal of Bioscience, Biochemistry and Bioinformatics 1: 148–52.

[28] Zhang, W., Z. Chen, H. Liu, L. Zhang, P. Gao and D. Li. 2011. Biosynthesis and structural characteristics of selenium nanoparticles by Pseudomonas alcaliphila. Colloids and Surfaces B: Biointerfaces 88(1): 196–201.

[29] Wangeline, A., J. Valdez, S.D. Lindblom, K. Bowling, F. Reeves and E. Pilon-Smits. 2011. Characterization of rhizosphere fungi from selenium hyperaccumulator and nonhyperaccumulator plants along the eastern Rocky Mountain Front Range. American Journal of Botany 98: 1139–47.

[30] Sarkar, J., P. Dey, S. Saha and K. Acharya. 2011. Mycosynthesis of selenium nanoparticles. Micro & Nano Letters, IET 6: 599–602.

[31] Zare, B., S. Babaie, N. Seyatesh and A.R. Shahverdi. 2012. Isolation and characterization of a fungus for extracellular synthesis of small selenium nanoparticles Extracellular synthesis of small selenium nanoparticles using fungi. Nanomed. J. 1: 14–20.

[32] Esmaeili, S., K. Khosravi, R. Pourahmad and R. Komeili. 2012. An experimental design for production of selenium-enriched yeast. World Applied Sciences Journal 19: 31–7.

[33] Ngoune, R., A. Peters, D. von Elverfeldt, K. Winkler and G. Pütz. 2016. Accumulating nanoparticles by EPR: A route of no return. Journal of Controlled Release 238: 58–70.

[34] Sung, H., J. Ferlay, R.L. Siegel, M. Laversanne, I. Soerjomataram, A. Jemal et al. 2021. Global Cancer Statistics 2020: GLOBOCAN estimates of incidence and mortality worldwide for 36 cancers in 185 countries. CA: A Cancer Journal for Clinicians 71(3): 209–49.

[35] Rajkumar, K., S. Mvs, S. Koganti and S. Burgula. 2020. Selenium nanoparticles synthesized using Pseudomonas stutzeri (MH191156) show antiproliferative and anti-angiogenic activity against cervical cancer cells. Int. J. Nanomedicine 15: 4523–40.

[36] Meng, Y., Y. Zhang, N. Jia, H. Qiao, M. Zhu, Q. Meng et al. 2018. Synthesis and evaluation of a novel water-soluble high Se-enriched Astragalus polysaccharide nanoparticles. Int. J. Biol. Macromol. 118(Pt B): 1438–48.

[37] Liao, G., J. Tang, D. Wang, H. Zuo, Q. Zhang, Y. Liu et al. 2020. Selenium nanoparticles (SeNPs) have potent antitumor activity against prostate cancer cells through the upregulation of miR-16. World Journal of Surgical Oncology 18(1): 81.

[38] Wadhwani, S.A., M. Gorain, P. Banerjee, U.U. Shedbalkar, R. Singh, G.C. Kundu et al. 2017. Green synthesis of selenium nanoparticles using Acinetobacter sp. SW30: optimization, characterization and its anticancer activity in breast cancer cells. Int. J. Nanomedicine 12: 6841–55.

[39] Vahidi, H., H. Barabadi and M. Saravanan. 2020. Emerging selenium nanoparticles to combat cancer: a systematic review. Journal of Cluster Science 31(2): 301–9.

[40] Yazdi, M.H., B. Varastehmoradi, E. Faghfuri, F. Mavandadnejad, M. Mahdavi and A.R. Shahverdi. 2015. Adjuvant effect of biogenic selenium nanoparticles improves the immune responses and survival of mice receiving 4T1 cell antigens as vaccine in breast cancer murine model. Journal of Nanoscience and Nanotechnology 15(12): 10165–72.

[41] Yazdi, M.H., M. Mahdavi, N. Setayesh, M. Esfandyar and A.R. Shahverdi. 2013. Selenium nanoparticle-enriched *Lactobacillus brevis* causes more efficient immune responses *in vivo* and reduces the liver metastasis in metastatic form of mouse breast cancer. Daru: Journal of Faculty of Pharmacy, Tehran University of Medical Sciences 21(1): 33.

[42] El-Batal, A., O. Abou Zaid, E. Noaman and E. Ismail. 2012. Promising antitumor activity of fermented wheat germ extract in combination with selenium nanoparticles. Int. J. Pharm Health Care 2(6): 1–22.

[43] Shoeibi, S., P. Mozdziak and A. Golkar-Narenji. 2017. Biogenesis of selenium nanoparticles using green chemistry. Topics in Current Chemistry 375(6): 88.

[44] Hosnedlova, B., M. Kepinska, S. Skalickova, C. Fernandez, B. Ruttkay-Nedecky, Q. Peng et al. 2018. Nano-selenium and its nanomedicine applications: a critical review. Int. J. Nanomedicine 13: 2107–28.

[45] Hariharan, H., N.A. Al-Dhabi, S.K. Rajaram and S. Arabia. (eds.). 2012. Microbial synthesis of selinium nanocomposite using *Saccharomyces cerevisiae* and its antimicrobial activity against pathogens causing nosocomial infection. Chalcogenide Letters December 2012, 9(12): 509–515.

[46] Kheradmand, E., F. Rafii, M. Yazdi, A. Akhavan Sepahi, A.R. Shahverdi and M. Oveisi. 2014. The antimicrobial effects of selenium nanoparticle-enriched probiotics and their fermented broth against Candida albicans. Daru : Journal of Faculty of Pharmacy, Tehran University of Medical Sciences 22: 48.

[47] Sasidharan, S., R. Sowmiya and R. Balakrishnaraja. 2015. Biosynthesis of selenium nanoparticles using citrus reticulata peel extract. World Journal of Pharmaceutical Research 4: 1322–30.

[48] Huang, T., J.A. Holden, D.E. Heath, N.M. O'Brien-Simpson and A.J. O'Connor. 2019. Engineering highly effective antimicrobial selenium nanoparticles through control of particle size. Nanoscale 11(31): 14937–51.

[49] Nicolas, J., S. Mura, D. Brambilla, N. Mackiewicz and P. Couvreur. 2013. Design, functionalization strategies and biomedical applications of targeted biodegradable/biocompatible polymer-based nanocarriers for drug delivery. Chemical Society Reviews 42(3): 1147–235.

[50] Huang, Y., L. He, W. Liu, C. Fan, W. Zheng, Y.-S. Wong et al. 2013. Selective cellular uptake and induction of apoptosis of cancer-targeted selenium nanoparticles. Biomaterials 34(29): 7106–16.

[51] Ashrafizadeh, H., S.R. Abtahi and A.A. Oroojan. 2020. Trace element nanoparticles improved diabetes mellitus; a brief report. Diabetes & Metabolic Syndrome: Clinical Research & Reviews 14(4): 443–5.

[52] Zhao, S.-J., D.-H. Wang, Y.-W. Li, L. Han, X. Xiao, M. Ma et al. 2017. A novel selective VPAC2 agonist peptide-conjugated chitosan modified selenium nanoparticles with enhanced anti-type 2 diabetes synergy effects. Int. J. Nanomedicine 12: 2143–60.

[53] Miroliaee, A.E., H. Esmaily, A. Vaziri-Bami, M. Baeeri, A.R. Shahverdi and M. Abdollahi. 2011. Amelioration of experimental colitis by a novel nanoseleniu-silymarin mixture. Toxicology Mechanisms and Methods 21: 200–8.

9

Strategies for Physicochemical Synthesis of Manganese Nanomaterials
A Present View

B. Panda, A. Lenka and *S.K. Dash**

1. Introduction

Manganese (Mn) nanomaterials (NMs) are unique by their physicochemical properties and applications such as composite synthesis [1], dye degradation [2, 3], metallic adsorption [4], construction of supercapacitors [5], batteries and solar cells [6], carrying drugs [7], scavenging of microbes [8, 9] and so on. Although these NMs are mostly synthesised as their oxides, they can also be produced as composite, alloys or doped with other metals [10–12]. Composites or alloys NMs exhibit synergistic properties of their counterparts and hence improved properties from their monometallic components [13]. On the contrary, doped-NMs do the same because their crystal defects and structural deformities resulted due to doping. However, all these forms of NMs have fascinated the researchers equally for their synthesis as they are unique by their properties and functions. Therefore, different groups have tried with different physicochemical and biological routes for the synthesis of these NMs either through top-down (milling, etching, sputtering, explosion, etc.) or bottom-up (sol-gel, spinning, flame spraying, laser or vapour deposition, etc.) approaches (Table 1). In the first case, bulk materials are first broken down into small mass and then those are converted into NMs, whereas in the latter case, atomic

Department of Zoology, Berhampur University, Odisha-760007, India.
* Corresponding author: dashsandipkumar@gmail.com

Table 1. Different physicochemical methods reported till date for the synthesis of Mn NMs.

Sl. No.	Type of NMs	Methods Used	Source	Shape	Size	Reference
01	Mn_3O_4	Mechanical milling	$MnAc_2 \cdot 4H_2O$	Tetragonal	~30 nm	[17]
02	MnO_2		$KMnO_4, MnCl_2$	Irregular Needle Rod	- D: < 10 nm D: 15–20 nm, L: Variable	[18]
03	$MnFe_2O_4$		$Mn(NO_3)_2 \cdot 6H_2O$	-	~10 nm	[19]
04			$MnCl_2 \cdot 4H_2O$	Spherical	7.6 nm	[20]
05			MnO_2 Powder	Spherical	20 nm	[21]
06			Mn-Ore	Spherical	117 ± 27 nm	[16]
07	$Ni_{51}Mn_{33.4}In_{15.6}$		Mn Element	-	30–200 nm	[22]
08	Mn_3O_4	Vapour deposition	Mn Powder	Square	42 nm	[23]
09	MnO, α-Mn, β-Mn, γ-Mn, Mn_3O_4, MnO_2			Irregular	≤ 80 nm	[24]
10	MnO_2 Mn_2O_3 Mn_2O_3/Mn_3O_4 Mn_3O_4		$Mn_2(CO)_{10}$	Rod Spherical	D: 10–15, L: $\geq$ 100 nm < 10 nm	[25]
11	Mn		$MnCl_2 \cdot 4H_2O$	Dendritic Tetragonal Polycrystalline	20–150 nm 20–50 nm 30–50 nm	[26]
12	Mn_5O_8		$Mn(NO_3)_2 \cdot 6H_2O$	-	~30 nm	[27]
13	γ-MnO_2		Mn Powder	Spherical	86.86 nm	[28]
14	Mn_5Si_3		Mn Metal	Hexagonal	~8.6 nm	[1]

No.	Material	Method	Precursor	Morphology	Size	Ref.
82	MnO_2		$MnSO_4 \cdot H_2O$	Needle Platelet	D: ~ 30, L: 300 nm; D: 200, T: ~ 20 nm	[95]
83	Mn_3O_4		$MnCl_2 \cdot 4H_2O$, $MnAc_2 \cdot 4H_2O$	Saucer	50–150 nm	[96]
84	α-MnO_2		$MnCl_2 \cdot 6(H_2O)$	Irregular	25–30 nm	[97]
85	Mn_3O_4		$Mn(NO_3)_2 \cdot 6H_2O$	Spherical	< 100 nm	[98]
86	Mn_2O_3		$MnCl_2 \cdot 4H_2O$	Cubic	10–30 nm	[99]
87	MnO_2		$MnSO_4 \cdot H_2O$	Spherical	10–30 nm	[100]
88	$(\gamma$-$Fe_2O_3)$-Mn		$FeCl_3/MnCl_2$	Spherical	~ 10–40 nm	[101]
89	$MnFe_2O_4$		$MnCl_2 \cdot 6H_2O$	Spherical	20–50 nm	[102]
90	MnO_2 $ZnMn_2O_4$		$KMnO_4$, $MnSO_4 \cdot H_2O$	Rod Hexagonal and Rod	L: 80–130 nm; D: ~ 100 nm (Hexagonal)	[103]
91	Fe-Mn		$MnSO_4 \cdot H_2O$	Spherical	10.33–17.48 nm	[104]
92	Mn_2O_3-Mn_3O_4			Spherical	20–30 nm	[105]
93	Mn_3O_4	Sonochemical	$MnCl_2 \cdot 4H_2O$	Tetragonal	5–10 nm	[106]
94	δ-MnO_2		$KMnO_4$	Needle Spherical Cubic	- 50–150 nm 0.2–1.0 μm	[107]
95	MnO_2		$KMnO_4$	Spherical	10–20 nm	[108]
96	α-MnO_2		$MnAc_2 \cdot 4H_2O$	Needle Spherical	10–30 nm -	[5]
97	MnO_2		$KMnO_4$	-	~ 02–03 nm	[109]

Table 1 contd. ...

...*Table 1 contd.*

Sl. No.	Type of NMs	Methods Used	Source	Shape	Size	Reference
98	Mn-Fe		$MnAc_2 \cdot 4H_2O$	Spherical	34–46 nm	[110]
99	$MnFe_2O_4$		$MnSO_4 \cdot H_2O$	Rods, Spherical	25 ± 0.5 nm, -	[111]
100	$SrMnO_3$		$KMnO_4$, $MnCl_2 \cdot 4H_2O$	Warts, Spherical	8–35 nm, 4–12 nm	[112]
101	$Mn_{0.5}Zn_{0.5}Dy_xEu_xFe_{1.8-2x}O_4$		$MnCl_2 \cdot 4H_2O$	Cubic	20 nm	[113]
102	$Mn_xZn_{1-x}Fe_2O_4$	Polyol Sonochemical	$MnCl_2 \cdot 4H_2O$	Spherical, Cube	7–23 nm, -	[114]
103	Mn_3O_4	Solvothermal	Mn Ore	Spherical	48 ± 12 nm	[115]
104	$CuMn_2O_4$		$MnSO_4 \cdot H_2O$	Rice	-	[116]
105	$MnFe_2O_4$, $MnFe_2O_3/C$		$MnSO_4 \cdot H_2O$	Polygonal, Spherical	10–30 nm, 06–30 nm	[117]
106	Fe-Mn:Phosphate		$Mn(NO_3)_2 \cdot 4H_2O$, $MnAc_2 \cdot 4H_2O$	Spherical	D: 20 nm	[118]
107	Sm_2NiMnO_6		$MnSO_4 \cdot H_2O$	Rod	-	[119]
108	OMS-2	Microwave-assisted	$KMnO_4$, $MnSO_4 \cdot H_2O$	Spherical	~ 200 nm	[120]
109	γ- MnO_2, α-MnO_2		$MnSO_4 \cdot H_2O$	Plates, Sea urchin	50 nm, 01–02 μm	[121]
110	Graphene sheet-Mn_3O_4		$MnAc_2 \cdot H_2O$	Spherical	20 nm	[122]
111	$LiMnPO_4/C$		$MnSO_4 \cdot H_2O$	Spindle	L: ~ 250, W: ~ 120 nm	[123]
112	$ZnMn_2O_4$		$Mn(NO_3)_2 \cdot 4H_2O$	Spinel	10–70 nm	[124]
113	$CoMn_2O_4$		$MnCl_2 \cdot 4H_2O$	Spherical	~ 51.42 nm	[125]

114	Mn_3O_4	Laser ablation	$Mn(OH)_2$	Tetragonal	7.1–9.2 nm	[126]
115	MnO_2		MnO_2 Powder	Spherical	100 nm	[127]
116	MnO, Mn_3O_4		Mn Disk	Tetragonal	7–11 nm	[128]
117	Mn_3O_4 $\alpha\text{-Mn}/Mn_3O_4$		Mn Pieces	Spherical, Irregular	20–90 nm	[129]
118	$Au\text{-}MnO_x$		Au-Mn Metal	-	4.8 ± 1.2 nm	[130]
119	$\alpha\text{-Mn}$	Chemical reduction	$MnCl_2 \cdot 4H_2O$	Spherical	13.1 ± 3.3 nm	[131]
120	$\gamma\text{-}MnO_2$		$KMnO_4$	Spherical	$\sim$ 10–18 nm	[132]
121	$\alpha\text{-}MnO_2$			Rod	D: 10, L: 50–100 nm	[133]
122				Rod	D: 15–50 nm, L: 1–3 μm	[134]
123	MnO_2/RGO		$MnSO_4 \cdot H_2O$	-	10–20 nm	[135]
124	$Mn_{0.5}Zn_{0.5}Fe_2O_4$		$Mn(NO_3)_2 \cdot 6H_2O$	Spherical	25 ± 3 nm	[136]
125	Ni_6MnO_8	Template Route	$MnAc_2 \cdot 4H_2O$	Spherical	-	[137]
126	Mn_3O_4	Electrochemical	Mn Metal	Rod Spherical	D: 100–200 nm, L: 02–06 μm 35 nm	[138]
127	$MnFe_2O_4$	Microemulsion, Co-precipitation	$MnAc_2 \cdot 4H_2O$	Cubic spinel	-	[139]
128	MnO_2	Selective etching	$Mn(NO_3)_2$	Hollow Spherical	D: 1–2 μm, T: 300 nm	[140]

D: Diameter; L: Length; T: Thickness and W: Width

or sub-atomic particles are first organized into clusters and then transformed into NMs. Although recent studies have campaigned for the biological synthesis of NMs considering them eco-friendly [14, 15], physicochemical synthesis is productive, time-saving, and comparatively specific in NM production [16]. Therefore, these are more popular and used commonly both for small and large-scale synthesis of Mn NMs. In the present chapter, we have discussed the different physicochemical approaches used for the synthesis of Mn NMs along with their merits and demerits.

2. Physical Methods

2.1 Mechanical Milling

Mechanical milling is one of the simple, economic, eco-friendly, but reliable top-down physical approach for synthesising pure, composite, and alloy Mn NMs. In this method, the metallic source is first ground into powder, inside a rotating abrasion-resistant hollow shell by repeated collision of the source onto metallic, alloy, ceramic or rubbers balls/rods, followed by blending them into NMs (Fig. 1) [16]. Furthermore, these mechanical mills are classified based on their mode of action: in case of planetary mills, the chambers rotate on a shaft, while in the case of tumblers, they rotate on their axes, causing the balls to fall to bottom from the top. Similarly, rod mills are different from the others as they rely on rods instead of balls. The morphology of the NMs produced in this method depend on the frequency, diameter, and time of rotation. The amount of heat produced during the process of synthesis is neutralized through cryo-cooling of the mills.

Abdul-Razaq and Wu [141] used this technique to synthesise MnO and Mn_3O_4 NPs in 2001 with the help of non-magnetic tungsten carbide vial and balls. In this process, the time of milling was varied at the range of 10, 20, 40, and 80 h, and found that size of particles depends reciprocally on the milling time. Gagrani et al. in 2018 [18] produced irregular or needle-shaped amorphous MnO_2 NMs from $KMnO_4$ and $MnCl_2$ in 4 h, using steel balls. Surprisingly, those amorphous particles got transformed into crystalline nanorods on heating them at 350°C for 1 h. In another study, Ochirkhuyag and group [142] utilized $MnCl_2.4H_2O$ and $KMnO_4$ as a NP source and in their finding, they saw that both MnO_2 and Mn_3O_4 NMs are produced on milling speed at 200 or 450 rpm, while on further increasing the speed to 600 rpm, only Mn_3O_4 NMs were produced. Several studies have also reported for the production of $MnFe_2O_4$ NMs using this method and their results have showed that crystal size of the NM directly depend on the annealing temperature of the synthesis. The foregoing process can also be used for the synthesis of alloy NMs from multiple metallic sources. Aslani et al. (2017) [22] prepared an alloy of such type, i.e., $Ni_{51}Mn_{33.4}In_{15.6}$. In spite of all the above utilities, there always exists a need for further improvement of this method mainly because of its time-consuming, noisy, contamination-prone, and energy-intensive nature.

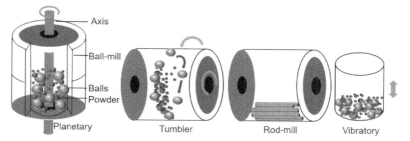

Fig. 1. Schematic presentation of different types of mechanical mills.

2.2 PVD Technique

PVD is another routinely used physical method of Mn NM synthesis, which basically involves vaporization of a Mn source and then deposition of the vapour onto a substrate through condensation. The process is classified further into vacuum evaporation (VE), ion plating (IP), and ionic sputtering (IS) based on the heating source used (Fig. 2). In the first two cases, the source is generally present on a filament or crucible which is heated under pressure by using induction, radiation, high energy electron beam or laser light [28], whereas in the third case, He^+, Ar^+ ions are collided onto the source under high pressure to produce plasma (secondary e^-s, reflected ions, the Mn atoms/ions, and photons) (Fig. 3a) [143]. The plasma is then localized on or around the source, using high frequency radio-waves (insulated IS) or powerful magnetic field (magnetron sputtering) [144]. The ions of Mn in the

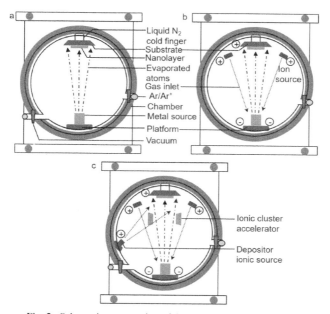

Fig. 2. Schematic presentation of the (a) VE, (b) IS, and (c) IP.

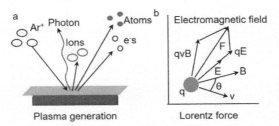

Fig. 3. Schematic presentation for (a) plasma and (b) Lorentz force imparted on a charged ion in an electromagnetic field.

plasma is imparted by Lorentz force (F) (Fig. 3b and equation 1), where, q, E, v, and B represent ion charge, electric field, potential gradient, and magnetic field, respectively [145]. The Mn vapours are then deposited onto a work piece in a single or multi-layer through condensation. The composition and thickness of deposition depend on the rate of evaporation of Mn source, applied pressure, reactive gas in the reaction chamber, sputtering yields, and/or distance between the source and the work-piece.

$$F = q\,(E + vB) \tag{1}$$

IP is a hybrid form of both VE and IS, taken together, in which the heating source can follow either of the two. However, sometimes, heating at high temperature may melt down the platform itself; therefore, e⁻ beams are used for target-specific heating of the source. Furthermore, to increase the rate of deposition and produce tuned NM, certain ion accelerators are used [27]. Chang et al. 2004 [23] used this PVD to synthesise ferromagnetic Mn_3O_4 NP in just 90 min and reported that size of the particle varies with temperature. Music and co-group in 2015 [146] produced MnO_2 NP nanolayer (9 mm) on Si, using a DC magnetron sputtering. After a year, the same approach was used but to deposit α-MnO_2 nanorods (length: 30 ± 5 nm) on Ni-coated anodic Al_2O_3 [147]. Researches have also reported for the synthesis of composite NMs; for example, Das et al. in 2016 [1] deposited a nanolayer of Mn_5Si_3 on the carbon surface through magnetron sputtering, while Nijam et al. in 2017 [28] fabricated a MgF_2/γ-MnO_2/α-Bi_2O_3/a-Si solar cell by depositing γ-MnO_2/α-Bi_2O_3 onto Si substrate. In another experiment, Fernandez-Barica and group in 2019 [148] electrodeposited a Fe-Mn layer of 300–500 nm onto Si, using DC-magnetron co-sputtering at room temperature (RT). Morphology and biocompatibility of the NMs are seen changing with the change in Mn:Fe ratio. Similarly, Mn oxide was deposited onto graphite foil to produce porous needle-like Mn_xO_y@graphite NMs for supercapacitor application [149].

Another type of PVD is laser ablation, which involves hitting the Mn source with a high-powered laser beam (in the UV spectrum) under ultra-high vacuum to form a plasma. The plasma is then condensed into liquid by colliding with an inert gas (Fig. 4a) [126]. The shape, size, and composition of the NM synthesised in this method depends on the source, chamber pressure, and laser type. Laser pyrolysis or laser assisted deposition is another type of PVD, in which non-reacting metallic

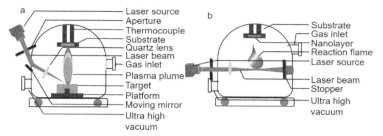

Fig. 4. Schematic presentation for (a) laser ablation and (b) laser pyrolysis technique.

sources are heat-decomposed and then reacted under ultra-high vacuum to form alloy NMs (Fig. 4b) [150].

Another simple but cost-effective PVD technique is electric arc deposition (EAD), which is used often to synthesise carbon nanotubes, but can also be used for preparing Mn NMs [24, 151]. When a current of high voltage is applied between two electrodes (1–2 mm gape) in vacuum, the Mn vapours get deposits at anode (Fig. 5) [150]. Although controlling the size and composition of the NMs is difficult in this process, the pressure and rate of discharge can do so to certain extent. This process is very common in producing thermal, chemical or mechanically resistant NMs. Kim et al. in 2013 [26] reported decreasing particle size with increasing discharge time for producing polycrystalline Mn NPs from the $MnCl_2 \cdot 4H_2O$. Further, the particle morphology also varied with time and concentration of surfactant. Without the addition of CTAB, the NPs produced between 10–40 min were of dendritic-shape, while after 50 min, they were of tetragonal-shape; with CTAB, the particles produced at initial stage were of spherical-shaped, while later, they appeared octahedral or whisker-shaped.

Zhang and group in 2010 [126] proposed tetragonal Mn_3O_4 NPs synthesis in MiliQ water at 1064 nm (pulse time 10 ns) for 30 min. At low temperature, the NPs exhibited ferromagnetism while at RT, they behaved as paramagnetic. After a year, Ganeev and group [152] synthesised Mn NPs in ethanol 50 ps laser in a laser ablation technique and observed a change in particle morphology with time. Particle size ranged from 6–50 nm at the beginning to 7–14 nm after 15 days. Similarly, the particles formed in the beginning were spherical-shaped, while towards end, they were triangle or square-shaped. In another study, $Au-MnO_2$ and $Au-Mn_2O_3$

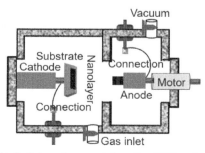

Fig. 5. Schematic presentation of an EAD method.

core-shell alloy nanolayers (~ 0.3–13 nm) were produced in 2 min using a laser beam of 238 nm in aqueous solution, pH-11. At 1064 nm, no core-shells were formed, rather simple Au and MnO_x NPs were formed [130]. Shukla et al. in 2016 [153] used 50 mJ/pulse for 15 min in polyvinyl alcohol and produced spherical $MnFe_2O_4$ NPs. The solvent not only controlled the size of the NPs, but also prevented agglomeration. Zhang et al. (2017) [154] produced $FeMn@FeMn_2O_4$ core-shell alloy, Mn_3O_4, and γ-MnO_2 NPs in C_2H_5OH, C_2H_5OH-H_2O, and H_2O, respectively. In 2019, Rahmat et al. [127] used laser at 1064 nm (pulse 5 ns) and power, 103 mJ cm^{-2} to manufacture MnO_2 nanocolloids from waste battery cell in H_2O and CH_3OH. Optical analysis of the particles revealed different properties of the NMs for different type of laser radiation used. Yang and co-workers, in the same year, synthesised irregular or spherical Mn_3O_4 and α-Mn/Mn_3O_4 composite NPs of size 20–90 nm at RT and ~ 20 psa using 1064 nm laser beam. α-Mn/Mn_3O_4 NPs showed antiferromagnetic characteristics, whereas Mn_3O_4 were ferrimagnetic [129]. NPs of different Mn oxides were produced recently in MiliQ water by changing the laser ablation period. At 10 min, both MnO and Mn_3O_4 were produced while, at 25–35 min, MnO was transformed into agglomerated Mn_3O_4 NPs (7–11 nm) [128]. In spite of all the above merits, this approach is replaced with other methods as this is time-consuming, expensive, and requires high temperature.

2.3 Microwave-assisted Synthesis

In a microwave-assisted method, the heat produced from dipole or ionic interactions of high frequency microwaves (3×10^5–3×10^8 Hz) with materials [155, 125] is used to enhance the reaction kinetics and nucleation of NM production [122] in fluids such as DMF, ethylene glycol (EG), C_2H_5OH, H_2O, and so on [155]. Opembe et al. in 2010 [120] synthesised cryptomelane-type MnO_x octahedral molecular sieve (OMS) from $MnSO_4 \cdot H_2O$ and $KMnO_4$ in the presence of dimethyl sulfoxide (DMSO) using continuous microwave flow. The effect of variation in power input, time, DMSO on the NP morphology was assessed and optimised. The results showed that, for synthesising NM crystals, 5% DMSO at 300 W and slow microwave is suitable. Zhang et al. [156] successfully produced MnO_2 nanostructures both in acidic and neutral condition but the NPs formed were smaller and γ-MnO_2, at pH~7, while at pH < 7, α-MnO_2 of larger of size was produced. In some other studies, microwave was used to assist other physicochemical methods for quicker and controlled synthesis of NMs. Using a microwave-assisted hydrothermal reaction, Li and co-workers [122] produced Mn_3O_4-graphene nanocomposite from $MnAc_2$ and graphite oxide. Similarly, Long et al. in 2017 [123] utilized microwave-assisted polyol method for the synthesis of spindle-shaped $LiMnPO_4/C$ structures at 130°C. In another study, microwave-assisted colloidal approach was employed, in which microwaves were irradiated at every 2 min interval for 4 h in C_2H_5OH to synthesise $ZnMn_2O_4$ NPs followed by drying at 500°C [124]. Microwave-assisted solvothermal method is another approach, adopted by Phuruangrat and group for synthesising crystalline ferromagnetic $MnFe_2O_4$ NPs (30 nm) from $Mn(NO_3)_2 \cdot 6H_2O$ in presence of EG in 30 min at 100°C [157].

3. Chemical Methods

3.1 Hydrothermal Method

In this process, hydrophilic inorganic compounds are heat-lysed at the hot end of a chamber under high pressure and then deposited onto the cool end on other side [75]. Ahmad and group [158] produced hexagonal (30 nm) and polycrystalline Mn_3O_4 nanoplates (100×10 nm^2) from $MnAc_2 \cdot 4H_2O$ in 14 h at 180°C in n-butylamine. In 2019, Li et al. [159] followed a two-step process involving $MnSiO_3$ as an intermediate to synthesise Mn_3O_4 NPs in the presence of NaOH. Besides the Mn_xO_y, studies have also reported for the synthesis of composite Mn NMs through this method. In 2019, Zhang and group [78] synthesised stable mesoporous and microporous $MnCo_2S_4$ NPs, while Akhtar and co-workers produced agglomerated spherical $Mn_{0.5}Zn_{0.5}Sm_xEu_xFe_{1.8-2x}O_4$ NPs (7–12 nm) at 180°C in 10 h [79]. In the same year, Ullrich et al. [77] synthesised core-shell cubes of $Mn_xFe_{3-x}O_4@FeO/MnO$ (21 ± 3 nm) from Mn (II)-oleate and Fe(III)-oleate, using Na-oleate and oleic acid (OA) as surfactants.

Shape and size of the NPs produced in hydrothermal method are influenced by temperature, pressure, time, solvent, ions, and surfactant [160]. A SDS-assisted hydrothermal approach was used for the synthesis of agglomerated MnO_2 nanorods, forming a sea urchin nanostructure [56]. α-MnO_2 sea urchin was also synthesised, using Al^{3+}, but when Fe^{3+} was used instead of Al^{3+}, clew-shaped ε-MnO_2 was produced [57].

Impact of time on the NP morphology was demonstrated by Subramanian and group in 2005 [55], while synthesising α-MnO_2 NPs at a constant temperature of 140°C. The results showed that at the beginning, both amorphous and crystalline NMs were produced, while later on, only crystalline NMs were produced. The shape of the particles produced also showed change with time, plate, plate/rod, and rod-like NMs at 1, 9, and 12 h of reaction, respectively. In a similar study, Wang et al., in 2018 [68] produced three different Mn NPs from same $MnAc_2 \cdot 4H_2O$ and CTAB, i.e., flower-like α-MnO_2 nanostructures (~ 500 nm), regular quadrilateral γ-MnOOH NPs ($\sim 20 \times 20$ nm), and quadrilateral Mn_3O_4 NPs after 3, 11, and 24 h, respectively. In 2020, Xiao et al. [76] had also observed that at 2 h, flower-like particles were produced, while at 4 h, needle-like α-MnO_2 NMs were produced from Mn-contaminated H_2O.

Hydrothermal temperature is another crucial parameter for determining the NM morphology [74]. In a study, Xiao et al. [59] produced vertical birnessite-MnO_2 microsphere/nanosheets, α-MnO_2 rods (2–3 µm), and α-MnO_2 nanotubes, at 100, 120, 140°C, respectively and on further heating, hollow α-MnO_2 nanostructures were formed. Similarly, in 2012, Hlaing and Win [61] found that, heating at 90°C for 2 h, α-MnO_2 nanorods were produced, while at 120°C both α and β-MnO_2 nanorods were produced. However, on heating the same for 8 h, some of the rods got aggregated into wires. Chu and co-researchers in 2017 [66] created nanoflower, urchin, and nanorods of MnO_2 at three distinct temperatures: 120, 140, and 160°C respectively. In a similar study, Venkata Swetha and group (2018) [67] used 150, 170, and 190°C to synthesise Mn oxide NPs from $KMnO_4$ in the presence of urea and CTAB. At 150°C, they observed mixed phage Mn_2O_3/Mn_3O_4 nanowires, while at 170°C, nanoflowers of the same were formed. On rising the temperature to 190°C, only single phage tetragonal Mn_2O_3 NPs were produced. In 2019, Selim et al. [70] found that heating $KMnO_4$ at 120°C for 10 h, γ-MnOOH was formed, which on calcination at 400 and 700°C, produced β-MnO_2 and α-Mn_2O_3 NPs, respectively. In 2020, Han et al. [73] used C_2H_5OH to make Mn_3O_4 NMs from $KMnO_4$. In their experiment, octahedron materials were produced at 170°C, while at 110°C, nanowires were produced.

In addition to the aforementioned factors, stabilizing agents also decide NM morphology in a hydrothermal method. Nguyen and co-workers in 2011 [161] used various concentrations of 6-aminohexanoic acid to produce $MnWO_4$ crystals (sphere, quasi-sphere, square, hexagonal, bar, and rod-shaped). In 2019, Shaik et al. [162] employed H_2O_2 to synthesise nanostructures of Mn_3O_4 from $MnCl_2 \cdot 4H_2O$ and observed that the particle size decreases with increasing the H_2O_2 concentration. They also observed particle morphology with changing H_2O_2 conc. At 1 M, 50-nm, agglomerated, spherical particles were formed, while at 2 and 3 M, flake-like and porous-shaped particles were produced, respectively. Although hydrothermal process is one of the widely accepted and adopted methods of NP synthesis, this method is quite expensive and accident prone.

3.2 Solvothermal Method

Solvothermal method is an one-step chemical process, used especially for the synthesis of composite NMs, which involves boiling of the solvents (H_2O, CH_3OH, C_2H_5OH, NH_4, CO_2, HCl, HF, etc.) in a autoclave under a pressure of > 1 bar [115,163,164]consequently, led to the nomenclature of phosphor-converted LEDs (pc-LEDs. Saravana and group (2017) [116] attempted to synthesise $CuMn_2O_4$ NPs in 12 h by heating at 120–160°C and found that 160°C as appropriate. However, crystallinity of the particles improved with increasing the temperature. Stoia et al. in 2017 [117] fabricated $MnFe_2O_4$ and $MnFe_2O_4/C$ nanocomposites from $MnCl_2.4H_2O$. Yue and group (2019) [165] synthesised porous Co-Mn nanosheets in 1 h and reported that with increasing the Co: Mn ratio, the length and thickness of the nanosheet also increased. Singh and Kumar [119] fabricated polycrystalline mesoporous Sm_2NiMnO_6 nanorods (diameter: 10 nm) from $Sm(NO_3)_3 \cdot 6H_2O$, $Ni(NO_3)_2 \cdot 6H_2O$, and $Mn(SO_4) \cdot 6H_2O$. Wang et al. [166] synthesised porous $MnFe_2O_4$ nanoflakes by heating $MnCl_2.4H_2O$ at 200°C for 12 h. Researchers have also utilized this method to synthesise metal-doped Mn NMs. In the same year, Liu et al. [118] prepared Co, Cu, Ni, and Fe-doped $Mn_3(PO_4)_2$ NPs, first by adding $Mn(NO_3)_2 \cdot 4H_2O$ to H_3PO_4 in the presence of olylamine and octadecene for 24 h at 180°C, followed by reaction with $Fe(NO_3)_2$ at 180°C. Among the different metallic-doped NPs produced, Fe-doped NPs showed the highest electrochemical activities. Like that of hydrothermal method, the morphology of the NPs produced in this method can also be controlled through temperature, time, and solvent concentration. Although both the hydrothermal as well as solvothermal methods are productive, they are time-consuming.

3.3 CVD Technique

This process entails the vaporisation of one or more chemicals either inside a hot chamber (hot wall CVD) or on a heated platform present in the chamber (cold wall CVD) and then reaction of the vapour before deposition onto the substrate (Fig. 6) [167, 168]. The composition of the NMs produced in this method depend on the chemicals reacted, heating temperature, and pressure in the chamber. In 2008, Higgins et al. [169] synthesised nanowires of $Mn_{19}Si_{33}$ from $Mn(CO)_5SiC_{13}$, using this method, and subsequently in 2011, they synthesised polyforms of the same NM with α-Mn_5Si_3, β-Mn_5Si_3, and β-Mn_3Si [170]. In the same year, Le and group [25] synthesised MnO_2, Mn_2O_3, Mn_2O_3/Mn_3O_4, Mn_3O_4 NPs by heating manganese carbonyl at 500, 700–1100, 1300, and 1500°C, respectively, in an electric furnace. A thin film of Mn oxide was deposited onto three substrates: glass, Si wafer, and carbon fibre paper from methylcyclopentadienyl manganese(I)tricarbonyl (MMT) [171]. Different parameters such as rate of plasma and H_2 flow, pressure in the chamber, MMT, and O_2 regulated the thickness and composition of NM film. The film thickness was calculated as 20 nm under a plasma flow of 500 W, chamber pressure of 80 Pa, and MMT, O_2, H_2 flow rate of 4.5×10^{-7} mol/min, 125 and 25 sccm, respectively, in the presence of Ar in an unoptimized condition. Plasma power $\geq$ 500 W and $\geq$ 53 Pa chamber pressure performed measurable deposition of film. A perfect, suitable deposited film was observed at MMT flow rate of 4.1×10^{-7} mol/min. Enhanced rate of flow of MMT precursor resulted in weak attachment of MnOx NP to surface. Barreca et al. 2018 [172] almost repeated the same experiment but by using fluorinated-Mn^{2+} as source. In their experiment, β-MnO_2 NPs were produced at a temperature of < 300°C but at ~ 400°C, both MnO_2 and Mn_3O_4 were produced.

In another study, aerosol-assisted CVD was used to deposit CdO-Mn_2O_3 nanocomposite from $[Cd(dmae)_2(OAc)_2]\cdot H_2O$ (dmae: dimethylaminoethanol, OAc: acetato) and $Mn(CH_3COO)_2$ (v/v 1:1) onto a fluorine (F)-doped TiO_2-SiO_2 substrate at 500°C in 45 mins in the presence of Ar. The thickness and morphology of the film varied with the type of solvent used. With tetrahydrofuran, an agglomerated and irregular NP film was formed, while in case of CH_3OH, a film of barren soil like small chips of agglomerated particles was formed. When C_2H_5OH was used as solvent, an agglomerated irregular brick-shaped structure having small spherical granules were observed [173]. A similar study was carried out to deposit β-MnO_2 thin films from fluorinated Mn (II)diamine diketonate onto F-doped TiO_2-SiO_2 at

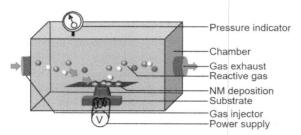

Fig. 6. Schematic representation of CVD based NMs synthesis.

100–400°C in the presence of Ar and O_2. The study showed variation in the morphology of NMs with variation in the temperature [174]. Recently, Bigiani and co-researchers (2020) [12] fabricated F-doped β-MnO_2 NP onto $MgAl_2O_4$, $YAlO_3$, and $Y_3Al_5O_{12}$ using Ar/O_2 plasma at 300°C using Mn(1,1,1,5,5,5-hexafluoro-2,4-pentanedione)$_2$ N,N,N,N-tetramethylethylenediamine (Mn(hfa)$_2$TMEDA) as precursor. Thus, although CVD approach is quite simple, economic, and dynamic, it sometimes produces harmful by-products.

3.4 Sol-gel Method

This is also a simple chemical approach, particularly for synthesis of pure or ultrapure NMs with a customized shape, size, and property. In this process, the precursor is first hydrolysed into an aqueous or non-aqueous solution, and then polymerized into a gel, either by olation or oxolation (Equations 2–4). These gels are then agitated and dried through spin/dip coating (xerogels), freezing (cryogels) or heating (aerogels) [43]. Finally, they are converted into powder through calcination (Fig. 7) [49]. The shape, size, and composition of the NPs synthesised by this method depend on the concentration of precursor, nature and pH of solvent, temperature and nature of the condenser, temperature and humidity of agitation, and/or calcination temperature [175].

$$M\text{-}OR + H\text{-}O\text{-}H \rightarrow M\text{-}OH + R\text{-}OH \tag{2}$$

$$M\text{-}OR + M\text{-}OH \rightarrow M\text{-}O\text{-}M + R\text{-}O \tag{3}$$

$$M\text{-}OH + M\text{-}OH \rightarrow M\text{-}O\text{-}M + H\text{-}OH \tag{4}$$

The M, R, O, H, M-OR, and M-OH in the equations denote metal, alkyl, oxygen, hydrogen, metal alkoxide, and metal hydroxides, respectively [40, 176]. This technique can be used to produce both Mn_xO_y as well as composite NMs with desirable size, shape, and properties. Zhang et al. in 2013 [44] adopted epoxide-based sol-gel technique to synthesise spherical mesoporous $NiMn_2O_4$ NPs. In their experiment, a mixture of $Ni(NO_3)_2 \cdot 6H_2O$ and $Mn(NO_3)_2 \cdot 6H_2O$ (1:2) was prepared in 12 h at RT and then CA and propylene oxide were added. The wet gel was dried using Sc-CO_2 and then calcinated at 200, 300, and 400°C for 5 h. In 2017, Zhao and group [177] produced Cu-Co alloy/Mn_2O_3-Al_2O_3 composite NP by gelating a mixture of two different solutions of Cu/Co and Mn/Al. Cu/Co was prepared by stirring a mixture of Cu $(NO_3)_2$ and $Co(NO_3)_2$ in CA at 50°C for 1 h, while the Mn/Al was prepared from Mn/Al [x:(8–x)] by using CA and PEG. Both the solutions were mixed dropwise and then gelated through continuous stirring for 2 h at 80°C. At the end, the gel was heated at 120°C for overnight and then calcinated at 320 and 400°C for 3 h each. In the next year, Dar and Varshney [178] synthesised both simple and metallic (Co, Ni, and Cu)-doped $Mg_{0.95}Mn_{0.05}O$ NPs (31–48 nm), at pH > 7, using CA. Finally, the gels were dried at 400°C for 4 h. Recently in 2020, Ismail and co-group [38] synthesised gels of Mn_3O_4 and Mn_3O_4/rGO nanocomposite. For the first one a mixture of CA and Mn $(CH_3CO_2)_2 \cdot 4H_2O$ was stirred at 500 RPM and 80°C for 5 h, while for the second one, two or five percentage of GO was added to the mixture of CA and Mn $(CH_3CO_2)_2 \cdot 4H_2O$, with other parameters being the

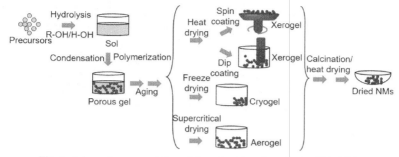

Fig. 7. Schematic representation of the sol-gel based synthesis of Mn NMs.

same. The gels were then dried at 110°C and calcined at 380°C for 12 h to produce corresponding NPs. The above steps yielded spherical and dispersed Mn_3O_4 NPs ($\sim$ 10 nm) with rGO sheets. The agglomeration and particle size decreased with increasing GO conc. Similarly, Ca-doped soft, porous and agglomerated $Mn_xFe_2O_4$ NPs were synthesised by sol-gel route from $Ca(NO_3)_2.4H_2O$ and $Mn(NO_3)_2 \cdot 4H_2O$ in the presence of CA and $C_6H_2O_7.H_2O$ (1:1) at 25–80°C and pH 7 [48]. The efficiency of different chelating agents: ethylenediaminetetracaetic acid (EDTA), CA, tartaric acid, and phthalic acid on the synthesis of Li_2MnO_3 NPs, was evaluated by Ranjeh and group in 2020 [45]. A mixture of metal ion, EG, and chelating agent (1:1:1) was used, of which EDTA produced the smallest (10–180 nm) but uniform NPs. Winiarska and group in 2012 [179] used a combinatorial approach of co-precipitation and sol-gel method to produce Mn-Zn Fe_2O_4 NPs, in which the Zn, Mn, and Fe sulphates were independently co-precipitated into their corresponding ions at 60°C with the help of either NaOH or ammonium oxalate. The precipitates were then filtered, dried, and heat-burnt in the presence of CA and HNO_3 to produce Mn-Zn Fe_2O_4 NPs. Their results showed that oxalate-derived particles were smaller and spherical but agglomerated, while sodium hydroxide-derived particles were heterogeneous in shape (spherical, dendritic, and polyhedral).

3.5 *Microemulsion Method*

Microemulsions are thermostable droplets (600–8000 nm) containing both polar and non-polar solvents separated by a surfactant and/or co-surfactant. These droplets can be oil in water (O/W) or water in oil (W/O). However, in some cases, W/Sc-CO_2 (supercritical CO_2) is used in place of W/O, particularly during NM synthesis in order to simplify the recovery step (Fig. 8). In a W/O nanoreactor, polar heads of the surfactants point inward with their hydrocarbon chains projecting outside. The synthesis follows either one microemulsion approach or one microemulsion plus reactant approach [180, 53]. In the first case, the chemicals present in the core of microemulsion is irradiated with a high energy ray to initiate the reaction (Equation 5) [139], while in the second case, chemicals contained in the different microemulsions are made to collide and exchange their contents along with reaction (Equation 6).

$$C_{aq} + Energy \rightarrow Solvent_{aq} + C_{NM} \qquad (5)$$

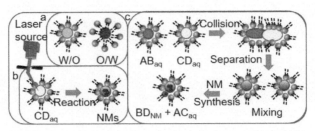

Fig. 8. Schematic representation for (a) microemulsions, (b) one microemulsion method, and (c) one microemulsion plus reactant method.

$$AB_{aq} + C_{aq} \rightarrow AC_{aq} + BD_{NM} \tag{6}$$

A hexanol oil phage-based W/O system with CTAB as surfactant was used by Kosak and group [50] for the synthesis of Mn-Zn-ferrite NPs. In 2011, Scano and co-group [51] synthesised $MnFe_2O_4$ NPs by thermal treatment of Mn and Fe oxohydride precursors in W/O. In another study, CTAB, 1-butanol (co-surfactant), and n-hexane were used to synthesise $La_{0.7}Sr_{0.3}Mn_{0.98}Ti_{0.02}O_3$ perovskite NPs which were then calcinated at 700°C for 4 h [54]. In 2017, Shahid et al. [181] produced Gd^{3+} and Co^{2+}-doped $MnFe_2O_4$ ($Mn_{1-x}Co_xFe_{2-y}Gd_yO_4$) NPs. Another group in 2015 used triton X-100/n-hexanol/cyclohexane system to synthesise Mn-Co-Ni-O NPs [182]. The NMs produced in this process were spherical at low temperatures, while tetragonal at 400°C, and on rising the temperature to 700°C, cubic spinel-shaped NPs were produced. A year later, Agarwal et al. [53] used pentanol and SDS to produce $Mn_3(PO_4)_2$ NPs and their study showed that size of the particles increase with increasing the temperature.

Although W/O system is the common microemulsion used for the synthesis of NMs, organic solvents used in this system can act as a pollutant, and also the yield is low, using this system. Therefore, O/W systems are used in place of the earlier. Pemartin et al. [52] used an O/W system to synthesise $Mn-Zn-Fe_2O_4$ NPs using tetramethylammoniumhydroxide and NaOH as precipitating agent and n-hexane as oil phage. They could find that particle size increased with increasing the conc. of oil phage and both size as well as crystallinity increased with the increase in the concentration of precipitating agent. Baig and co-workers in 2019 [139] used paraffin, dodecanol, and toluene as oil phage and CTAB, SDS, and Triton X-100 as surfactants for the synthesis of $MnFe_2O_4$ NPs, and reported paraffin oil/W to be cheap and best.

3.6 Polyol Method

Polyol method basically involves hydrolysis of metal ions in a polyol such as EG, butylene glycol, propylene glycol, diethylene glycol (DG), triethylene glycol, tetraethylene glycol or polyethylene glycol (PEG) at a specific refluxing temperature [85]. These solvents act both as reducing as well as stabilizing agent for NM synthesis [123]. Diao et al. (2014) [183] used DEG to synthesise $K-MnO_2$ and $LiMn_2O_4$ NPs from $KMnO_4$ in 10 min at 70°C, while Li et al. 2018 [184] employed PEG to produce hydrophilic MnO NPs from $Mn(NO_3)_2 \cdot 4H_2O$. Composite NMs have also been produced using the above technique. Ono and group [84] described one such study in which $PtAc_2$ was initially reduced by 1,2-tetradecanediol at RT followed by increase in the temperature. When the temperature attained 100°C, $Mn_2(CO)_{10}$ in n-dioctyl ether containing OA, and oleylamine was added to the precipitate and on further rising the temperature, black particles appeared at 250°C. The particles were then characterized to be ferromagnetic face cantered cubic (Fcc)-shaped $Mn_{52.5}Pt_{47.5}$ alloy NPs. Liu and co-workers [185] used PEG to make powdered Li_2MnSiO_4 from $Si(OC_2H_5)_4$, $LiAc_2 \cdot H_2O$ and $MnAc_2 \cdot 4H_2O$. Sucrose was then used as a carbon source to coat the powder through ball milling. In two different studies, DG was used as reducing as well as stabilizing agent to synthesize $Mg_{0.8}Mn_{0.2}Fe_2O_4$ [88] and $MnFe_2O_4$ NPs [85] from $Mn(NO_3)_2$ and $Mn(Ac)_2$, respectively. In this method, particle morphology also relies on the time and temperature for reduction, which also played crucial roles in determining the shape and size of the NMs [87, 83]. Rhadif et al. [81] showed that $Mn(Ac)_2 \cdot 4H_2O$ produced oval-shaped Mn_3O_4 NPs at 2 h, while at 5 and 16 h, rhombohedron-shaped particles were formed. Sicard et al. [82] also proved the same by producing spherical yet oval-shaped Mn_3O_4 NPs at 5–30 min, while rhomboidal-shaped particles at 2 h of reaction time. In another study, hollow, spherical, ferromagnetic $MnFe_2O_4$ and $ZnFe_2O_4$ NPs were synthesised, using EG and $NaAc \cdot 3H_2O$ at RT which turned into superparamagnetic, simply by increasing the temperature [186]. Using the same reducing agent, the group also reported spinel-shaped Mn, Co, and Ni ferrite NPs from their respective precursors [86].

3.7 Co-precipitation Method

Co-precipitation method is a simple, effective, and low-cost technique for the synthesis of metal NPs [187]. In this procedure, the metallic ions are precipitated in the form of hydroxides, carbonates, oxalates or citrates with the help of certain reagents and then calcinated into nano-powders [188]. Many research groups have employed this method for synthesising Mn_xO_y [89, 189]. MnO_2 being the most prevalent of these oxides, researchers have attempted to synthesise these NMs using NaOH [93], SDS [95], etc. from MnC_2O_4 [91], $MnSO_4$, [100], and so on. Shaker and Abdasalam used KOH instead of NaOH to produce Mn_3O_4 and Mn_2O_3 NPs [97]. In another report, Jamil et al. [96] used $MnCl_2$ and MnAc$_2$ to prepare saucer-shaped crystalline Mn_3O_4 NPs. Vignesh and co-workers [102] used $MnCl_2 \cdot 6H_2O$ and $FeCl_3 \cdot 9H_2O$ to prepare electrochemically stable $MnFe_2O_4$ NPs. In an attempt to synthesise Fe-Mn alloy NMs, Buccolieri et al. [101] used different combination of $FeCl_3$ and $MnCl_2$. At high concentration of $MnCl_2$, no NMs were produced, while at low concentration, porous, spherical NPs (10–40 nm) were formed. Eslami and group [190] used an aeration-coprecipitation method for an increased rate of oxidation. This method produced spherical NMs with 29.36% Mn_2O_3 and 49.83% Fe_2O_3. Another experiment showed that treating $MnSO_4 \cdot H_2O$ with NaOH at RT followed by calcination at 600°C for 2 h produced spherical composite NM of Mn_2O_3-Mn_3O_4 [105].

Morphology of the particles produced through this method is pH dependent. The size of the cubic Mn_2O_3 NPs produced by Najjar et al. in 2019 [99] was found to shrink with increasing the pH from 10 to 13. Zainab and Sadeq [191] used two capping agents: CTAB and polyvinyl alcohol (PVA) to synthesise Mn_2O_3 NPs, in which CTAB created plate-like NMs (36–44 nm), while the other created non-uniform nanofibers (30–37 nm). Several groups have compared this method with other methods with regard to their efficacy and sensitivity and it was found to be superior than ultrasonic irradiation [98] and micro-emulsion [139]. Kafshgari et al. [49] synthesised $MnFe_2O_4$ NPs from $Mn(NO_3)_2 \cdot 4H_2O$ and $Fe(NO_3) \cdot 9H_2O$ using co-precipitation, sol-gel, and hydrothermal processes, and found that co-precipitation yielded 36-nm spherical NPs, while sol-gel and hydrothermal processes produced 45-nm reticular structured NPs and 16-nm nanosheets, respectively. Despite all of these, this method fails to synthesise pure or ultra-pure NPs, and also the method is time-taking.

3.8 Sonochemical Method

Sonochemical method is a kind of novel chemical approach for the synthesis of NMs that uses ultrasonic sound energy for accelerating the rate of hydrolysis [192, 193]. As compared to other methods, this method is preferred for producing small but pure and eco-friendly NPs. The technique can be grouped into primary and secondary sonochemistry depending on the precursor they use: the first method uses volatile precursors, while the second one uses non-volatile precursors [194]. Gnana Sundara Raj et al. [108] and Rajrana et al. [109] synthesised MnO_2 NPs from $KMnO_4$, using a sonochemical approach with PEG as reducing agent. Wang and group [195] synthesised PVP-coated $MnFe_2O_4$ NPs in 2018. $Mn_{0.5}Zn_{0.5}Dy_xEu_xFe_{1.8-2x}O_4$ NPs (20 nm) in aggregated cubic grain were synthesised by Rehman et al. [113]. Amulya and co-workers produced rod-shaped $MnFe_2O_4$ NPs from $MnSO_4$ quite recently [2].

Lei et al. [106] succeeded in producing uniform-sized tetragonal colloidal Mn_3O_4 NPs from $MnCl_2$ in ethanolamine at 40–100°C without even using any surfactant or extra nucleating component. Their findings revealed that, with increasing the temperature, size of the particle also increases. In another report, Dharmarathna and co-workers [196] synthesised octahedral molecular sieve (OMS) of Mn-ferrite from $KMnO_4$ and $MnSO_4 \cdot H_2O$ at RT by using a mixed phage of water/acetone. The NPs morphology also depended on sonication time and calcination temperature. A similar trend of the results was observed from Goswami et al. [110] for synthesising $MnFe_2O_4$ NPs from $MnAc_2$. On increasing the temperature from 923 to 1223 K, particle size increased from 34 to 46 nm. Along with size, the shape of the particles also changed from spherical to rod-type. Excluding these factors, pH also plays a crucial role in deciding the particle morphology, which was proved from the study of Abulizi et al. in 2014 [107]. They could synthesise sheet/needle, spherical, and cubic/polyhedron-shaped δ-MnO_2 NPs in just 20 min, from the same precursor, i.e., $KMnO_4$ in the presence of PEG by simply varying the pH to 2.2, 6.0, and 9.3, respectively.

Comparison study between the present method and other physicochemical methods has also been done. Mn-Zn ferrite ($Mn_xZn_{1-x}Fe_2O_4$) NPs were synthesised from $MnCl_2$ and $MnSO_4$ via both polyol and sonochemical methods. From $MnCl_2$, the polyol method produced polydispersed tiny, aggregated, and low crystalline spherical NPs, while sonochemical route yielded monodispersed, cube-like, highly crystalline NPs. Similarly, $MnSO_4$ created tiny NPs via the sonochemical approach, while the polyol method produced chain like circular NPs. Overall, the sonochemical method was proven to be more effective than the other [114]. Gholamrezaei and Salavati-Niasari [112] used ultrasonic, microwave, hydrothermal, and co-precipitation method to synthesise $SrMnO_3$ NPs from $KMnO_4$ and $MnCl_2 \cdot 4H_2O$. Except sonochemistry, in all the other approaches, the NPs formed were of aggregated, destructured and indetermined form. Simultaneously, the surfactants also decided the particle morphology. PEG 600 produced wart-shaped agglomerated 8–35 nm NPs, while SDS produced, 4–12 nm spherical NPs. In spite of all, the main limitations of this method are low yield and inefficiency.

3.9 Chemical Reduction

This is nothing but oxidoreduction approach, in which the source of Mn is chemically reduced using a reducing agent. Air stable α-Mn NPs was synthesized by Bondi et al. [131] through Schlenk and Glove box technique, using n-butyllithium as a strong reducing agent and oleic acid as stabilizer. The NPs produced showed paramagnetic properties. In 2011, Hu and co-group leached Zn-Mn batteries and then burnt them in the presence of iron shells and citrate-nitrate precursors to prepare $Mn_{0.5}Zn_{0.5}Fe_2O_4$ NPs [136]. In the same year, Qian et al. [135] employed polymer-assisted chemical reduction to synthesise MnO_2/RGO nanocomposites from $MnSO_4 \cdot H_2O$; in this process, the source of Mn itself acted as a catalyst. Le and Phuc [132] synthesised γ-MnO_2 NPs from $KMnO_4$ in C_2H_5OH in 4 h at RT. In another study, instead of C_2H_5OH, deep eutectic solvent was used for synthesising rods and sheets of α-MnO_2 at 60, 70, and 80°C [133].

4. Additional Approaches

In addition to the above physicochemical approaches, researchers have also explored other strategies for the synthesis of Mn NMs. Sui et al. [197] used molten salts of KNO_3 and mixture of $NaNO_3$ and $LiNO_3$ to synthesise α-MnO_2 wires and β-MnO_2 rods, respectively, from $MnSO_4 \cdot H_2O$. In the first case, reaction mixture was heated at 380°C for 2 h, while in the other for 3 h. The products were washed, recovered, and cooled to RT. However, increasing the temperature to above 400°C, Mn_2O_3 was produced in both the cases. Furthermore, the NMs produced at the beginning were found to be amorphous type while towards late, crystal NMs were formed. In another study, Wang et al. [137] followed a templet approach to make mesoporous Ni_6MnO_8 nanospheres from $Mn(CH_3COO)_2 \cdot 4H_2O$. Yang et al. (2019) [138] produced Mn_3O_4 NPs through electrochemical scanning and observed a change in the morphology of the synthesised particles with the change in scan rate. Surprisingly, at 5 and 200 V/s, spherical and rod-shaped particles, respectively, were formed, while at 50 V/s both the type of particles were produced.

5. Summary

Manganese NMs have drawn the interest among researchers due to their novel properties and applications. However, since metal-doped, composite, alloy, polymetallic Mn NMs are better and superior than their counterparts, researchers are more inclined towards these NMs. For synthesising these NMs *in vitro*, different physicochemical or biological approaches are used but the Former is common and specific.

Acknowledgement

Ms. Bandita Panda would like to acknowledge S&T Department, Odisha for providing BPRF while writing the chapter. The authors would also like to thank HOD, Zoology for providing infrastructure and timely suggestions.

References

[1] Das, B., B. Balasubramanian, P. Manchanda, P. Mukherjee, R. Skomski, G.C. Hadjipanayis and D.J. Sellmyer. 2016. Nano Lett. 16: 1132.

[2] Amulya, M.A.S., H.P. Nagaswarupa, M.R.A. Kumar, C.R. Ravikumar and K.B. Kusuma. 2021. J. Phys. Chem. Solids. 148: 109661.

[3] Wang, Y., C. Hou, X. Lin, H. Jiang, C. Zhang and G. Liu. 2021. Appl. Phys. A. 127: 277.

[4] Wan, S., J. Wu, S. Zhou, R. Wang, B. Gao and F. He. 2018. Sci. Total Environ. 616–617: 1298.

[5] Ghasemi, S., S.R. Hosseini and O. Boore-talari. 2018. Ultrason. Sonochem. 40: 675.

[6] Dessie, Y., S. Tadesse, R. Eswaramoorthy and B. Abebe. 2019. J. Sci.: Adv. Mater. Devices. 4: 353.

[7] Poon, K., Z. Lu, Y.D. Deene, Y. Ramaswamy, H. Zreiqat and G. Singh. 2021. Nanoscale. Adv. 3: 4052.

[8] Ogunyemi, S.O., M. Zhang, Y. Abdallah, T. Ahmed, W. Qiu, Md.A. Ali, C. Yan, Y. Yang, J. Chen, and B. Li. 2020. Front. Microbiol. 11: 3099.

[9] Shaik, M.R., R. Syed, S.F. Adil, M. Kuniyil, M. Khan, M.S. Alqahtani, J.P. Shaik, M.R.H. Siddiqui, A. Al-Warthan, M.A.F. Sharaf, A. Abdelgawad and E.M. Awwad. 2021. Saudi J. Bio. Sci. 28: 1196.

[10] Hoseinpour, V. and N. Ghaemi. 2018. J. Photochem. Photobiol B: Biol. 189: 234.

[11] Souri, M., V. Hoseinpour, A. Shakeri and N. Ghaemi. 2018. IET Nanobiotechnol. 12: 822.

[12] Bigiani, L., C. Maccato, A. Gasparotto, C. Sada, E. Bontempi and D. Barreca. 2020. Nanomat. (Basel) 10: E1335.

[13] Huynh, K.-H., X.-H. Pham, J. Kim, S.H. Lee, H. Chang, W.-Y. Rho and B.-H. Jun. 2020. Int. J. Mol. Sci. 21: 5174.

[14] Dewi, N. and Y. Yulizar. 2020. Mater. Today: Proc. 22: 199.

[15] Amatya, S., S. Shrestha and S. Amatya. 2021. Asian J. Phy. Chem. Sci. 9: 1.

[16] Sukmarani, G., R. Kusumaningrum, A. Noviyanto, F. Fauzi, A.M. Habieb, M.I. Amal and N.T. Rochman. 2020. Journal of Materials Research and Technology 9: 8497–8506.

[17] Chen, D., B. Yang, Y. Jiang and Y. Zhang. 2018. Chem. Select. 3: 3904.

[18] Gagrani, A., J. Zhou and T. Tsuzuki. 2018. Ceramics International. 44: 4694.

[19] Aslibeiki, B., P. Kameli, H. Salamati, M. Eshraghi and T. Tahmasebi. 2010. J. Magn. Magn. Mater. 322: 2929.

[20] Bellusci, M., C. Aliotta, D. Fiorani, A. La Barbera, F. Padella, D. Peddis, M. Pilloni and D. Secci. 2012. J. Nanopart. Res. 14.

[21] Chen, D., Y. Zhang and Z. Kang. 2013. Chem. Eng. J. 215–216: 235.

[22] Aslani, A., M. Ghahremani, M. Zhang, L.H. Bennett and E. Della Torre. 2017. IEEE Trans. Magn. 53: 1.

[23] Chang, Y.Q., X.Y. Xu, X.H. Luo, C.P. Chen and D.P. Yu. 2004. J. Cryst. Growth. 1–3: 232.

[24] Si, P.Z., E. Brück, Z.D. Zhang, O. Tegus, W.S. Zhang, K.H.J. Buschow and J.C.P. Klaasse. 2005. Mater. Res. Bull. 40: 29.

[25] Le, H.A., S. Chin, E. Park, L.T. Linh, G.-N. Bae and J. Jurng. 2011. Chem. Vap. Depos. 17: 228.

[26] Kim, H.-G., H. Lee, S.-J. Kim, D.-H. Kim, J.-S. Kim, S.-Y. Kang and S.-C. Jung. 2013. J. Nanosci. Nanotechnol. 13: 6103.

[27] Aghazadeh, M., M. Ghannadi Maragheh, M.R. Ganjali and P. Norouzi. 2017. Inorg. Nano-Met. Chem. 47: 1085.
[28] Najim, A., M. Muhi, K. Gbashi and A. Salih. 2017. Plasmonics 13: 1.
[29] Kang, Y. and C.B. Murray. 2010. J. Am. Chem. Soc. 132: 7568.
[30] Lee, J.-G., P. Li, C.-J. Choi and X.-L. Dong. 2010. Thin Solid Films 519: 81.
[31] Al-Hada, N.M., H.M. Kamari, A.H. Shaari and E. Saion. 2019. Results Phys. 12: 1821.
[32] Wang, X., X. Wang, W. Huang, P.J. Sebastian and S. Gamboa. 2005. J. Power Sources 140: 211.
[33] Gnanam, S. and V. Rajendran. 2011. J. Sol-Gel Sci. Technol. 58: 62.
[34] Tang, W., X. Shan, S. Li, H. Liu, X. Wu and Y. Chen. 2014. Mater. Letters 132: 317.
[35] Chen, B., G. Rao, S. Wang, Y. Lan, L. Pan and X. Zhang. 2015. Mater. Letters 154: 160.
[36] Bui, P.T.M., J.-H. Song, Z.-Y. Li, M.S. Akhtar and O.-B. Yang. 2017. J. Alloys Compd. 694: 560.
[37] Ahn, M.-S., R. Ahmad, J.-Y. Yoo and Y.-B. Hahn. 2018. J. Colloid Interface Sci. 516: 364.
[38] Ismail, M., S. Hemaanandhan, M. Durai, M. Arivanandhan, G. Anbalagan and R. Jayavel. 2020. J. Sol-Gel Sci. Technol. 93.
[39] Blinov, A.V., A.A. Kravtsov, S.O. Krandievskii, V.P. Timchenko, A.A. Gvozdenko and A.A. Blinova. 2020. Russ. J. Gen. Chem. 90: 283.
[40] Kanagesan, S., S.B.A. Aziz, M. Hashim, I. Ismail, S. Tamilselvan, N.B.B.M. Alitheen, M.K. Swamy and B.P.C. Rao. 2016. Molecules 21: 312.
[41] Ashwini, K., H. Rajanaika, K.S. Anantharaju, H. Nagabhushanad, P. Adinarayana Reddy, K. Shetty and K.R.V. Mahesh. 2017. Mater. Today: Proc. 4: 11902.
[42] Bhandare, S.V., R. Kumar, A.V. Anupama, H.K. Choudhary, V.M. Jali and B. Sahoo. 2017. J. Magn. Magn. Mater. 433: 29.
[43] Mary Jacintha, A., V. Umapathy, P. Neeraja, and S. Rex Jeya Rajkumar. 2017. J. Nanostruct. Chem. 7: 375.
[44] Zhang, M., S. Guo, L. Zheng, G. Zhang, Z. Hao, L. Kang and Z.-H. Liu. 2013. Electrochimica Acta. 87: 546.
[45] Ranjeh, M., M. Masjedi-Arani, M. Salavati-Niasari and H. Moayedi. 2020. J. Mol. Liq. 300: 112292.
[46] Pál, E., V. Zöllmer, D. Lehmhus and M. Busse. 2011. Colloids Surf. A: Physicochem. Eng. Asp. 384: 661.
[47] Quraishi, M.A.M. and M.H.R. Khan. 2013. Ind. J. Mater. Sci. 2013: e910762.
[48] Noor, A., M.N. Akhtar, S.N. Khan, M.S. Nazir and M. Yousaf. 2020. Ceram. Int. 46: 13961.
[49] Kafshgari, L.A., M. Ghorbani and A. Azizi. 2019. Part. Sci. Technol. 37: 904.
[50] Košak, A., D. Makovec, M. Drofenik and A. Žnidaršič. 2004. J. Magn. Magn. Mater. 272–276: 1542.
[51] Scano, A., G. Ennas, F. Frongia, A. La Barbera, M.A. López-Quintela, G. Marongiu, G. Paschina, D. Peddis, M. Pilloni and C. Vázquez-Vázquez. 2011. J. Nanopart. Res. 13: 3063.
[52] Pemartin, K., C. Solans, J. Alvarez-Quintana and M. Sanchez-Dominguez. 2014. Colloids. Surf. A: Physicochem. Eng. Asp. 451: 161.
[53] Agarwal, S., I. Tyagi, V.K. Gupta, M. Jafari, M. Edrissi and H. Javadian. 2016. J. Mol. Liq. 219: 1131.
[54] Soleymani, M. and M. Edrissi. 2016. Bull Mater Sci. 39: 487.
[55] Subramanian, V., H. Zhu, R. Vajtai, P.M. Ajayan and B. Wei. 2005. J. Phys. Chem. B. 109: 20207.
[56] Song, X., Y. Zhao and Y. Zheng. 2007. Cryst. Growth Des. 7: 159.
[57] Yu, P., X. Zhang, D. Wang, L. Wang and Y. Ma. 2009. Cryst. Growth Des. 9: 528.
[58] Ahmed, K.A.M., Q. Zeng, K. Wu and K. Huang. 2010. J. Solid State Chem. 3: 744.
[59] Xiao, W., D. Wang and X.W. Lou. 2010. J. Phys. Chem. C. 114: 1694.
[60] Zhang, X., Y. Chen, P. Yu and Y. Ma. 2010. J. Nanosci. Nanotechnol. 10: 7711.
[61] Hlaing, A.A. and P.P. Win. 2012. Adv. Nat. Sci: Nanosci. Nanotechnol. 3: 025001.
[62] Haoran, Y., D. Lifang, L. Tao and C. Yong. 2014. Sci. World J. 2014: e791672.
[63] Harichandran, G., P. Parameswari, D.S. Amalraj and P. Shanmugam. 2014. Int. J. Innov. Res. Sci. Eng. 443.
[64] Dinh, V.-P., N.-C. Le, T.-P.-T. Nguyen and N.-T. Nguyen. 2016. J. Chem. 2016: e8285717.
[65] Ahmad, K., A. Mohammad and S.M. Mobin. 2017. Electrochimica. Acta. 252: 549.

[66] Chu, J., D. Lu, J. Ma, M. Wang, X. Wang and S. Xiong. 2017. Mater. Letter. 193.

[67] Venkata Swetha, J., H. Parse, B. Kakade and A. Geetha. 2018. Solid State Ion. 328: 1.

[68] Wang, L., G. Duan, S.-M. Chen and X. Liu. 2018. J. Alloys Compd. 752: 123.

[69] Racik, K.M., K. Guruprasad, M. Mahendiran, M. Joseph, T. Maiyalagan and V. Antony Raj. 2019. J. Mater. Sci.: Mater. Electron. 30.

[70] Selim, M.S., Z. Hao, Y. Jiang, M. Yi and Y. Zhang. 2019. Mater. Chem. Phys. 235: 121733.

[71] Shaik, D.P.M.D., P. Rosaiah and O.M. Hussain. 2019. J. Electroanal. Chem. 851: 113409.

[72] Xia, A., W. Yu, J. Yi, G. Tan, H. Ren and C. Liu. 2019. J. Electroanal. Chem. 839: 25.

[73] Han, R., M. Chen, X. Liu, Y. Zhang, Y. Xie and Y. Sui. 2020. Nanomater. (Basel) 10: 461.

[74] Kumar, Y., S. Chopra, A. Gupta, Y. Kumar, S.J. Uke and S.P. Mardikar. 2020. Mater. Sci. Energy Technol. 3: 566.

[75] Mothkuri, S., S. Chakrabarti, H. Gupta, B. Padya, T.N. Rao and P.K. Jain. 2020. Materials Today: Proc. 26: 142.

[76] Xiao, Y., Y. Wang, Y. Xie, H. Ni, X. Li, Y. Zhang and T. Xie. 2020. Environ. Technol. 41: 2037.

[77] Ullrich, A., M.M. Rahman, P. Longo and S. Horn. 2019. Sci. Rep. 9: 19264.

[78] Zhang, F., M. Cho, T. Eom, C. Kang and H. Lee. 2019. Ceram. Internation. 45: 20972.

[79] Akhtar, S., S. Rehman, M.A. Almessiere, F.A. Khan, Y. Slimani and A. Baykal. 2019. Nanomater. (Basel) 9: 1635.

[80] Balakumar, V., J.W. Ryu, H. Kim, R. Manivannan and Y.-A. Son. 2020. Ultrason. Sonochem. 62: 104870.

[81] Rhadfi, T., J.-Y. Piquemal, L. Sicard, F. Herbst, E. Briot, M. Benedetti and A. Atlamsani. 2010. Appl. Catal. A: Gen. 386: 132.

[82] Sicard, L., J.-M. Le Meins, C. Méthivier, F. Herbst and S. Ammar. 2010. Journal of Magnetism and Magnetic Materials 322: 2634–2640.

[83] Goikolea, E., B. Daffos, P.L. Taberna and P. Simon. 2013. Mater. Renew Sustain Energy 2: 16.

[84] Ono, K., R. Okuda, Y. Ishii, S. Kamimura and M. Oshima. 2003. J. Phys. Chem. B. 107: 1941.

[85] Ghutepatil, P.R., A.B. Salunkhe, V.M. Khot and S.H. Pawar. 2019. Chem. Pap. 73: 2189.

[86] Iacovita, C., G.F. Stiufiuc, R. Dudric, N. Vedeanu, R. Tetean, R.I. Stiufiuc and C.M. Lucaciu. 2020. Magnetochem. 6: 23.

[87] Kim, T.R., D.H. Kim, H.W. Ryu, J.H. Moon, J.H. Lee, S. Boo and J. Kim. 2007. J. Phys. Chem. Solids 68: 1203.

[88] Sabale, S., V. Khot, V. Jadhav, X. Zhu and Y. Xu. 2014. Acta Metallurgica Sinica (Eng. Lett.) 27: 1122.

[89] Chen, Z.W., J.K.L. Lai and C.H. Shek. 2006. Scripta Materialia 55: 735.

[90] Kumar, H., S.P. Manisha and P. Sangwan. 2013. Int. J. Chem. Chem. Eng. 3: 155.

[91] Sagadevan, S. 2015. J. Material Sci. Eng. 4.

[92] Guo, S., W. Sun, W. Yang, Q. Li and J. Ku Shang. 2015. RSC Adv. 5: 53280.

[93] Cherian, E., A. Rajan and Dr. B. Gurunathan. 2016. Int. J. Mod. Sci. Technol. 01: 17.

[94] Gnanasekaran, L., R. Hemamalini, R. Saravanan, K. Ravichandran, F. Gracia, S. Agarwal and V.K. Gupta. 2017. J. Photochem. Photobiol. B: Biol. 173: 43.

[95] Moazzen, E., E.V. Timofeeva and C.U. Segre. 2017. J. Mater. Sci. 52: 8107.

[96] Jamil, S., S.R. Khan, B. Sultana, M. Hashmi, M. Haroon and M.R.S.A. Janjua. 2018. J. Clust. Sci. 29: 1099.

[97] Shaker, K. and A. AbdAlsalm. 2018. Eng. Technol. J. 36: 946.

[98] Tholkappiyan, R., A.N. Naveen, K. Vishista, and F. Hamed. 2018. J. Taibah Univers. Sci. 12: 669.

[99] Najjar, R., R. Awad, and A.M. Abdel-Gaber. 2019. J. Supercond Nov. Magn. 32: 885.

[100] Soam, A. and R. Kumar. 2020. Surf. Rev. Lett. 27: 1950199.

[101] Buccolieri, A., A. Serra, G. Maruccio, A.G. Monteduro, S. Kunjalukkal, A. Licciulli, V. Bonfrate, L. Salvatore, D. Manno, L. Calcagnile and G. Giancane. 2017. J. Anal. Methods Chem. 2017.

[102] Vignesh, V., K. Subramani, M. Sathish and R. Navamathavan. 2018. Colloids Surf. A: Physicochem. Eng. Asp. 538: 668.

[103] Zia, J., E.S. Aazam and U. Riaz. 2020. J. Mater. Res. Technol. 9: 9709.

[104] Eslami, H., M.H. Ehrampoush, A. Esmaeili, A.A. Ebrahimi, M.T. Ghaneian, H. Falahzadeh and M.H. Salmani. 2019. Mater. Chem. Phys. 224: 65.

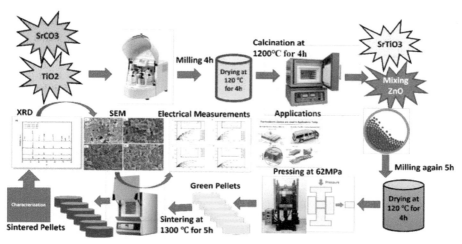

Fig. 1. The schematic of the solid-state process for preparation of Strontium Titanate.

top-down approach or bottom-up approach. The ceramic nanoparticles can be processed by applying pressure ranging from 3000 Psi to 10000 Psi, pressing it into pellets, obtaining powders from the mixing of ball mills, and then heating at high temperatures to get the required product [1–4].

The compositions prepared from the solid-state method in the form of cylindrical pellets can be characterized by several techniques as Scanning Electron Microscopy, X-Ray diffraction, Fourier transform infrared spectroscopy, and chemical analysis techniques [5–9].

This chapter focuses on the special case for the synthesis of ceramic nanomaterials by solid-state route, incorporating defects in the materials, milling the particles in either wet or dry medium. The particles were milled at high rotation per minute to reduce the size from micrometer to nanometer scale. The rate of diffusion can be increased by the temperature and pressure. The reactants having the same crystal structure enhance the nucleation rate which ultimately affects the composition prepared [10, 11]. There will be an increase in the mechanical, electrical, magnetic, properties that can be explained in detail in this chapter.

2. Methods of Solid-State Synthesis

2.1 Stoichiometric Calculations

The precursors are weighted stoichiometry according to balanced chemical equations. The charge balance should be maintained for the reactants as well as for the products. The carbonates, nitrates, and oxides of the metals are used for this purpose. The commonly used precursors are metallic oxides that are FeO, Fe_2O_3, TiO_2, CuO, ZnO, MgO_2, Li_2O, Bi_2O_3. The other precursors are carbonates of sodium, potassium, and calcium such as $NaCO_3$, KCO_3, and $CaCO_3$. The carbon dioxide, ammonia, and water obtained in the products are sometimes not written in the balanced chemical equations.

Some of the synthesis chemical equations can be explained below.

1. The equation for the synthesis of Barium Titanate

$$BaCO_3 + TiO_2 \rightarrow BaTiO_3 + CO_{2(\uparrow)} \tag{1}$$

2. The equation for the synthesis of Strontium Titanate

$$SrCO_3 + TiO_2 \rightarrow SrTiO_3 + CO_{2(\uparrow)} \tag{2}$$

3. The equation for the synthesis of Bismuth Ferrite

$$Bi_2O_3 + Fe_2O_3 \rightarrow 2BiFeO_3 \tag{3}$$

There are compositions that can be prepared by mixing the two precursors together and then balancing the equations. The powders should be used in nanometer (nm) size as the wet milling step will further decrease the particle size and the physical mixing of the precursors. Some of the equations below explain the synthesis of the Barium Calcium Zirconium Titanate (BCZT), the most common lead-free ceramic material. Besides this, there are many other compositions that can be prepared with replacing lead oxide (PbO$_2$) like Na$_{0.5}$K$_{0.5}$NbO$_3$-LiSbO$_3$-BiFeO$_3$, (1–x) Na$_{1/2}$Bi$_{1/2}$TiO$_3$-xBiFeO$_3$, Na$_{0.5}$K$_{0.5}$NbO$_3$-BiFeO$_3$.

4. The equation for the synthesis of Barium Calcium Zirconium Titanate

$$0.85BaCO_3 + 0.15CaCO_3 + 0.1ZrO_2 + 0.9TiO_2 \rightarrow (Ba_{0.85}Ca_{0.15})(Zr_{0.1}Ti_{0.9})O_3 + CO_{2(\uparrow)} \tag{4}$$

2.2 Milling

A ball plant is a sort of mixing/reduction of powder size, and it is utilized to grind powders by two forces: (I) shear force between the two balls (II) impact force of the balls from the height of the jar. The particle size is reduced to an amazing limit for use in mineral dressing forms, paints, fireworks, and pottery. The rotations per minute (rpms) of the ball mill can be adjusted from 200–400 rpm. The oxides that are hard ceramics required more rotations per minutes (rpm) and time while it takes less rpm and time for soft ceramic powders. The medium used for the mixing, grinding, and sizing is ethanol/methanol/acetone or any other inert solvent that may not react with the powder particles. The medium provide the slurry to create a force i–e impact force and shear force. Various materials are utilized as media, including zirconia balls, stone rocks, and stainless-steel balls. An inside falling impact diminishes the material to a fine powder. The distinction in speeds between the balls and granulating containers creates a connection among frictional and sway powers, which discharges high unique energies. The interchange between these powers creates the high and exceptionally viable level of size decrease of the planetary ball mill. The parameters involved in the milling are listed below:

1. Milling speed
2. Milling medium
3. Balls/powder ratio
4. Size of the powders

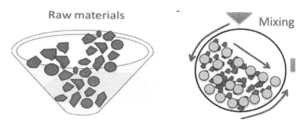

Fig. 2. The mixing of raw materials and milling by shear and impact forces.

2.3 Drying and Sieving

After milling the slurry obtained must be dried in the oven at 80–100°C. The drying process was done to evaporate the ethanol from the jars and the remaining powders were cleaned from the zirconia ball for the process of calcination. In case of water milling, it should be dried at a temperature of 100°C to evaporate water from the slurry. Increasing the temperature increases decreases the drying time. Once the powder dried it must be sieved properly. The recovery of the product can be done by the polyethylene spatulas, spoons, stirrer, and giving some amount of energy to the powders.

2.4 Calcination

The process of removal of small molecules like CO_2, H_2O, and others at a temperature below their melting point to change the phase from one to another is called calcination; it is done in the oven or a low heating furnace by heating from room temperature to the required temperature. The removal of volatile particles occurs and the powders' color, density, weight, and sometimes size may be changed due to heating cycle which confirms that the process is in the right way. Calcination is to be differentiated from roasting, in which progressively complex gas-strong responses occur between the furnace environment and the solids. Calcination is the process of thermal decomposition at a particular temperature or the progress (transition) temperature (for stage changes) to remove small molecules like water, ammonia and carbondioxide. This temperature is generally characterized by the Gibbs free energy in response to the material value that is equivalent to zero.

The calcination temperatures can be found from the Thermogravimetric Analysis (TGA), i.e., heating material by changing the weight loss of the sample. The calcination temperatures of ceramic nanomaterials range from 600–800°C. The highest calcination temperature is of BCZT, BZT, and BT groups. While the ferrites groups are calcined at lower temperatures, so that the intermediates formed Fe_xO_y-M can be avoided.

2.5 Pressing of Pellets

The pressing of the ceramic nano powders is done by applying a pressure of 4000 Psi to 10000 Psi in the required time. The morphology of the powder must be studied before pressing and if there is the diversity of the particles in the powder like circular, angular, spherical, etc., the pellets obtained are fine. If there are the

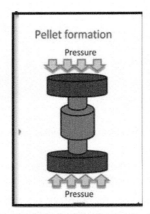

Fig. 3. The pressure is applied on the die to make a cylindrical pellet.

same type of particles in the powders, there will be spaces in the interlocking of the particles that may be removed by adding some additive. Hydrostatic pressing with stainless steel die is used to press the powder in cylindrical pellets. Sometimes there should be the application of lubricant to properly bind the material while applying pressure simultaneously.

2.6 Sintering

As the heat is applied to the pressed pellets, the densification mechanism activated and the normal grain size expands; this process is called sintering of ceramic nano-materials. The fundamental grain growth happens when it is given time called "holding time". The process requires helps to form single phase. Sintering intends to deliver sintered parts with reproducible and, if conceivable, structured microstructure through control of the sintering factors [12, 13].

To get the maximum densification sintering parameters (time, temperature and heating rate) must be adjusted according to the needs. Sintering temperature varies with the thickness. The temperature rate must be adjusted for the compositions as the heating and cooling cycles must be kept in mind so that the material may not be burned or may not stick with the substrate. The sintering of the pellets can be done at a higher temperature, as the group of lead-free ceramics is sintered at higher temperatures usually at 1000°C to 1400°C.

3. Conclusions

The solid state route is applied to synthesize the ceramic nanoparticles into pellets by a series of steps-from stoichiometric calculations to the sintering and obtaining the final product. The composition prepared can be tested by number of characterizations to study the details of the materials. The cylindrical pellets are further characterized to study the application-based effects of the materials.

References

[1] Jaffe, B. 2012. Piezoelectric ceramics. Vol. 3.: Elsevier.

[2] Smith, B.C. 2011. Fundamentals of Fourier Transform Infrared Spectroscopy. CRC Press.

[3] Singh, K. et al. 2011. Room temperature long range ferromagnetic ordering in $(BiFeO_3)1-x$ $(PbTiO_3)x$ nanocrystallites. Vol. 109: 123911–123911.

[4] Carter, C. 2007. MG Norton Ceramic Material Science and Engineering. Springer Science and Business Media, New York.

[5] Butz, B. 2011. Yttria-doped zirconia as solid electrolyte for fuel-cell applications: Fundamental aspects. Suedwestdeutscher Verlag fuer Hochschulschriften.

[6] Rai, R. et al. 2010. Ferroelectric and Ferromagnetic Properties of Gd-Doped $BiFeO_3$-$BaTiO_3$ Solid Solution. 119: 539–545.

[7] Lloyd, J. and J. Mitchinson. 2010. QI: The Book of General Ignorance-The Noticeably Stouter Edition. Faber & Faber.

[8] Hamilton, S. 2007. An Analog Electronics Companion: Basic Circuit Design for Engineers and Scientists. Cambridge University Press.

[9] Vilarinho, P.M., Y. Rosenwaks and A. Kingon. 2006. Scanning Probe Microscopy: Characterization, Nanofabrication and Device Application of Functional Materials: Proceedings of the NATO Advanced Study Institute on Scanning Probe Microscopy: Characterization, Nanofabrication and Device Application of Functional Materials, Algarve, Portugal, 1–13 October 2002. Vol. 186. Springer Science & Business Media.

[10] Stuart, B. 2005. Infrared Spectroscopy. Wiley Online Library.

[11] Moulson, A.J. and J.M. Herbert. 2003. Electroceramics: Materials, Properties, Applications. John Wiley & Sons.

[12] Yanagida, H., K. Kōmoto and M. Miyayama. 1996. The Chemistry of Ceramics. John Wiley & Son Ltd.

[13] Buchanan, R.C. 1986. Ceramic Materials for Electronics: Processing, Properties, and Applications. Marcel Dekker, Inc.

11

Nanofabrication of Porous Structures

Solution Combustion Synthesis of Advanced Electrode Materials in Energy Storage Devices

Parameshwar Kommu,[1,2,]* *Divya Velpula,*[1]
Shilpa Chakra Chidurala,[1,]* *Shireesha Konda,*[1]
Rakesh Kumar Thida,[1] *Vikash Kumar,*[2] *Madhuri Sakaray,*[1]
G.P. Singh[2,]* and *Arnab Shankar Bhattacharyya*[2,]*

1. Introduction

The increasing depletion of fossil fuels and greenhouse gas emissions have urged people to develop energy storage systems [1, 2]. Energy storage systems play a major role in extracting energy from various sources and transforming it into the energy forms necessary for utility, manufacturing, construction, and electric vehicles (EV) applications. Energy sources like fossil fuels provide power based on consumer demand, easily stored while not in use. However, as new resources, such as solar and wind energy, become accessible, they must be captured and stored [3]. Energy storage is a viable option. Energy systems provide numerous advantages, including enhanced renewable energy distribution and improved economic performance

[1] Center for Nano Science and Technology, Institute of Science and Technology, JNTU Hyderabad, India-500085.
[2] Department of Nanotechnology, Central University of Jharkhand, Ranchi, India-835205.
* Corresponding author: shilpachakra.nano@jntuh.ac.in, gpsinghcuj@gmail.com, 2006asb@gmail.com

[4]. Power storage is also essential for electrical systems because it allows load leveling and peak shaving, frequency management, energy oscillation damping, and improved power quality and reliability [3]. Electrochemical and battery energy storage, thermal and thermochemical energy storage, flywheel energy storage, and compressed gas energy storage are the most frequent energy storage methods. Pump/magnetic/chemical/hydrogen energy storage are all options for storing energy. Batteries and capacitors can be used to store electrical energy. Batteries are high-capacity, high-voltage energy storage devices with high power densities. Lithium-ion (LIB), sodium ion (SIB), lithium sulphur (LiS), lithium-air (Li-O$_2$), zinc ion (ZIB), and zinc-air batteries are only a few of the several varieties. Supercapacitors or ultra-capacitors (UCs), have the highest capacitance per unit volume due to their porous electrode structure [5]. They are categorized as electrostatic electrolytic capacitors and electrochemical capacitors [6]. Many new electrode materials and electrolytes have been investigated and proposed to enhance the cost, energy density and power density, cycle life, and battery safety [7]. In this chapter, porous structured electrode material focuses on solution combustion synthesis process for advanced electrode material in energy storage device applications.

1.1 Combustion Synthesis

Combustion synthesis (CS) is a well-known, efficient, and appealing synthesis process. It's utilized to make powders, ceramics, composites, and functional materials. Merzanov et al. were the first to develop this approach (1970) [8]. The CS is also a self-propagating, high-temperature synthesis as exothermic combustion reactions will form the desired inorganic matter [9]. The CS technique has been used in various academic and industrial applications [10–15]. Due to its unique approach, excellent benefits at a low cost, and a way that saves energy and time, this approach has garnered more visibility and accuracy in a short period. With these benefits, combustion synthesis has shown to be the most acceptable synthesis process for commercial adaption. The combustion synthesis is separated into two stages: self-transmitting high-temperature synthesis (SHS), and the thermal blast mode, although the phrase "combustion synthesis" is now generally used to refer to all of those self-sustaining and self-transmission illumination reactions [16]. According to the existing reports, carbide, nitride, boride, sulfate, and alumina nitride materials are made by the combustion synthesis method [17–22]. The combustion method has been divided into solid-state combustion and solution combustion in recent years. Combustion synthesis is the ideal option for a fast reaction and energy-saving.

The following are a few critical steps in the combustion synthesis process:

Step 1. The precise proportion of fuel to the oxidizer is vital in combustion synthesis, and stoichiometric balance is also essential.

Step 2. The fuel to oxidizer ratio should be equal to 1.

Step 3. The oxidizer and fuel are combined and agitated to form a homogenous solution using a solvent.

Step 4. The resulting homogenous solution must be kept on a hot plate or in a muffle furnace with the temperature adjusted to prevent the solution from burning with flames. Once the combustion process starts, it is self-propelled by an exothermic redox chemical reaction.

Step 5. When the entire homogenous mixture has been uniformly heated, it can be removed from the hot plate or furnace and crushed thoroughly in a mortar pestle to obtain powder form.

2. Classification of Combustion Synthesis

Solid-state combustion and solution combustion are the two most common types of combustion synthesis. The synthesis of solid-state combustion is further separated into two groups.

1. Linear or self-propagating high-temperature synthesis (SHS) and
2. Bulk or volume combustion synthesis (VCS).

While the solution combustion synthesis can occur in various modes as we can see Fig. 1 [23], a detailed discussion of all combustion synthesis protocols is provided as follows.

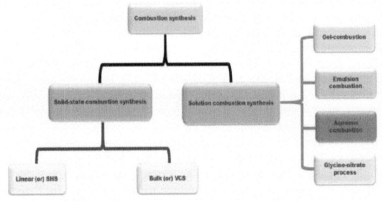

Fig. 1. Different types of process are involved in Combustion Synthesis Process.

2.1 Solid-state Combustion Method (SSCs)

The SSCs synthesis technique has been subject to chemical reactions and products in the solid-state [16]. The product created explodes the reactants, which are primarily pellets. Solid-state combustion produces borides, carbides, nitrides, and oxides, among other compounds [10].

2.1.1 Self-Propagating High-Temperature Synthesis

The SHS is an effective method for producing borides, carbides, and oxide powders directly from the reactions that exist in a reactive process [10, 23]. The process develops quickly by initiating and self-propagating extreme heatwaves generated from exothermic redox chemical reactions. The waves transfer at high speeds from high-temperature results to low-temperature factors, allowing the reactants to be heated to high temperatures in a short period and leading to the highly pure and fine nanopowder or nanoparticles [23–27].

There are many complex and interdependent parameters for self-propagating high-temperature synthesis, viz. the amount, composition and nano particle size, reaction purity, gas phase pressure, type, and amount of fuel of nanoparticles [23, 25]. In addition, other conditions are required here for the self-propagation high-temperature synthesis reactions of the critical reaction temperature (> 1500°C) [23].

To know the chemical reaction of Linear or SHS response, it is important to understand the nature of chemical reactions as SHS reactions are of the redox probes [23, 26]. Reducers such as iron, zinc and magnesium will reduce others by donating electrons [10, 23, 24]. The oxidizer in the SHS reaction is an electron receptor, while the fuel is an electron donor [26].

2.1.2 Volume Combustion Synthesis (VCS)

VCS is a established method for planning a wide range of materials due to its effortlessness, wide niche range, and potential to effectively obtain elements in an ideal structure. VCS is less controlled and is used for miserable exothermic reactions that require pre-heating. VCS involves a reaction in a homogeneous aqueous oxidizer-fuel setting, heated continuously by an external bioenergy source [28].

2.2 Solution Combustion Synthesis

The solution combustion synthesis (SCS) methods have drawn much interest in the scientific world as it is straightforward, simple, efficient, and fast process for the synthesis of porous structure nanomaterials. It can produce ceramics, metal oxides, sulfides, intermetallics, composites, and advanced functional materials in the range of 1–100 nm [29, 30]. The oxidizer, fuel, and temperature are three crucial components in the SCS process. As shown in Fig. 2, the process comprises of an exothermic chemical reaction between an oxidizer (metal nitrates) and a fuel (urea, glycine, sucrose, polyvinyl alcohol, etc.) combined in an aqueous solution and heated on hot plate [13, 31]. The fuels are rich in carbon and hydrogen and facilitate heat release by forming CO_2 and H_2O during the combustion process. In addition, they efficiently form complexes with metal ions, thereby improving the mixing level and preventing separation [11, 16, 23, 25, 32]. Forming a precursor in viscous liquid or gel is essential to mix the basic ingredients at the molecular level and prevent accidental redox reactions between the oxidizer and the fuel [23]. On the other hand, the fuel is expected to start combustion with an oxidizer at low ignition temperatures. The fuel, the amount of fuel, the pH of the starting solution, and the fuel/oxidizer ratio are critical parameters that affect the properties of the precursor [23]. The second stage in nanoparticles synthesis by SCS is automatic or auto-ignition, which derives from the highly exothermic nature of the reactions between glycine nitrate reactants, that facilitates the hot crystal generated during combustion. The crystallization and phase

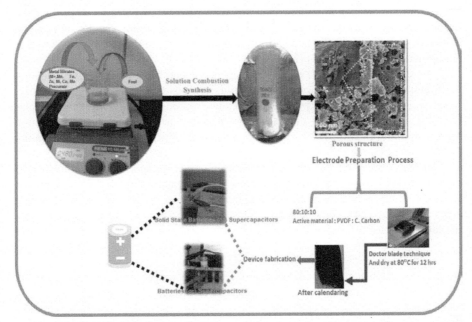

Fig. 2. Details of Solution combustion synthesis process to evaluate porous structure powder and electrode fabrication for energy storage applications.

formation occur in most of the cases of SCS, but it can increase crystal size, stiffness and specific surface area [23].

The advantages of solution combustion synthesis are:

1) Pure phase formation and high crystallinity
2) Controlled morphology
3) Porous nature
4) High surface area
5) Low temperature
6) Simple, cost effective and easily to handle while synthesizing nano materials
7) High yield (80–90%) and scalable nano powder

2.3 Fuels

The nanomaterials can be synthesized with the help of fuels (reducer) and metal nitrates (oxidizer) [28, 30, 33]. The fuel is an important component for preparing the porous structure of nano materials using solution combustion. The inorganic and organic fuels affect the properties of the final compound. The decrease in decomposition temperatures is also important due to the evolution of large amounts of gases. These gases help to produce enough heat distribution to create excess material porosity, good crystallinity, and cell aggregation [28, 29]. For example, porous structured $ZnMn_2O_4$ and $ZnMn_2O_4/rGO$ nanopowder were synthesized

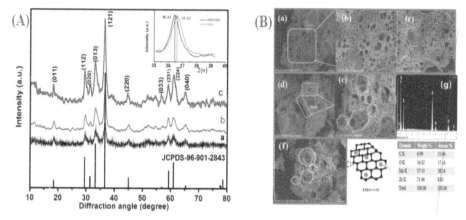

Fig. 3. (A and B) Reprinted with permission (Parameshwar Kommu et al. 2020). Copyright (2020) Material Science and Engineering B 261 (2020) 114647.

by SCS using sucrose as fuel. The crystallographic and morphological analysis confirms the formation of porous $ZnMn_2O_4$ and $ZnMn_2O_4/rGO$ nanopowder as is given in Fig. 3 (A&B) [34]. Here, the fuel is an important factor for changing the mechanism and dynamics of solution combustion synthesis. The choice of oxidant (metal nitrates) for the fuel ratio is the extremely crucial step that affects the behavior of the nanomaterials formed. The ratio of fuel to oxidizer is called "Ψ", which is defined as [10, 28, 35–37]

$$\Psi = \frac{Reducing\ valences(fuel)}{oxidizing\ valences(Metal\ Nitrate)} \quad (1)$$

$$X(NO_3)_2.\ XH_2O\ (oxidizing)\ +\ Fuel\ (reducing)\ \rightarrow\ XnO\ (Product)\ +\ CO_2(g)\ +\ N_2(g)\ +\ H_2O(g) \quad (2)$$

Here, "X" is metal nitrates (X = Li, Mn, Fe, Zn, Co, Mo, Ti, Sn, and Ce, etc.). Fuel can be urea, glycine, citric acid, sucrose, starch, or thiourea, etc., the solvent is water. The concentration of fuel plays a crucial role in controlling particle size, morphology, and specific surface area. The various types of fuels used in SCS method are given in Table 1. The reaction between zinc nitrate (Zn $(NO_3)_2.6H_2O$) and urea (NH_2-CO-NH_2) is provided in equation (3). Herein, elemental valency of Zn, Mn, C, H, N and O is +2, +4, +1, 0 and –2, as calculated based on propellant chemistry. Accordingly, the oxidizing valency of zinc nitrate and reducing valiancy of urea are –10 and +6, respectively. The stoichiometric equilibrium combustion reaction is expressed by the equation (3) [38].

$$Zn(NO_3)_2 + \frac{5}{3}\Psi NH_2 - CO - NH_2 + 5(\Psi - 1)O_2 \rightarrow ZnO + \frac{5\Psi + 3}{3}N_2(g) + \frac{5}{3}\Psi CO_2 + \frac{10}{3}\Psi HO_2(g) \quad (3)$$

Where, $\Psi = 1$ is stoichiometric state, $\Psi < 1$ and $\Psi > 1$ indicates fuel-lean and fuel-rich, respectively [29, 30]. The porous structure electrode material makes it very useful in electrochemical energy storage systems such as LIB, SIB and UCs. However, Li^+,

Table 1. Various types of fuels are used in SCs method.

Fuel	Chemical formula	Reducing valence
Sucrose	$C_{12}H_{22}O_{11}$	48
Glucose	$C_6H_{12}O_6$	24
Urea	$NH_2-CO-NH_2$	6
Hexamethylenetetramine	$C_6H_{12}N_4$	36
Glycine	$C_2H_5NO_2$	9
Ascorbic acid	$C_6H_8O_6$	20
Citric acid	$C_6H_8O_7$	18
Ethylene glycol	$C_2H_6O_2$	10
Hydrazine	N_2H_4	4
Hexamethylenetetramine	$C_6H_{12}N_4$	36
Alanine	$C_3H_7NO_2$	15
Acrylamide	C_3H_5NO	15
Aspartic acid	$C_4H_7NO_4$	15
Tartaric acid	$C_4H_6O_6$	10
Carbohydrazide	CH_6N_4O	8
Tryptophan	$C_{11}H_{12}N_2O_2$	52
Phenylalanine	$C_9H_{11}NO_2$	43
Arginine	$C_6H_{14}N_4O_2$	34
Triethanolamine	$C_6H_{15}NO_3$	33
Valine	$C_5H_{11}NO_2$	27
Glutamic acid	$C_5H_9NO_4$	21

Na^+, and K^+, etc. ions could allow more ions to adsorb onto electrode surface area and enhance charge-discharge performance of batteries and supercapacitors. Few porous structure electrode materials are given in Table 2.

Table 2. Porous structures' advanced electrode materials synthesis by solution combustion synthesis.

Fuel	Material	Structure	Applications	Ref.
Urea	$LiFePO_4/C$	Porous	Li-ion battery	[39]
CTAB and glycine as fuel	$LiFePO_4$	Hierarchical porous	Li-ion battery	[40]
Sucrose	$ZnMn_2O_4$ and $ZnMn_2O_4/rGO$	Porous	Li-ion battery and Supercapacitors	[34]
Glycine	$FeNi_3/NiFe_2O_4$	Microstructure with macropores	Hybrid capacitors	[41]
Glycine	NiS/rGO	Porous with spherical nanoparticles	Supercapacitors	[42]
Citric acid	Li_2MnO_3	Spongy morphology with pores	Li-ion battery	[43]
D-(+)-glucose	Co_3O_4	Porous	Li-ion battery	[44]

2.4 Oxidizers

A metal precursor contains a specific metal cation that adds metallic components to the final product by introducing that element into the combustion mixture. Oxynitrates, chlorides, and oxychlorides are more metal precursors. Chlorides should not be used since they may adsorb or seep into the powder, polluting it; instead, chlorides can be dissolved in concentrated nitric acid and heated to remove the chlorine produced by the procedure. Metal precursors for SCS might include oxalates, acetates, hydroxides, acetylacetonates, and alkoxides. At higher temperatures, metal sulphates and phosphates are stable, but they do not provide enough oxygen to burn. They are rarely regarded precursors to combustion processes for this reason [13]. Metal precursors are salts that contain oxidants, reducers, or neutrals as counter anions. An oxidant is a moiety that serves as an energy source in combustion and redox processes. Hydrated nitrates are an excellent choice for oxidants because of their high oxidizing power (negative charge), solubility in water and polar organic solvents, and low breakdown temperature. Metal precursors commonly contain oxidizing moieties in the form of counter anions [45]. Commercial nitrates, water-soluble and inexpensive, are the metal precursors of choice. As a reduction, the metal cation has a significant impact on the chemical makeup of the final product (positive charge). The counter anion (NO_3), on the other hand, acts as an oxidizing agent. The metal precursor utilized to introduce the metal into the combustion mixture impacts the combustion process, phase composition, and even the morphological features of the resultant powder. The following Table 3 lists some metal precursors for creating metal oxides utilized in combustion synthesis.

Table 3. Various types of oxidizers involved in SCs method.

Metal Oxidizer	Fuel	Material	Temp (°C)	Structure	Particle/ Crystallite Size (nm)	Ref.
$Co(NO_3)_2 \cdot 6H_2O$	Citric Acid	Co_3O_4	350	Nanoparticles	20	[46]
$(Fe(NO_3)_3 \cdot 9H_2O$	Glycine/Glucose	$\alpha\text{-}Fe_2O_3$	500	Nanosheets	18	[47]
$Mg(NO_3)_2$, $Mg(OH)_2$	Ethylene Glycol	MgO	600	Nano-size bubble-like holes	50 W, 200 L	[48]
$Ni(NO_3)_2 \cdot 6H_2O$	Glycine	NiO	470	Nanofoam	30	[49]
NH_4VO_3	Glycine/Citric Acid	V_2O_5	-	Nanospheres	200	[50]
$Fe(NO_3)_3$	Glycine	Fe_2O_3	300	Nanoneedles	100	[51]
$(NH_4)_6Mo_7O_{24} \cdot 4H_2O$	Urea	$\alpha\text{-}MoO_3$	200–600	Nanorods	50	[52]

3. Conclusion

Solution combustion synthesis is one of the simplest, cost-effective technique for producing various nanomaterials. Significantly, the production of nanostructured materials using solution combustion protocol was studied extensively. The applications of nanomaterials synthesized by combustion methodology were discussed briefly. Further, fuel and oxidizers' importance in combustion synthesis is explained with suitable examples.

Credit Authorship Contribution Statement

Parameshwar Kommu: Writing. **Divya Velpula, Shireesha Konda, Madhuri Sakaray and Rakesh Kumar Thida:** Data curation, Formal analysis. **Shilpa Chakra Chidurala, GP Singh, Arnab Shankar Bhattacharyya:** Supervisions, Conceptualization

Acknowledgements

One of the authors Parameshwar Kommu is thankful to Department of Nanotechnology, Central University of Jharkhand, India for financial support during PhD work. The authors also gratefully acknowledge F.No. CRG/2019/007040, DST SERB; File No: SP/YO/2019/1599, DST SYST and sanction no. SR/WOS-A/CS-13/2019, DST Women Scientist (WOS-A), New Delhi.

References

[1] V, D., S. K. and S. Chakra Ch. 2021. Impact of synthetic strategies for the preparation of polymers and metal-polymer hybrid composites in electrocatalysis applications. Synth Met. 282. https://doi.org/10.1016/j.synthmet.2021.116956.

[2] Ritchie, A.G. 2004. Recent developments and likely advances in lithium rechargeable batteries. J. Power Sources 136: 285–289. https://doi.org/10.1016/j.jpowsour.2004.03.013.

[3] Koohi-Fayegh, S. and M.A. Rosen. 2020. A review of energy storage types, applications and recent developments. J. Energy Storage 27: 101047. https://doi.org/10.1016/j.est.2019.101047.

[4] Divya, V., S. Mondal and M.V. Sangaranarayanan. 2018. Shape-controlled synthesis of palladium nanostructures from flowers to thorns: electrocatalytic oxidation of ethanol. J. Nanosci. Nanotechnol. 19: 758–769. https://doi.org/10.1166/jnn.2019.15752.

[5] Rakesh Kumar, T., C.H. Shilpa Chakra, S. Madhuri et al. 2021. Microwave-irradiated novel mesoporous nickel oxide carbon nanocomposite electrodes for supercapacitor application. J. Mater Sci. Mater. Electron. 32: 20374–20383. https://doi.org/10.1007/s10854-021-06547-5.

[6] Shireesha, K., V. Divya, G. Pranitha et al. 2021. A systematic investigation on the effect of reducing agents towards specific capacitance of NiMg@OH/reduced graphene oxide nanocomposites. Mater Technol 00: 1–13. https://doi.org/10.1080/10667857.2021.1995933.

[7] Shireesha, K., T.R. Kumar, T. Rajani et al. 2021. Novel NiMgOH-rGO-based nanostructured hybrids for electrochemical energy storage supercapacitor applications: Effect of reducing agents. Crystals 11. https://doi.org/10.3390/cryst11091144.

[8] Varma, A. and A.S. Mukasyan. 2004. Combustion synthesis of advanced materials: Fundamentals and applications. Korean J. Chem. Eng. 21: 527–536. https://doi.org/10.1007/BF02705444.

[9] Liu, G., J. Li and K. Chen. 2013. Combustion synthesis of refractory and hard materials: A review. Int. J. Refract Met. Hard Mater. 39: 90–102. https://doi.org/10.1016/j.ijrmhm.2012.09.002.

[10] Patil, K.C., S.T. Aruna and S. Ekambaram. 1997. Combustion synthesis. Curr. Opin. Solid State Mater Sci. 2: 158–165. https://doi.org/10.1016/s1359-0286(97)80060-5.

the researchers focus mainly on inexhaustible renewable solar energy and carbonous materials, because carbon is the most abundant and extensively available component after oxygen in the biosphere, which offers a foundation for the storage of renewable energy in the form of carbohydrates and other biopolymers. The current demand is for the development of advanced high-performance with cost-effective materials for practical use in energy storage devices like battery or supercapacitor and other means of energy storage/conversion. Meanwhile, a carbon based composite materials played a vital role in the development of renewable energy storage process and energy conversion like hydrogen storage, fuel cells, and as an effective electrode material for the Lithium ion battery and supercapacitor, respectively [3–5].

The conventional method for the development of carbonous materials (e.g., graphene, carbon nanotubes and activated carbon) was based on coal or petroleum products through tedious synthetic process and extensive energy consumption. Generally, activated carbon is produced from coal or other renewable resources via different process such as steam/CO_2 activation or by applying chemicals like $ZnCl_2$, H_3PO_4 and KOH, etc. The carbon nanotubes and graphene is produced by chemical vapor deposition or electric-arc-discharge techniques. The practical implication of using above mentioned techniques cannot be implicated as it requires high temperature and tedious chemical process which restricts the large-scale production and industrial application. Since it is highly expensive and also not suitable for environment, it is the demand of scientific community to develop a new technique/method for the production of carbonous material in cost-effective manner. The feedstock materials for the production of biochar is cost-effective and abundant with respect to other materials. The production of biochar requires less energy consumption, is economically viable and robust which not only fulfills the requirement of energy but also reduces the environmental stress [6, 7]. Therefore, the biochar carbon materials are considered as potential replacement of above-mentioned carbon materials (graphene and CNT, etc.) due to their abundant availability and renewable nature. However, there is no fundamental difference between the activated carbon and biochar materials as both have amorphous matrix with huge porosity as well. The basic difference between them is the existence of enormous functional group at the surface of biochar as compared to the other carbon materials. The conventional method employed for the production of carbon from fossils emitted huge amount CO_2 that can be mitigated by the production of biochar from biomass. Generally, biomass is composed of cellulose, hemicellulose, pentoses, hexoses and uronic acid, etc. The biomass can easily be pyrolyzed at low temperature and it starts decomposing at the temperature ranges from 200–260°C. However, researchers reported that the biochar obtained at low temperature is not suitable for energy storage and conversion field including Li/Na ion batteries and so on due to the low surface area and poor pore volume [1]. Before their practical implication, the surface has to be functionalized and activated by addition of suitable reagents or techniques.

During last few decades, biochar-based materials attracted attention in field of energy storage and other means of conversion because the surface chemistry and porosity can easily be tuned up. Ample researchers provide a mechanism that

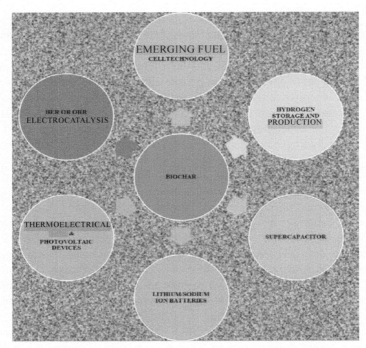

Fig. 1. Schematic representation of biochar based functional material for probable electrochemical storage application and conversion field.

energy storage and conversion involves mainly physical and chemical interaction between the interface and surface. As activity of energy storage is very much dependent on the surface morphology and porosity of materials, biochar plays an important role in developing new and advanced electrode material for energy storage system. The surface functional groups greatly influence the thermodynamics of the heterogeneous reaction that occurs at the interface when the transition of phases is taking place whereas the porosity can limit the extent of kinetics and rate of physical and chemical reaction. The biochar-based electrode materials are not only used in the supercapacitor or lithium-ion batteries but it can also be used as the other means of energy storage like hydrogen storage and production, fuel cells and oxygen production, respectively. The potential application of biochar-based nanocomposite materials is enlisted in Fig. 1.

2. Working Principles of Ball Milling and Its Parameters

Ball milling is a class of grinder that works on the impact and attrition used to grind the materials for the defect formation and size adjustment of solid materials. A ball mill consists of hollow cylindrical shell rotating about its axis and is partially filled with the requisite mass of balls. The solid can be adjusted into small size through grinding media which may be made of stainless steel, ceramics, zirconia, tungsten carbide, etc. In research, it is basically used for the adjustment of size of solid grain particle in nanoscale ranges. During the course, a high-energy mill is employed and specific powder charge is placed along with milling medium. The mass of sample and balls are fixed in specific ratio to maintain the size of particles. The kinetic energy produced during the motion is responsible for breaking of chemical bond in powder and reducing the particles' size. Several chemicals, including melamine, carboxylic acid, ammonium bicarbonate, magnesium, hexane, yttrium carbon dioxide, dry ice, etc., have been used to mill together with carbon powder in order to affect the properties of the biochar when functionalized moieties are applied. The parameters which govern the process of ball milling are types of mills (i.e., planetary ball mills, tumbler ball mills, vibratory and attrition mill), which decide the intensity of kinetic energy executed over the carbonous powder. The different types of ball mills are shown in Fig. 2(b). The major advantages of this process are as follows: -

i) It can be performed at room temperature.

ii) It can be used for both wet and dry sample.

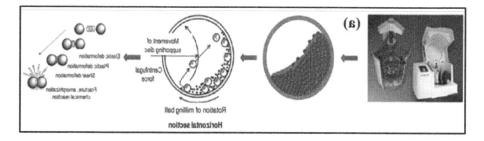

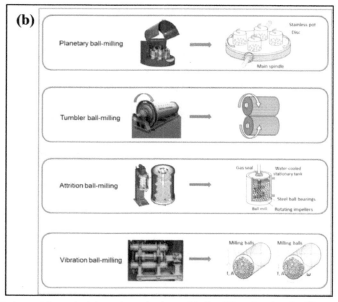

Fig. 2. (a) Basic working principle and mechanism of ball milling (reprinted with permission [8]). (b) Different types of ball mills (reprinted with permission [8]).

iii) It is used for grinding the toxic materials and can be performed in inert atmosphere as well.

iv) The heat generated during grinding is much less than that of other chemical approaches.

v) The grinding speed and time are the influencing factors on properties of catalyst in the ball milling method and also problems like caking, overheating, and high temperature safety do not exist in this method.

Along with all the advantages, this process has several disadvantages also, like it is a noisy machine, very slow process, and it cannot be employed for the soft, tacky and fibrous materials. The general working principle and mechanism of ball milling is presented in Fig. 2(a).

3. Synthesis/Preparation of Biochar Using Ball Mill

The properties and functionalities of the materials are determined by compositional and structural characteristics. The percentage of carbon content depends upon the environment. In the oxygen restricted mode, the biochar material comprises of high carbon content produced by pyrolysis of feedstock with specific temperature ranges of 300 to 1000°C. From the reported data, it has been concluded that the different feedstock treated with varying temperature comprises of different chemical composition and structure [6]. Feedstock has been classified into three different group, i.e., non-traditional material, agricultural waste, and forestry. The preparation of biochar is generally carried out by using agricultural waste and forestry waste due to its easy availability and cost-effectiveness. The residue like wood chips, rice husk, rice-straws, corn straws, and other biowaste are produced each year by agricultural and human activities. The researchers have reported that low-cost biochar is synthesized by the biomass origin consisting of large number of lignin and cellulose content. The preparation of biochar by using different feedstock has been presented in Fig. 3.

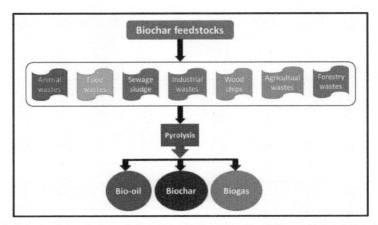

Fig. 3. Schematic representation of formation of biochar using different feedstock (reprints with permission) [6].

The emerging interest for applying biochar in various application has drawn its great attention to the researchers for the conversion of biomass to biochar. In lieu of this, ball milling is the most suitable and economically viable process for the production of biochar as it does not require any external sources of energy and tedious process. It is an energy efficient and ecofriendly procedure to synthesize nanomaterials including biochar. From the report, it is assumed that carbon-based materials treated in ball milling have higher absorption capability, functional groups and environmental concern. The surface functional group of biochar can be tuned by ball milling process which help in the wide area of application. The surface properties and stability of the biochar can be tuned by introducing suitable heteroatom having excess of functional group. The process of optimization of ball milling parameters has great importance for the synthesis of biochar or biochar-based composite materials for customizing the functionality and performances. The particle size of the biochar can be tuned by controlling the speed of balling and reaction time. Thus, the selection of ball milling process condition should take into consideration the desired properties of biochar products, interaction with solvent and stabilizer as well as cost and environmental impact.

4. Biochar-based Composite Materials for Batteries

In the past few decades, tremendous development has taken place in the research on renewable energy production systems and their efficient storage. These renewable energy systems mitigate the eco-hazards and uphold the environmental sustainability. With this perspective, several renewable energy storages have been developed and these are lithium-ion, lead-acid, zinc-bromine, lithium-polymer, and solid-state batteries. Among them, superior attention has been devoted to the lithium-ion batteries' (LIBs) research that successfully meets the commercial perspective in numerous portable as well as electrical devices. In addition to that, there has been further growth in the development of sodium-ion (SIBs) and lithium-sulfur batteries (Li-S) as well, which can be considered as a superior alternate system compared to LIBs [9–11]. The electrochemistry of SIBs is similar to the LIBs. Li-S system also exhibits excellent energy density than the LIBs. Most of the commercial LIBs contain graphite, Li-based metal oxides/phosphates and 1 M $LiPF_6$ in carbonate solvents, which are used as anode, cathode and electrolyte, respectively. It is noteworthy that to attain full performance of both LIBs and SIBs, contribution from anode part is imperative and efficient. However, few risk are yet to be researched further at anode section such as safety accidents due to the formation of dendrite, and strict volume changes in charging/discharging process. This can be attributed to the in-homogeneity in surface of active anode via cracks and voids, etc. [12, 13]. Moreover, exploitation of conventional graphite as anode in LIBs is incessantly increasing, which will lead to a shortage of graphite resources in future. Thereby, price of the same will be improved and comes under the critical supply risk material. In order to address these challenges, extensive research has been proposed on the synthesis of bio-char and related materials as a proficient anode in upcoming storage operations. Hence offering a fresh alternative and suggestions for the development of biochar anodes with better storage capabilities. For instance, Li and co-workers [9] have attempted to modify the porous and surface tuning properties of the charcoal via ball-milling approach with thermal treatment. The modified charcoal is utilized as anode for both SIBs and LIBs and delivers the supreme charge storage behavior. They have attained higher specific capacity of 257 mAhg^{-1} and 109 mAhg^{-1} for LIBs and SIBs, respectively. Both LIBs and SIBs demonstrate the sufficient capacity retention of 97.6% and 92.7%, which substantiates impact of tailoring the charcoal surface in order to obtain good cycling performance. On the one hand, cost-effective and environmental benefit biochar from chitin biopolymer is successfully obtained and elucidated by Magnacca et al. [11]. As-prepared biochar is investigated as positive electrode material in Li-S batteries and also delivers the higher specific surface area of 333 m^{2}g^{-1}. From the galvanostatic charging/discharging measurements, highest discharge capacity of 905 mAhg^{-1} is obtained and also reveals the stable storage performance over several cycles. The stable electrochemical properties might be due to the rest of oxygen and nitrogen functionalities, and have strong chemisorption affinity for lithium polysulphides. The conductivity tuning of lignin feedstock-based biochar material is studied by Seth Kane and co-workers [14]. The lignin biochar is expected to demonstrate nearly equal electrical conductivity value compared to carbon black. They have analyzed the electrical conductivity with the use of three different biomass sources including wheat stem and cellulose with different experimental condition. As prepared biochar materials have the similar range of electrical conductivity and the range is 0.002 to 18.5 S/m. In order to further increase the conductivity of lignin biochar, content of oxygen percentage has to be reduced. More interestingly, miscanthus based biocarbon material is prepared by pyrolysis and ball milling route. As milled biocarbon shows that the heterogeneous shape and average size of particle has been reduced to less than 1 μm at higher milling time. Also, specific surface area of miscanthus biocarbon is doubled and the value is found to be 300 m^{2}g^{-1}. The ball milled biocarbon displays the thermal conductivity of 0.116 W/mK [15]. More importantly, nitrogen (N) doped chitosan based biochar is synthesized by Nistico and workers [16]. The low-cost N-rich chitosan derived biochar material is thermally, morphologically and electrochemically studied with several analytical techniques. Finally, it plays a role as cathode host in Li-S batteries. The test result indicates that the biochar/sulfur cathode shows the superior initial discharge capacity (1330 mAhg^{-1}) and good rate capability strength. The obtained biochar electrochemical result is consistent with the reference MWCNT substrate performance. This enhanced storage property is due to encapsulation of sulfur compound into active N-rich biochar via porous system, thereby presenting a good homogeneity of the same. Reproducible N-doped agaric biochar with low-cost and extremely porous structure is synthesized and reported by Gu and co-workers [17]. The N-doped agaric carbon reveals the higher specific surface area of 1568.2 m^{2}g^{-1} and further assists the Li-ion storage properties. Thus, it helps to attain maximum reversible capacity of 875 mAh/g at 0.2 C over multiple cycles and retention capacity of 620 mAh/g at 2 C rate, which substantiates the reversibility and rate capability of the Li-S device. The overwhelmed storage might be ascribed to the porous nature of N-doped biochar thereby accommodating more ions as well as active sulfur and polysulfides. Also, construction of conducting carbon skeletal network of N-doped agaric biochar supplies the constructive migration pathways and superior transportation of ions and electrons. Likewise, milled silica particles incorporated into chitosan based biocarbon material have been implemented as anode in LIBs, reported by Prasanna et al. [18]. As prepared biocarbon embedded with silica particles reveals higher performance than the bare silica material. The highest discharge capacity of 942.4 mAhg^{-1} at 0.1 C rate, and columbic efficiency of 97% after several cycles is obtained. Lyu et al. [19] have reported that the ball-milled biochar exhibits the electrical conductivity of 9210 μScm^{-1} whereas unmilled biochar delivers the conductivity of 1054 μScm^{-1}. The ball-milled biochar presents superior conductivity which is nine times greater than the unmilled biochar. As a matter of fact, ball-milled and thermally assisted eggshell collagen has been employed as additive material in LIBs, investigated by Chang Won Ho and co-workers [20]. Here, eggshell membrane is effectively converted into eco-friendly biochar material for storage applications. Eggshell derived N-doped biochar is also prepared via solid-state route and thermal treatment. The N-doped biochar is fruitfully coated on the lithium iron phosphate cathode, thereby revealing the excellent ionic and electronic conductivity due to synergetic effect of the same. Thus, it contributes to the sufficient transport kinetics of Li-ion and lesser charge transfer resistance. As a result, stable discharge capacity of 125 mAhg^{-1} is achieved for N-doped biochar/cathode whereas bare cathode shows the lower value of capacity (110 mAhg^{-1}). Based on these findings, research on biochar materials provide new guidance to global communities to use as an alternate as well as promising material for futuristic greener storage devices as shown in Fig. 4.

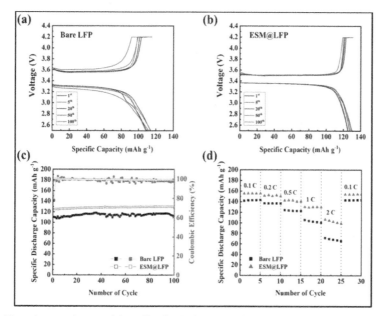

Fig. 4. The galvanostatic potential profiles for (a) bare LFP, (b) ESM@LFP, (c) cycling performance profiles showing discharge capacity and its columbic efficiency of bare LFP and ESM@LFP for 100 cycles between the voltage window of 2.5–4.2 V at a current rate of 1C, and (d) rate capability profiles of bare LFP and ESM@LFP. Reprinted with permission [20].

5. Biochar-based Composite Materials for Supercapacitor

Supercapacitor is the energy storage device, which offers promising approach towards the storage of clean and renewable energy. It is also known as ultracapacitor which attracts a considerable attention due to its long life-cycle, high power and energy density with an excellent reversibility [21, 22]. The numerous researchers/scientific community have well demonstrated about the biochar based composite materials as electrode for supercapacitor application with different process. Currently, researchers are very much keen on the recent development of biochar based composite materials from agricultural waste by using ball milling process as it is economically viable and eco-friendly in nature for the industrial development. The biochar based composite material has drawn attention towards the development of suitable electrode in the field of electrochemistry [23]. Herein, the biochar based composite materials as supercapacitor have been discussed. In search of this, Thines et al. [24] developed biochar based composite materials as high-performance supercapacitor. They have developed high porosity use of biochar by impregnating with three different metallic salts at temperature 800°C for 25 minutes. They have fabricated biochar-based electrode materials for supercapacitor by support of PANI (polyaniline). The electrochemical study has been done by using conventional three-electrode system where they found an ultra-specific capacitance of 615 F/g at the scan rate of 10 mV/s with energy density of 76.88 Wh/kg. The ultrahigh specific capacitance comprises of the synergistic effect of biochar and PANI. Tulakarn Ketwong and co-workers demonstrated CuO loaded biochar electrode materials and its comparative study with different electrolyte (KOH, Na_2SO_4). The electrochemical study of this composite has been performed in conventional three-electrode system using 2 M KOH and 1 M Na_2SO_4. The electrochemical properties of electrode materials showed better results in 2 M KOH than that of Na_2SO_4. The electrode materials exhibited an excellent specific capacitance of 495 and 274 Fg^{-1} for 2 M KOH and 1 M Na_2SO_4 respectively. They have also examined the cyclic stability/retention of electrode materials in 5000 cycles where 92.7% capacitance retention is observed. Similarly, Nirmaladevi and co-workers [25] developed wood-based biochar supported MnO_2 nanorods for high energy asymmetric supercapacitor. The successful formation and surface morphology of the prepared composite has been characterized with the help of various physico-chemical techniques. FESEM (Field emission scanning electron microscope) spectroscopic techniques reveal that the composite material has porous nature and bundle of nanorod like morphologies. The high surface area and morphologies are suitable for the electrochemical application. Hence, they have also tuned the electrochemical performances of composite by using three electrode system in 1 M Na_2SO_4 as electrolytic solution. In three electrode system. The specific capacitance in a three electrode system is 512 Fg^{-1} at 0.5 Ag^{-1} with an outstanding cyclic stability of 93% after 10,000 cycles. On the basis of three electrode results, they have also examined electrochemical performances in two electrode system. They have assembled asymmetric device which delivers huge energy density of 74.3 $Whkg^{-1}$ and power density of 1996 Wkg^{-1}. On the basis of observed electrochemical properties, the biochar based composite

[6] Zhao, Y., S.A. Qamar, M. Qamar, M. Bilal and H.M.N. Iqbal. 2021. Sustainable remediation of hazardous environmental pollutants using biochar-based nanohybrid materials. J. Environ. Manage. 300: 113762.

[7] Ahmed, M.J. and B.H. Hameed. 2020. Insight into the co-pyrolysis of different blended feedstocks to biochar for the adsorption of organic and inorganic pollutants: A review. J. Clean. Prod. 265: 121762.

[8] Kumar, M., X. Xiong, Z. Wan, Y. Sun, D.C.W. Tsang, J. Gupta, B. Gao, X. Cao, J. Tang and Y.S. Ok. 2020. Ball milling as a mechanochemical technology for fabrication of novel biochar nanomaterials. Bioresour. Technol. 312: 123613.

[9] Li, M., W.-Y. Tsai, B.P. Thapaliya, H.M. Meyer, III, B.L. Armstrong, H. Luo, S. Dai, J. Nanda and I. Belharouak. 2021. Modified coal char materials with high rate performance for battery applications. Carbon N. Y. 172: 414–21.

[10] Li, M., Du, Z., Khaleel, M.A. and Belharouak, I. 2020. Materials and engineering endeavors towards practical sodium-ion batteries. Energy Storage Mater. 25: 520–36.

[11] Magnacca, G., F. Guerretta, A. Vizintin, P. Benzi, M.C. Valsania and R. Nisticò. 2018. Preparation, characterization and environmental/electrochemical energy storage testing of low-cost biochar from natural chitin obtained via pyrolysis at mild conditions. Appl. Surf. Sci. 427: 883–93.

[12] Perumal, P., P. Sivaraj, K.P. Abhilash, G.G. Soundarya, P. Balraju and P.C. Selvin. 2020. Green synthesized spinel lithium titanate nano anode material using Aloe Vera extract for potential application to lithium ion batteries. J. Sci. Adv. Mater. Devices 5: 346–53.

[13] Perumal, P., T. Kiruthika, P. Sivaraj, D. Lakshmi and P.C. Selvin. 2020. Tamarind seed polysaccharide biopolymer-assisted synthesis of spinel zinc iron oxide as a promising alternate anode material for lithium-ion batteries. J. Mater. Sci. Mater. Electron. 31: 10593–604.

[14] Kane, S., R. Ulrich, A. Harrington, N.P. Stadie and C. Ryan. 2021. Physical and chemical mechanisms that influence the electrical conductivity of lignin-derived biochar. Carbon Trends 5: 100088.

[15] Wang, T., A. Rodriguez-Uribe, M. Misra and A.K. Mohanty. 2018. Sustainable carbonaceous biofiller from miscanthus: Size reduction, characterization, and potential bio-composites applications. BioResources 13: 3720–39.

[16] Nistico, R., F. Guerretta, P. Benzi and G. Magnacca. 2020. Chitosan-derived biochars obtained at low pyrolysis temperatures for potential application in electrochemical energy storage devices. Int. J. Biol. Macromol. 164: 1825–31.

[17] Gu, X., H. Li, H. Wen, Y. Zhou, H. Kang, H. Liao, M. Gao, Y. Wang, L. Deng and X. Yi. 2020. From agaric hydrogel to nitrogen-doped 3D porous carbon for high-performance Li–S batteries. J. Mater. Sci. 55: 1136–47.

[18] Prasanna, K., T. Subburaj, Y.N. Jo, P. Santhoshkumar, S.K.S.S. Karthikeyan, K. Vediappan, R.M. Gnanamuthu and C.W. Lee. 2019. Chitosan complements entrapment of silicon inside nitrogen doped carbon to improve and stabilize the capacity of Li-ion batteries. Sci. Rep. 9: 1–13.

[19] Lyu, H., Z. Yu, B. Gao, F. He, J. Huang, J. Tang and B. Shen. 2019. Ball-milled biochar for alternative carbon electrode. Environ. Sci. Pollut. Res. 26: 14693–702.

[20] Ho, C.W., N. Shaji, H.K. Kim, J.W. Park, M. Nanthagopal and C.W. Lee. 2022. Thermally assisted conversion of biowaste into environment-friendly energy storage materials for lithium-ion batteries. Chemosphere 286: 131654.

[21] Raj, B., R. Oraon, M. Mohapatra, S. Basu and A.K. Padhy. 2020. Development of SnO₂@ rGO hybrid nanocomposites through complexometric approach for multi-dimensional electrochemical application. J. Electrochem. Soc. 167: 167518.

[22] Raj, B., A.K. Padhy, S. Basu and M. Mohapatra. 2020. Futuristic direction for R&D challenges to develop 2D advanced materials based supercapacitors. J. Electrochem. Soc. 167: 136501.

[23] Norouzi, O., F. Di Maria and A. Dutta. 2020. Biochar-based composites as electrode active materials in hybrid supercapacitors with particular focus on surface topography and morphology. J. Energy Storage 29: 101291.

[24] Thines, K.R., E.C. Abdullah, M. Ruthiraan, N.M. Mubarak and M. Tripathi. 2016. A new route of magnetic biochar based polyaniline composites for supercapacitor electrode materials. J. Anal. Appl. Pyrolysis 121: 240–57.

[25] Nirmaladevi, S., R. Boopathiraja, S.K. Kandasamy, S. Sathishkumar and M. Parthibavarman. 2021. Wood based biochar supported MnO_2 nanorods for high energy asymmetric supercapacitor applications. Surfaces and Interfaces 27: 101548.

[26] Kiminaitė, I., A. Lisauskas, N. Striūgas and Ž. Kryževičius. 2022. Fabrication and characterization of environmentally friendly biochar anode. Energies 15: 112.

[27] Yu, J., Y. Zhao and Y. Li. 2014. Utilization of corn cob biochar in a direct carbon fuel cell. J. Power Sources 270: 312–7.

[28] Wu, H., J. Xiao, S. Hao, R. Yang, P. Dong, L. Han, M. Li, F. Yu, Y. Xie and J. Ding. 2021. *In-situ* catalytic gasification of kelp-derived biochar as a fuel for direct carbon solid oxide fuel cells. J. Alloys Compd. 865: 158922.

[29] Xie, Y., J. Xiao, Q. Liu, X. Wang, J. Liu, P. Wu and S. Ouyang. 2021. Highly efficient utilization of walnut shell biochar through a facile designed portable direct carbon solid oxide fuel cell stack. Energy 227: 120456.

[30] Qiu, Q., M. Zhou, W. Cai, Q. Zhou, Y. Zhang, W. Wang, M. Liu and J. Liu. 2019. A comparative investigation on direct carbon solid oxide fuel cells operated with fuels of biochar derived from wheat straw, corncob, and bagasse. Biomass and bioenergy 121: 56–63.

[31] Lobato-Peralta, D.R., E. Duque-Brito, H.I.V. Vidales, A. Longoria, P.J. Sebastian, A.K. Cuentas-Gallegos, C.A. Arancibia-Bulnes and P.U. Okoye. 2021. A review on trends in lignin extraction and valorization of lignocellulosic biomass for energy applications. J. Clean. Prod. 126123.

[32] Sevilla, M. and R. Mokaya. 2014. Energy storage applications of activated carbons: supercapacitors and hydrogen storage. Energy Environ. Sci. 7: 1250–80.

[33] Mohan, M., V.K. Sharma, E.A. Kumar and V. Gayathri. 2019. Hydrogen storage in carbon materials—A review. Energy Storage 1: e35.

[34] Yeboah, M.L., X. Li and S. Zhou. 2020. Facile fabrication of biochar from palm kernel shell waste and its novel application to magnesium-based materials for hydrogen storage. Materials (Basel) 13: 625.

[35] Arshad, S.H.M., N. Ngadi, A.A. Aziz, N.S. Amin, M. Jusoh and S. Wong. 2016. Preparation of activated carbon from empty fruit bunch for hydrogen storage. J. Energy Storage 8: 257–61.

[36] Heo, Y.-J. and S.-J. Park. 2015. Synthesis of activated carbon derived from rice husks for improving hydrogen storage capacity. J. Ind. Eng. Chem. 31: 330–4.

[37] Ramesh, T., N. Rajalakshmi and K.S. Dhathathreyan. 2015. Activated carbons derived from tamarind seeds for hydrogen storage. J. Energy Storage 4: 89–95.

13

Nanofabrication Using Natural Flavonoids for Biomedical Applications

Prasanti Sharma,[1] *Neelima Sharma,*[1,*] *Trishna Bal*[1] and
Gayatri Thapa[2]

1. Introduction

The recent decade has seen tremendous progress in the field of nanotechnology, especially in the biomedical field. Nanofabrication has taken amazing strides with respect to drug delivery and therapeutics along with providing solutions to a number of obstacles in the area of science and research. Compared to their bulk form, nanoparticles (NPs) have higher catalytic and biological activity, thermal conductivity, non-linear optical performance, and chemical stability because of their huge surface area to volume ratio. Owing to these properties, NPs are used in various sectors such as medicine [1], food technology [2], space [3], chemistry [4], cosmetic industries [5] and agriculture [6]. Nanoparticle synthesis can be done in a variety of ways, including physical, chemical, and biological approaches. Chemical methods include sol-gel technique, redox and hydrothermal processes. Physical methods include sonication, laser ablation, radiation and electro deposition while biological methods include nanoparticles synthesized from plants and micro-organisms [7]. The chemical and physical approaches are appropriate for the production of large amounts of particles within a short span of time with predetermined shapes and sizes, but they have the disadvantage of being difficult, costly, inefficient and out of date. These techniques pose a threat of toxicity and pollution as they emit harmful

[1] Department of Pharmaceutical Sciences and Technology, Birla Institute of Technology, Mesra-835215, India.

[2] Department of Pharmacology, Himalayan Pharmacy Institute, Sikkim-737136, India.

* Corresponding author: nsharma@bitmesra.ac.in, neelimarsharma@hotmail.com

by-products that are potentially detrimental to the environment [8]. Furthermore, NPs synthesized using such hazardous procedures are unsuited for medical use.

To overcome these issues, recent years have witnessed a surge in interest towards developing techniques that do not involve the generation of hazardous by-products as part of the fabrication process. This task was achieved by implementing procedures that involve the use of green chemistry as a replacement for physical and chemical methods—a concept now known as "green synthesis".

Green nanosynthesis involves the use of naturally derived plants, plant extracts and their by-products such as proteins, lipids, alkaloids, and flavonoids and microorganisms (viruses, bacteria, fungi, and algae) for the development of safe and non-toxic nanoparticles by applying different biotechnology tools and techniques [9–13]. Green technology creates NPs that are superior than those generated by conventional methods because of a number of factors that include the use of cost-effective chemicals, less energy expenditure and the production of ecologically friendly products and by-products [14, 15]. Green synthesis of NPs uses a bottom-up approach involving the reducing and stabilizing agents. It is based on a redox mechanism in which an organism, plant, plant extract or its phytoconstituent reduces metal ions to stable NPs. There are three main factors that need to be taken into account while considering green nano-synthesis: the selection of a solvent medium, an environmentally safe and benign reducing agent and a nontoxic substance as a capping agent to stabilize the manufactured NPs [16]. Even though living organisms, such as fungi, algae, bacteria and plants can be exploited for the synthesis of NPs *in vivo*, plant extract-mediated *in vitro* green synthesis of NPs has gained appeal due to its simplicity, low cost, environmentally benign nature and ease of scale-up. The number of papers on green-synthesized nanoparticles is currently expanding at an exponential rate. The synthesis of NPs can be achieved using plant extracts as well as isolated components. The ability of plant extracts to reduce metal ions may be explained by the widespread presence of phenolic compounds as part of the extract. In context of the importance of plant extracts in mediating the synthesis of NPs, this chapter attempts to highlight and summarize the current state and prospective uses of the green synthesis with special emphasis on plant flavonoids contributing to the process.

2. Techniques Used for Nanofabrication

2.1 Conventional Approaches

There are two main conventional approaches for the synthesis of nanomaterials:

2.1.1 Top-down Approach

The top-down approach begins with macroscopic structures. It is a destructive process that begins with larger particles being reduced to nanoparticles after a series of procedures applied to them. The larger molecules (bulk material) are decomposed into smaller molecules and then the smaller particles are transformed into nanosized particles. The main disadvantages of these technologies are that they require vast installations and a lot of money to set up. The methods are highly costly and unsuitable for large-scale production; thus, they are often used

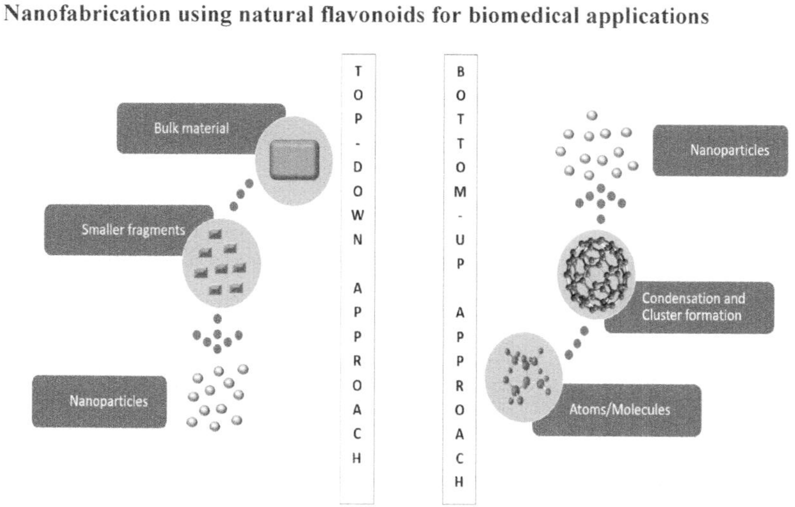

Nanofabrication using natural flavonoids for biomedical applications

Fig. 1. Approaches of nanoparticle synthesis.

primarily in laboratory experiments. These methods are not suitable for soft samples. Figure 1 provides the graphical representation of this approach. Examples of methods in top-down approach are mechanical milling, lithography, thermal decomposition, etching, laser ablation, sputtering and electro-explosion, etc.

2.1.2 Bottom-up Approach

Bottom-up approach of nanomaterial synthesis is a constructive process that constitutes miniaturization of materials to the atomic level consequently leading to the development of nanostructures. The method is principally based on the principle of molecular recognition (self-assembly). Figure 1 provides a graphical representation of this approach. Many of these approaches are still in development or are only starting to be employed for commercial nanoparticle synthesis. The methods used in bottom-up approach include sol-gel synthesis, pyrolysis, colloidal precipitation, hydrothermal synthesis, organometallic chemical route, electrodeposition, chemical reduction and green synthesis, etc.

2.2 Physical Methods

2.2.1 Mechanical Milling

Mechanical milling is a low-cost approach for fabricating nanoscale structures from bulk materials. Planetary, vibratory, rod and tumbler are the forms of mills employed. Hard steel or carbide balls are enclosed in the container. This process is used to make nanocrystalline Co, Cr, W, and Ag-Fe. The ball-to-materials ratio is 2:1. The container is filled with inert gas or air and rotated rapidly around its axis. The materials are pushed between the container›s walls and the balls. Milling speed and time are important factors in producing nanoparticles of the right size [17, 18].

2.2.2 Pulse Laser Ablation

Nanoparticles are produced utilizing a powerful laser beam that hits the target material. The precursor or target vaporizes due to the high intensity laser irradiation, resulting in nanoparticle formation. This process can develop a wide variety of nanomaterials, including metal nanoparticles, carbon nanomaterials, oxide composites and ceramics [19, 20].

2.2.3 Arc Discharge Method

It is a physical method that is most extensively used for producing metal nanoparticles. A pulsated current vaporizes a metal wire, resulting in a vapour that is then cooled by ambient gas to process nanoparticles. This scheme has a high fabrication speed and high energy productivity [21, 22].

2.2.4 Sputtering

Sputtering is a technique for making nanomaterials that involves hitting solid surfaces with high-energy particles like plasma or gas. Sputtering can be accomplished in a variety of methods, including using a magnetron, a radio-frequency diode or a DC diode. Sputtering is typically carried out in an evacuated chamber into which the sputtering gas is injected. Free electrons collide with the gas and form gas ions when a high voltage is supplied to the cathode target. The positively charged ions move rapidly in the electric field towards the cathode target, which they repeatedly strike, causing atoms to be ejected off the target's surface. The sputtering technique is intriguing because the composition of sputtered nanomaterials is similar to that of the target material while containing fewer contaminants [23–25].

2.3 Chemical Methods

2.3.1 Sol-gel Method

Sol-gel is a method for producing solid materials from small molecules. It is a wet-chemical method for creating several types of high-quality metal-oxide based nanoparticles. In this chemical procedure, the sol (or solution) is the liquid precursor that leads to the production of a gel-like diphasic system with both a liquid and solid phase, with the morphologies of the nanoparticles formed ranging from discrete particles to a continuous polymer network. Metal alkoxides are commonly used as precursors in the sol–gel process for the creation of nanomaterials. The sol–gel method for production of nanoparticles can be performed in multiple steps that mainly comprises of hydrolysis, condensation, aging, drying and finally calcination [26, 27].

2.3.2 Hydrothermal Synthesis

One of the most well-known and widely used processes for producing nanostructured materials is the hydrothermal process. Nanostructured materials are created using the hydrothermal process, which involves a heterogeneous reaction in an aqueous medium at high pressure and temperature near the critical point in a sealed vessel. The solvothermal technique is similar to the hydrothermal technique. The only distinction is that it takes place in a non-aqueous environment. Hydrothermal and solvothermal methods are appealing because it can be used for creating various nano-geometries of materials, such as nanowires, nanorods, nanospheres and nanosheets [28, 29].

2.3.3 Co-precipitation Method

Nucleation, growth, coarsening, and/or agglomeration processes all occur at the same time in coprecipitation reactions. In this approach, the precursors are usually inorganic salts (nitrate, chloride, sulphate, and so on) that are dissolved in water or any other appropriate media to generate a homogenous solution with ion clusters. To drive such salts to precipitate as hydroxides or oxalates, the solution is treated to pH modification or evaporation. The concentration of salt, temperature, the actual pH, and the rate of pH change all influence crystal formation and aggregation. The solid nanomaterials thus formed are then collected after precipitation, cleaning and progressive drying by heating to the medium's boiling point. The washing and drying techniques used for co-precipitated hydroxides have an impact on the degree of agglomeration in the final powder [30, 31].

2.3.4 Inert Gas Condensation

Metal nanoparticles are mostly made using this method. This is an inactive gas compression technique which produces fine nanoparticles by dispersing a metallic source in an inert gas. Metals are vaporized at an acceptable pace at a temperature that can be reached. Metal nanoparticles are synthesized inside a chamber containing argon, helium, or neon (inert gases) where the vaporization of metal atoms takes place thereby forming nanoparticles of the respective metal used for dispersion. Liquid nitrogen cools the gases, forming nanoparticles of the metal being considered in the range of 2–100 nm [31].

2.3.5 Sonochemical Synthesis

It is based on acoustic cavitations that involve the development, growth and implosive collapse of bubbles in liquids. Bubbles in solutions are implosively deflated by acoustic fields where they are exposed to severe ultrasonic irradiation. At the centres of the bubbles, high-temperature and high-pressure fields are created. The implosive collapse of the bubbles causes adiabatic compression or shock wave production within the gas phase of the falling bubbles, resulting in a localized hotspot. In certain circumstances, the end product is nano amorphous particles, whereas in others, it is nanocrystalline. The temperature in the ring region where the reaction occurs determines type of end product formed [32].

2.4 Biological Methods

2.4.1 Synthesis Using Microorganisms

This method utilizes multicellular and unicellular organisms like bacteria [33], fungi [34], viruses [35], algae [36] and yeasts [37] for the formation of nanoparticles. There are two techniques of nanofabrication using micro-organisms: extracellular and intracellular biosynthesis. The synthesis of nanoparticles by various microbes is a consequence of development of resistance mechanisms to a specific metal that may result in them becoming less toxic. This happens through two processes: bioreduction and biosorption. For example, the bacterium *Rhodopseudomonas capsulata* was reported to fabricate gold nanoparticles (10–20 nm in size) extracellularly through NADH-dependent reductase enzyme released by the bacterium [38]. Another bacterium *Bacillus licheniformis* was seen to produce silver nanoparticles intracellularly [39]. However, the major drawback with intracellular nanosynthesis is the difficulty in extraction and purification, therefore extracellular synthesis is preferred.

2.4.2 Synthesis Using Plants and Plant Extracts

Plants are believed to be more suitable for green nanoparticle manufacturing than microorganisms because they are non-pathogenic and the method of synthesis is extremely simple. For making nanoparticles from plant extracts, simply mix the extract with a metal salt solution at room temperature, and the reaction begins within minutes. Plant extracts containing bioactives have been used for the synthesis of a wide spectrum of nanoparticles. The leaf extract of *Acacia nilotica* resulted in the production of gold nanoparticles within 5 mins (as seen by the appearance if a pinkish red colour) with no need for additional stabilizing or capping agents. Homogenous particles ranging in size from 6 to 12 nm were formed with storage stability of several months [40]. Similarly, the bark extract of *Pinus eldarica* exhibited the ability to synthesize silver nanoparticles of size range 10–40 nm [41]. Gold and silver are the most commonly synthesized metals; however, plant extracts have been investigated and successfully reported to form nanoparticles of copper [42], copper oxide [43], platinum [44], palladium [45], titanium dioxide [46] and iron [47]. Bimetallic nanostructures are also being synthesized using extracts of certain plants such as *Azadirachta indica* [48], *Anacardium occidentale* [49] and *Swietenia mahagony* [50]. The major mechanism of metal nanoparticle formation using plant extract is the high reduction potential of metals that can be reduced to metal atoms by the polyphenolic components present in the extract. This results in the subsequent oxidation of polyphenols to their corresponding quinones. Further, the metal atoms collide with each other forming metal nanoparticles that is then stabilized by the resultant quinone or other phytoconstituents present in the extract. The stabilizing agent prevents the aggregation of formed nanoparticles [40]. Factors such as nature of the plant extract, concentration of the reactants, reaction time, pH and temperature affect the shape, size, yield and stability of the biosynthesized nanoparticles [51]. Nanoparticles have been fabricated *in vivo*, inside living plants and tissues [52]. Alfafa plants grown in gold enriched soil were found to show the presence of pure gold nanoparticles within the size range of 4 nm [10]. ZnO nanoparticles were synthesized within *Physalis alkekengi* with a mean size of 72.5 nm [53]. Similarly, growth of Sesbania seedlings in chloroaurate solution resulted in the formation and accumulation of stable gold nanoparticles within plant tissues. Secondary metabolites found within the cells are thought to catalyze the reduction of metal ions [54].

2.4.3 Synthesis Using Isolated Phytochemicals

Numerous chemical constituents have been extracted from plants that have shown much promise in the synthesis of nanoparticles through the process of bio-reduction. Tannic acid is a plant derived polyphenol used for the synthesis of gold [55], silver [56] and palladium nanoparticles [57]. The presence of several phenolic groups renders it a good reducing property and stabilizes the formed nanoparticles [58]. Glucose and gallic acid mediated metal nanoparticles have also been synthesized but the former possesses weak reducing ability while poor stabilizing potential of the later leads to the aggregation of the formed nanoparticles [59, 60]. The use of ascorbic acid both as a reducing and capping agent resulted in the production of copper nanoparticles in aqueous medium with average particle size less than 2 nm [61]. Polysaccharides, flavonoids, terpenoids and active glycosides are some other phytoconstituents that have been investigated with the aim of producing stable nanoparticles [62]. The current chapter mainly focuses on the use of flavonoids for the biosynthesis of nanoparticles, the possible mechanism involved, along with the likely biomedical application. Table 1 lists the various physical, chemical and biological methods that are used for nanoparticle synthesis.

Table 1. Various methods of nanofabrication.

Methods of nanoparticle synthesis		
Physical methods	**Chemical methods**	**Biological methods**
Mechanical method	Sol-gel method	Micro-organism mediated synthesis
Pulse laser ablation	Hydrothermal synthesis	Plants and plant extract mediated synthesis
Arc discharge method	Co-precipitation method	Phytochemical mediated synthesis
Sputtering	Inert gas condensation method	
	Sonochemical synthesis	

2.5 *Shifting of Nanofabrication Techniques to Green Synthesis*

Phyto-nanotechnology is a novel method for the synthesis of nanoparticles that are environmentally acceptable, pure and involves cost-effective production techniques. Scalability, formation of non-toxic and bio-compatible products and by-products are the major advantages of green synthesis that facilitate its biomedical use. While the physical and chemical methods of nanoparticle synthesis are still in practice, they possess certain drawbacks such as the presence of impurities in the synthesized product, high energy consuming procedures, the use of toxic organic solvents and surfactants, time consuming processes, high cost of production, safety issues, requirement of expensive reactants, and toxic by-products, which have diverted the interest of researchers towards green synthesis [8, 63]. Green synthesized nanoparticles have a higher therapeutic potential, smaller size, superior mono-dispersity and are biologically non-toxic [15]. Major limitations to the commercial production of green synthesized nanoparticles are difficulty in scale-up, variability in the source of plant extracts and variability in experimental conditions [64]. Despite these shortcomings, green synthesis has been proposed as an alternative to the traditional methods of nanofabrication that aims to reduce the use of hazardous chemicals, is environmentally friendly and produces non-toxic nanomaterials.

3. Flavonoid Mediated Nanofabrication

Plant extracts have been extensively investigated for the purpose of nanosynthesis that have shown outstanding results especially with regard to metal nanofabrication. The phytoconstituents present in these extracts are responsible for the reduction of metal ions to their respective nano-formulations. This has fascinated researchers to further investigate individual components of the plant extracts and look deeper into the mechanism of phyto-nanosynthesis. Flavonoids are one of the most ubiquitously present phytochemicals that are most commonly reported and predicted to participate in the nanofabrication of metal ions with some noteworthy results. Here we have emphasized on the most frequently studied flavonoids and their role in the green synthesis of nanoparticles.

3.1 Nanofabrication Using Different Flavonoids

Anthocyanins, flavone, flavonol, flavanone, chalcones, and isoflavone derivatives are all members of the flavonoid family of natural polyphenols. Flavonoids have a skeleton made up of two phenyl rings (A and B) joined by an oxygenated heterocycle ring C, which is hydroxylated in multiple places [65]. Because they engage in the response to biotic and abiotic stressors, these chemicals play a vital function in plants [66]. Natural flavonoids have received a lot of interest because of their metal chelating and antioxidative effects, which are necessary for plant physiology and favourable for human health. Flavonoids operate as a catalytic centre for the Fenton reaction where these molecules chelate metal ions and the resultant metal-flavonoid complex has been reported to act as an acceptor of hydroxyl radical, consequently exhibiting free radical scavenging potency. The antioxidant activity of flavonoid-metal complexes has been found to be higher than that of free flavonoid compounds [67]. Flavonoids are capable of actively chelating and reducing metal ions into nanoparticles through various functional groups. The tautomeric conversions of flavonoids from enol to keto form may release reactive hydrogen atoms that can convert metal ions to nanoparticles. Green synthesis of Ag NPs was achieved by Jain and Mehata [11] utilizing *Ocimum sanctum* leaf extract and a flavonoid (quercetin) contained in the extract. Their findings demonstrated that Ag NPs formed from both the extract as well as quercetin had identical optical, morphological, and antibacterial properties, indicating that quercetin was involved in NP formation. It was hypothesized that upon reaction with silver salt, quercetin was able to reduce two silver ions through a redox reaction in which the flavonoid underwent a tautomeric change from enol to keto form thereby releasing two protons that reduces silver ions into silver nanoparticles [11]. Quercetin also possesses potent chelating activity since it can chelate metals at three positions, i.e., the hydroxyl, carbonyl and catechol groups. These groups are capable of chelating several divalent and trivalent metal ions such as Fe^{2+}, Fe^{3+}, Cu^{2+}, Zn^{2+}, Al^{3+}, Cr^{3+}, Pb^{2+} and Co^{2+} [68]. After the reduction of metal ions, the subsequent adsorption of flavonoids onto the surface of formed nanoparticles provides stability against agglomeration. Apiin a natural flavonoid, present abundantly in celery, parsley and banana leaves was isolated from the leaves of *Lawsonia inermis* and used for the synthesis of gold and quasi-spherical silver nanoparticles. The mechanism involved the binding of metal ions to the carbonyl group of the flavonoid resulting in the bio-reduction of gold and silver ions to nanoforms and then a layer of apiin accumulated over the metal ions prevented the formation of nanoparticle clusters [69]. Kaempherol, a dietary flavonoid, produced gold nanoparticles from chloroauric acid through a rapid redox reaction. The formation of nanoparticles began within 15 secs that was seen through a change in the colour of the reaction medium. The hydroxyl group in the B ring of the flavonoid was believed to play a role the reduction of Au^{3+} to Au^0 [70]. In another study, kaempferol mediated nanogold exhibited potent anti-neoplastic activity against A549 lung cancer cells [71]. Green synthesis of silver nanoparticles using *Withania somnifera* leaf extract produced particles ranging from 70–110 nm in size. The major phytochemicals trapped within the metal complex as identified by HPLC-UV were catechin, p-coumarin and luteolin-7-glucoside [72]. Three flavonoids hesperidin, naringin and diosmin found in citrus fruits and Mentha species were used for the synthesis of silver nanoparticles. Hesperidin and Naringin produced homogenously dispersed nanoparticles while diosmin derived particles showed the occurrence of agglomeration. This indicated that the presence of an unsaturated pyran ring in diosmin decreases the number of reducing functional groups thereby affecting its stabilizing ability. The FTIR spectrum revealed a decrease in the concentration of the -O-H groups in the reaction medium containing silver ions. This further confirms that the hydroxyl groups in flavonoids are responsible for the reduction of Ag^+ ions consequently leading to the formation of Ag-nanoparticles [73]. This study is in accordance with another report by Stephen et al. where stable spherical nanoparticles of silver were produced in the size range of 20–40 nm using hesperidin [74]. The green synthesis of gold nanoparticles using epigallocatechin-3-gallate, resveratrol and fisetin reported the formation of stable nanoparticles exhibiting enhanced anti-oxidant, anti-proliferative and apoptotic activities [75]. Another study evidenced that epigallocatechin gallate is a very efficient reducing and stabilizing agent capable of reducing tetrachloroaurate to its corresponding nanoparticle [76]. Dihydromyricetin mediated the synthesis of gold nanoparticles through the reduction of metal ions and self-oxidation of hydroxyl to carbonyl groups. pH dependent formation of uniform spherical particles was seen [77]. Likewise, interaction of the flavonoid Rutin with chloroauric acid led to the formation of gold nanoparticles in the following steps: first, rutin forms a salt with $HAuCl_4$, then charge transfer between a hydroxyl group of rutin and $AuCl_4^-$ occurs forming an auric chloride-rutin complex with the loss of a water molecule. Next, the complex is reduced with the addition of $2H^+$ ions thereby releasing Au atoms which aggregates to form gold nanoparticles. Further, rutin molecules adsorb onto the surface of gold nanoparticles thereby stabilizing the formed nanoparticles [78]. Analogous to this study, silver nanoparticles were formed from silver nitrate using rutin through a rather simple redox reaction where rutin reacts with Ag^+ through the hydroxyl atoms at 3' and 4' carbon of the B ring. The enol groups are consequently oxidized to keto forms and Ag^+ is reduced to Ag^0. Silver nanoparticles approximately 1 nm in size are initially formed which slowly coalesce resulting in the formation of larger particles within the size range of 40–90 nm [79]. Zinc oxide nanoparticles were biosynthesized via a simple precipitation technique using the flavonoid quercetin isolated from *Combretum ovalifolium*. The synthesized nanoparticles showed significant antioxidant behaviour and catalytic degradation of methylene blue dye [80]. Gokul et al. synthesized copper nanoparticles utilizing quercetin. The isolated flavonoid acts as a reducing, capping and stabilizing agent to produce particles of 295.4 nm having good anti-oxidant and anti-cancer properties [81]. Rajkumari et al. reported the synthesis of Baicalein mediated gold nanoparticles and confirmed their enhanced antibacterial activity [82]. Stolarczyk et al. observed that genistin, a naturally occurring isoflavonoid, reduces ionic gold to neutral gold nanocrystals. The nanoparticles formed exhibited high toxicity against human melanoma cells [83]. All of the above mentioned green synthesized nanoparticles were reported to be highly bioactive and biocompatible. An overview of the various flavonoid mediated nanoparticles and their investigated bioactivities have been provided in Table 2. Figure 2 provides the structures of commonly studied flavonoids involved in green synthesis.

Table 2. List of flavonoids used for the fabrication of metal nanoparticles and their investigated bioactivities.

Flavonoids	Plant species	Nanoparticle	Size (nm)	Bio-activity reported	Ref.
Quercetin	*Ocimum Sanctum*	Ag	12	Anti-bacterial	[12]
Apiin	*Lawsonia inermis*	Au Ag	21 39		[70]
Kaempherol	-	Au	18.24	Anti- Leishmanial	[71]
Kaempherol	-	Au	1–3	Anti-cancer	[72]
Catechin, p-coumaric acid, Luteolin-7-glucoside	*Withania somnifera*	Ag	70–10	Anti-microbial	[73]
Diosmin, Hesperidin, Naringin	-	Ag	20–80 5–50 5–40	Anti-bacterial, Cytotoxicity	[74]
Hesperidin	-	Ag	20–40	-	[75]
Epigallocatechin-3-gallate (EGCG) Resveratrol Fisetin	-	Au	25.55 14.55 9.76	Antioxidant, Antiproliferative, Apoptotic	[76]
EGCG	-	Au	15–45	Cellular internalization, cytotoxicity	[77]
Dihydro-myricetin	-	Au	-	-	[78]
Rutin	-	Au	16–60	-	[79]
Rutin	-	Ag	40–90	-	[80]
Quercetin	*Combretum ovalifolium*	ZnO	31.24	Antioxidant	[81]
Quercetin	*Thespesia populnea*	Cu	295.4	Antioxidant, Anti-cancer	[82]
Baicalein	-	Au	26.5	Anti-microbial	[83]
Genistin	-	Au	14–33	Anti-cancer	[84]

3.2 Mechanism of Flavonoid-mediated Green Synthesis

Many plant species are capable of synthesizing and storing nanoparticles in their cells [84]. This is facilitated by the presence of several phytoconstituents that function

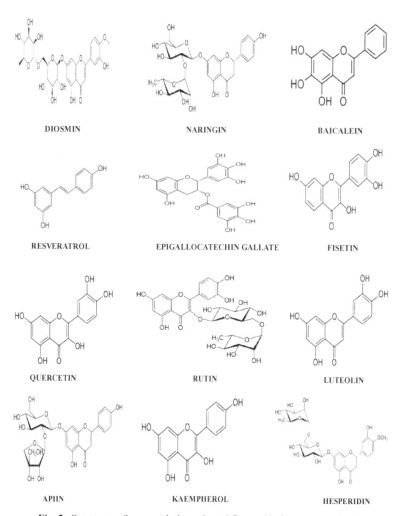

Fig. 2. Structures of commonly investigated flavonoids for green synthesis.

through bio-reduction resulting in the synthesis of nanoparticles. The entire process takes place in three phases:

i) **Reduction** of metal ions to atoms- where the charged ions accept electrons from the reducing agents to form high energy metal-flavonoid complexes.

ii) **Nucleation** and growth phase- where the highly energized complexes spontaneously aggregate and conform to their lower energy states that are thermodynamically stable.

iii) **Termination**- In this phase, the nanoparticles acquire their most favorable conformation, highly influenced by the stabilizing ability of the phytochemical [85].

The ability of flavonoid molecules to chelate metal ions through their hydroxyl and carbonyl functional groups catalyzes the formation of nanoparticles [68]. Flavonoids act as phyto-reductants that donate electrons to the metal ions and transform them to nanoparticles. These nanoparticles exist at a high energy state and tend to covert to their low energy conformations by aggregating with each other. The size of the nanoparticles thus formed depends on the nature and ability of the flavonoid to act both as a reducing and stabilizing agent. Flavonoids with strong stabilizing potential result in the formation of smaller sized nanoparticles by exerting strong repulsive forces between the metal-flavonoid complex.

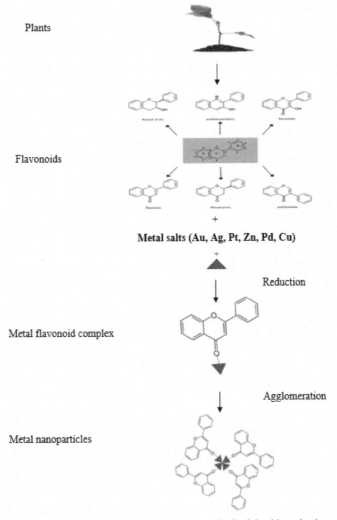

Fig. 3. Schematic representation of metal nanoparticles synthesized by bio-reduction using natural flavonoids. The metal ions bind to the carbonyl/hydroxyl groups of flavonoids and undergo reduction. The resultant metal-flavonoid complex coalesces to form small nanoparticles.

Metal-binding activity is influenced by the quantity of hydroxyl groups and the structure of flavonoids. Metal ions may be accepted in one coordination pocket between the 4-carbonyl group and the 5-hydroxyl group in simple aglycones like chrysin and apigenin. Divalent metal ions are therefore bound by two flavonoid ligands in a 1:2 (metal:ligand) stoichiometry while trivalent ions with a 1:3 (metal:ligand) stoichiometry [86, 87]. The flavonoid baicalein has three potential bidentate binding sites, making it a highly bioactive flavonoid (4-carbonyl and three hydroxyl groups at carbons number 5, 6, 7). With a 1:1 and 1:2 stoichiometry, either hydroxyls at 5- and 6-carbon atoms or 6-hydroxyl-7-hydroxyl are suitable binding sites for Fe^{2+} and Fe^{3+} ions. The Fe-baicalein complexes have significant antioxidant characteristics [88, 89]. Similarly, two potential bidentate binding sites are present in the luteolin structure and both sites can bind Al^{3+} ions in the molar ratio 2:1 (metal:ligand) [90]. Quercetin has three potential bidentate binding places rendering it a very strong chelating ability. For a wide range of metal ions, stable complexes of quercetin have been reported [68].

It may be inferred that the number of free hydroxyl and carbonyl groups in flavonoids determines it metal chelating, reducing and stabilizing potencies. Figure 3 provides a schematic representation of the metal nanoparticles synthesized by bio-reduction using natural flavonoids.

4. Biomedical Applications of Flavonoid Mediated Nanoparticles

Green nanoparticles can be used in a variety of biomedical applications. They could be employed for medication delivery, biosensing, bio-imaging, and disease treatments. Because of their antimicrobial qualities, nanoparticles are also used in everyday items such as cosmetics, toothpaste, deodorants, water purification systems, and humidifiers (Fig. 4).

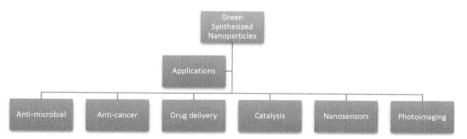

Fig. 4. Applications of green synthesized nanoparticles.

4.1 Anti-microbial Potential

The rise in antibiotic resistance amongst harmful bacteria has drawn attention to nanoparticles' antibacterial characteristics and their potential as novel medical tools. The antimicrobial activity of green synthesized gold and silver nanoparticles is well-known and is utilized in multiple medical preparations against infectious diseases. Silver nanoparticles exhibit antibacterial activity against gram-negative and gram-positive bacteria [91]. Anti-microbial studies have shown that metal oxide nanoparticles can cause significant membrane damage and DNA toxicity upon cellular uptake [92]. Copper nanoparticles have shown antibacterial efficacy against common pathogenic bacteria like *E. coli* [42].

4.2 Anti-cancer Activity

Because of their cytotoxic effect against certain tumour cells, silver nanoparticles have been extensively studied for their anti-tumorigenic properties. Cu nanoparticles made using the stem latex of *Euphorbia nivulia* was found to curb the growth of cancerous cells in the lungs. This emphasises that green synthesized nanoparticles are as efficient as conventionally synthesized copper nanoparticles as potent chemotherapeutic agents in the field of oncology [93]. The small size of nanoparticles enables them to penetrate cancer cells for targeted treatment. Gold nanoparticles have shown increased anti-neoplastic efficacy towards cancer cell lines [94].

4.3 Drug Delivery Applications

Metal nanoparticles serve as useful tools for targeted delivery of not only small molecules but they are also capable of delivering large biomolecules and phytochemicals [95]. Site specific delivery of drugs not only increases the therapeutic potential of the drug but also helps reduce systemic toxicity [96]. Delivery of flavonoid encapsulated metal nanoparticles is beneficial in enhancing the pharmacokinetic and dynamic properties of the sensitive molecules [97]. Several metals formulated as nanoparticles have been investigated as drug carriers of not just biomolecules and phytoconstituents but also of existing synthetic drugs in an attempt to reduce their toxicity and amplify therapeutic activity.

4.4 Bio-sensing Applications

Gold nanoparticles have been utilized in biosensing applications as they can be conjugated with recognition molecules such as antibodies. Metal nanoparticles can provide sensitivity for the detection of cancerous cells, blood glucose levels, pathogens and biological molecules [98].

Besides the above-mentioned applications, nanoparticles are extensively used in food, cosmetic and agriculture. They are also used as catalysts for the fast and efficient catalysis of several reactions [99].

5. Conclusion and Future Perspective

The current chapter illustrates the various methods of nanoparticle synthesis that includes chemical, physical and biological methods used in the fabrication of nanomaterials. The physical and chemical methods of nanofabrication possess limitations associated with the use of toxic chemicals during synthesis and the production of environmentally and biologically harmful byproducts. Green synthesis serves as an eco-friendly and cost-effective alternative to produce biologically suitable nanoparticles. Phytochemicals isolated from plants, especially flavonoids, are capable of efficiently reducing metal ions to their respective nanoforms. Upon investigation of the mechanism behind this phenomenon, it was revealed that the hydroxyl and carbonyl groups present in these compounds are responsible for their metal chelating and reducing ability. Flavonoids are capable of synthesizing stable nanoparticles without any requirement of additional surfactants, stabilizing or capping agents. Therefore, several flavonoids are being studied with regard to the nanoformulation of metals including gold, silver, platinum, copper, palladium, iron and zinc. Exploitation of these natural compounds provides an opportunity for the rapid, facile, economically viable and eco-friendly approach of nanofabrication. Since the green synthesized nanomaterials are free from toxic impurities, they have shown increased therapeutic potential and has opened up avenues for use in drug delivery, bioimaging and therapeutics. Despite the obvious advantages of using green nanosynthesis, issues pertaining to the large scale bio-synthesis and an exhaustive understanding of the molecular mechanism of bioreduction still exist. As a result, further research is needed to analyse and comprehend the plant-dependent process, as well as to investigate its applications, particularly in the biomedical field.

References

[1] Joob, B. and V. Wiwanitkit. 2017. Nanotechnology for health: A new useful technology in medicine. Med. J. DY Patil Univ. 10: 401.

[2] Singh, T., S. Shukla, P. Kumar, V. Wahla, V.K. Bajpai and I.A. Rather. 2017. Application of nanotechnology in food science: perception and overview. Front. Microbiol. 8: 1501.

[3] Meyyappan, M. and M. Dastoor. 2004. Nanotechnology in space exploration. Rep. Nat. Nanotechnol. Initiative Workshop. 2: 24–26.

[4] Mohan, S., G. Govindankutty, A. Sathish and N. Kamaraj. 2021. *Spirulina platensis*-capped mesoporous magnetic nanoparticles for the adsorptive removal of chromium. Can. J. Chem. Eng. 99: 294–305.

[5] Fytianos, G., A. Rahdar and G.Z. Kyzas. 2020. Nanomaterials in cosmetics: Recent updates. Nanomaterials 10: 979.

[6] Prasad, R., A. Bhattacharyya and Q.D. Nguyen. 2017. Nanotechnology in sustainable agriculture: Recent developments, challenges, and perspectives. Front. Microbiol. 8: 1014.

[7] Cele, T. 2020. Preparation of Nanoparticles. Engineered Nanomaterials - Health and Safety 14.

[8] Romania, E.M. and A.G. Modan. 2020. Advantages and disadvantages of chemical methods in the elaboration of nanomaterials. Metallurg. Mater. Sci. 43: 53–60.

[9] Bala, N., S. Saha, M. Chakraborty, M. Maiti, S. Das, R. Basu and P. Nandy. 2015. Green synthesis of zinc oxide nanoparticles using *Hibiscus subdariffa* leaf extract: effect of temperature on synthesis, anti-bacterial activity and anti-diabetic activity. RSC Adv. 5: 4993–5003.

[10] Gardea-Torresdey, J.L., J.G. Parsons, E. Gomez, J. Peralta-Videa, H.E. Troiani, P. Santiago and M.J. Yacaman. 2002. Formation and growth of Au nanoparticles inside live Alfalfa plants. Nano Lett. 2: 397–401.

[11] Jain, S. and M.S. Mehata. 2017. Medicinal plant leaf extract and pure flavonoid mediated green synthesis of silver nanoparticles and their enhanced antibacterial property. Sci. Rep. 7: 15867.

[12] Kumar, V. and S.K. Yadav. 2009. Plant-mediated synthesis of silver and gold nanoparticles and their applications. J. Chem. Technol. Biotechnol. 84: 151–157.

[13] Narayanan, K.B. and N. Sakthivel. 2010. Biological synthesis of metal nanoparticles by microbes. Advances in Colloid and Interface Science 156: 1–13.

[14] Gómez-Graña, S., M. Perez-Amemeiro, X. Vecino, I. Pastoriza-Santos, J. Perez-Juste, J. Cruz and A. Moldes. 2017. Biogenic synthesis of metal nanoparticles using a biosurfactant extracted from corn and their antimicrobial properties. Nanomaterials 7: 139.

[15] Sudhasree, S., A. Shakila Banu, P. Brindha and G.A. Kurian. 2014. Synthesis of nickel nanoparticles by chemical and green route and their comparison in respect to biological effect and toxicity. Toxicological & Environmental Chemistry 96: 743–754.

[16] Marslin, G., K. Siram, Q. Maqbool, R. Selvakesavan, D. Kruszka, P. Kachlicki and G. Franklin. 2018. Secondary metabolites in the green synthesis of metallic nanoparticles. Materials 11: 940.

[17] Muñoz, J.E., J. Cervantes, R. Esparza and G. Rosas. 2007. Iron nanoparticles produced by high-energy ball milling. J. Nanopart. Res. 9: 945–950.

[18] Prasad Yadav, T., R. Manohar Yadav and D. Pratap Singh. 2012. Mechanical milling: a top down approach for the synthesis of nanomaterials and nanocomposites. Nanosci. Nanotechnol. 2: 22–48.

[19] Amendola, V. and M. Meneghetti. 2009. Laser ablation synthesis in solution and size manipulation of noble metal nanoparticles. Phys. Chem. Chem. Phys. 11: 3805.

[20] Zhang, J., M. Chaker and D. Ma. 2017. Pulsed laser ablation-based synthesis of colloidal metal nanoparticles for catalytic applications. Journal of Colloid and Interface Science 489: 138–149.

[21] Jones, J.M., R.P. Malcolm, K.M. Thoma and S.H. Bottrell. 1996. The anode deposit formed during the carbon-arc evaporation of graphite for the synthesis of fullerenes and carbon nanotubes. Carbon 34: 231–237.

[22] Zhang, D., K. Ye, Y. Yao, F. Liang, T. Qu, W. Ma, B. Yang, Y. Dai and T. Watanabe. 2019. Controllable synthesis of carbon nanomaterials by direct current arc discharge from the inner wall of the chamber. Carbon. 142: 278–284.

[23] Ayyub, P., R. Chandra, P. Taneja, A.K. Sharma and R. Pinto. 2001. Synthesis of nanocrystalline material by sputtering and laser ablation at low temperatures. Journal of Appl. Phys. 106: 67–73.

[24] Nie, M., K. Sun and D.D. Meng. 2009. Formation of metal nanoparticles by short-distance sputter deposition in a reactive ion etching chamber. Journal of Applied Physics 106: 054314.

[25] Wender, H., P. Migowski, A.F. Feil, S.R. Teixeira and J. Dupont. 2013. Sputtering deposition of nanoparticles onto liquid substrates: Recent advances and future trends. Coordination Chemistry Reviews 257: 2468–2483.

[26] Bokov, D., A. Turki Jalil, S. Chupradit, W. Suksatan, M. Javed Ansari, I.H. Shewael, G.H. Valiev and E. Kianfar. 2021. Nanomaterial by sol-gel method: synthesis and application. Advances in Materials Science and Engineering 2021: 1–21.

[27] Parashar, M., V.K. Shukla and R. Singh. 2020. Metal oxides nanoparticles via sol–gel method: a review on synthesis, characterization and applications. J. Mater Sci: Mater Electron 31: 3729–3749.

[28] Jiang, Y., Z. Peng, S. Zhang, F. Li, Z. Liu, J. Zhang, Y. Liu and K. Wang. 2018. Facile *in-situ* solvothermal method to synthesize double shell $ZnIn_2S_4$ nanosheets/TiO_2 hollow nanosphere with enhanced photocatalytic activities. Ceramics International 44: 6115–6126.

[29] Meng, L.-Y., B. Wang, M.-G. Ma and K.-L. Lin. 2016. The progress of microwave-assisted hydrothermal method in the synthesis of functional nanomaterials. Materials Today Chemistry 1: 63–83.

[30] Das, S. and V.C. Srivasatava. 2016. Synthesis and characterization of ZnO–MgO nanocomposite by co-precipitation method. Smart Science 4: 190–195.

[31] Srivastava, R. 2012. Synthesis and characterization techniques of nanomaterials. International J. Green Nanotech. 4: 17–27.

[32] Xu, H., B.W. Zeiger and K.S. Suslick. 2013. Sonochemical synthesis of nanomaterials. Chem. Soc. Rev. 42: 2555–2567.

[33] Husseiny, M.I., M.A. El-Aziz, Y. Badr and M.A. Mahmoud. 2007. Biosynthesis of gold nanoparticles using *Pseudomonas aeruginosa*. Spectrochimica Acta Part A: Molecular and Biomolecular Spectroscopy 67: 1003–1006.

[34] Mukherjee, P., A. Ahmad, D. Mandal, S. Senapati, S.R. Sainkar, M.I. Khan, R. Parishcha, P.V. Ajaykumar, M. Alam, R. Kumar and M. Sastry. 2001. Fungus-mediated synthesis of silver nanoparticles and their immobilization in the mycelial matrix: A novel biological approach to nanoparticle synthesis. Nano Lett. 1: 515–519.

[35] Aljabali, A.A.A., J.E. Barclay, G.P. Lomonossoff and D.J. Evans. 2010. Virus templated metallic nanoparticles. Nanoscale 2: 2596.

[36] Hamida, R.S., N.E. Abdelmeguid, M.A. Ali, M.M. Bin-Meferij and M.I. Khalil. 2020. Synthesis of silver nanoparticles using a novel cyanobacteria *Desertifilum* sp. extract: Their antibacterial and cytotoxicity effects. Int. J. Nanomed. 15: 49–63.

[37] Agnihotri, M., S. Joshi, A.R. Kumar, S. Zinjarde and S. Kulkarni. 2009. Biosynthesis of gold nanoparticles by the tropical marine yeast *Yarrowia lipolytica*. Materials Letters 63: 1231–1234.

[38] He, S., Z. Guo, Y. Zhang, S. Zhang, J. Wang and N. Gu. 2007. Biosynthesis of gold nanoparticles using the bacteria *Rhodopseudomonas capsulata*. Materials Letters 61: 3984–3987.

[39] Kalimuthu, K., R. Suresh Babu, D. Venkataraman, Mohd. Bilal and S. Gurunathan. 2008. Biosynthesis of silver nanocrystals by *Bacillus licheniformis*. Colloids and Surfaces B: Biointerfaces 65: 150–153.

[40] Majumdar, R., B.G. Bag and N. Maity. 2013. *Acacia nilotica* (Babool) leaf extract mediated size-controlled rapid synthesis of gold nanoparticles and study of its catalytic activity. Int. Nano. Lett. 3: 53.

[41] Iravani, S. and B. Zolfaghari. 2013. Green synthesis of silver nanoparticles using *Pinus eldarica* bark extract. BioMed Research International 5: 1–5.

[42] Lee, H.-J., J.Y. Song and B.S. Kim. 2013. Biological synthesis of copper nanoparticles using *Magnolia kobus* leaf extract and their antibacterial activity. J. Chem. Technol. Biotechnol. 88: 1971–1977.

[43] Thekkae Padil, V.V. and M. Černík. 2013. Green synthesis of copper oxide nanoparticles using gum karaya as a biotemplate and their antibacterial application. Int J. Nanomed. 8: 889–898.

[44] Song, J.Y., E.-Y. Kwon and B.S. Kim. 2010. Biological synthesis of platinum nanoparticles using Diopyros kaki leaf extract. Bioprocess Biosyst. Eng. 33: 159–164.

[45] Kumar Petla, R., S. Vivekanandhan, M. Misra, A. Kumar Mohanty and N. Satyanarayana. 2012. Soybean (*Glycine max*) leaf extract based green synthesis of palladium nanoparticles. J. Biomater. Nanobiotechnol. 3: 16695, 6 pages

[46] Sundrarajan, M. and S. Gowri. 2011. Green synthesis of titanium dioxide nanoparticles by *Nyctanthes Arbor-Tristis* leaves extract. Chalcogenide Lett. 8: 447–451.

[47] Pattanayak, M. and P.L. Nayak. 2013. Green synthesis and characterization of zero valent iron nanoparticles from the leaf extract of *Azadirachta indica* (Neem). World J. NSci. Tech. 2: 6–9.

[48] Shankar, S.S., A. Rai, A. Ahmad and M. Sastry. 2004. Rapid synthesis of Au, Ag, and bimetallic Au core–Ag shell nanoparticles using Neem (*Azadirachta indica*) leaf broth. Journal of Colloid and Interface Science 275: 496–502.

[49] Sheny, D.S., J. Mathew and D. Philip. 2011. Phytosynthesis of Au, Ag and Au–Ag bimetallic nanoparticles using aqueous extract and dried leaf of *Anacardium occidentale*. Spectrochimica Acta Part A: Molecular and Biomolecular Spectroscopy 79: 254–262.

[50] Mondal, S., N. Roy, R.A. Laskar, I. Sk, S. Basu, D. Mandal and N.A. Begum. 2011. Biogenic synthesis of Ag, Au and bimetallic Au/Ag alloy nanoparticles using aqueous extract of mahogany (*Swietenia mahogani* JACQ.) leaves. Colloids and Surfaces B: Biointerfaces 82: 497–504.

[51] Mittal, A.K., Y. Chisti and U.C. Banerjee. 2013. Synthesis of metallic nanoparticles using plant extracts. Biotechnology Advances 31: 346–356.

[52] Rodriguez, E., J.G. Parsons, J.R. Peralta-Videa, G. Cruz-Jimenez, J. Romero-Gonzalez, B.E. Sanchez-Salcido, G.B. Saupe, M. Duarte-Gardea and J.L. Gardea-Torresdey. 2007. Potential of *Chilopsis linearis* for gold phytomining: Using XAS to determine gold reduction and nanoparticle formation within plant tissues. International Journal of Phytoremediation 9: 133–147.

[53] Qu, J., X. Yuan, X. Wang and P. Shao. 2011. Zinc accumulation and synthesis of ZnO nanoparticles using *Physalis alkekengi* L. Environmental Pollution 159: 1783–1788.

[54] Sharma, N.C., S.V. Sahi, S. Nath, J.G. Parsons, J.L. Gardea-Torresde and T. Pal. 2007. Synthesis of plant-mediated gold nanoparticles and catalytic role of biomatrix-embedded nanomaterials. Environ. Sci. Technol. 41: 5137–5142.

[55] Aswathy Aromal, S. and D. Philip. 2012. Facile one-pot synthesis of gold nanoparticles using tannic acid and its application in catalysis. Physica E: Low-dimensional Systems and Nanostructures 44: 1692–1696.

[56] Sivaraman, S.K., I. Elango, S. Kumar and V. Santhanam. 2009. A green protocol for room temperature synthesis of silver nanoparticles in seconds. Current Science 97: 6.

[57] Meena Kumari, M., S.A. Aromal and D. Philip. 2013. Synthesis of monodispersed palladium nanoparticles using tannic acid and its optical non-linearity. Spectrochimica Acta Part A: Molecular and Biomolecular Spectroscopy 103: 130–133.

[58] Ahmad, T. 2014. Reviewing the tannic acid mediated synthesis of metal nanoparticles. Journal of Nanotechnology 2014: 1–11.

[59] Liu, J., G. Qin, P. Raveendran and Y. Ikushima. 2006. Facile "Green" synthesis, characterization, and catalytic function of β-D-glucose-stabilized Au nanocrystals. Chem. Eur. J. 12: 2131–2138.

[60] Martínez-Castañón, G.A., N. Niño-Martínez, F. Martínez-Gutierrez, J.R. Martinez-Mendoza and F. Ruiz. 2008. Synthesis and antibacterial activity of silver nanoparticles with different sizes. J. Nanopart. Res. 10: 1343–1348.

[61] Xiong, J., Y. Wang, Q. Xue and X. Wu. 2011. Synthesis of highly stable dispersions of nanosized copper particles using l-ascorbic acid. Green Chem. 13: 900.

[62] Park, Y., Y.N. Hong, A. Weyers, Y.S. Kim and R.J. Linhardt. 2011. Polysaccharides and phytochemicals: A natural reservoir for the green synthesis of gold and silver nanoparticles. IET Nanobiotechnol. 5: 69.

[63] Rane, A.V., K. Kanny, V.K. Abitha and S. Thomas. 2018. Methods for synthesis of nanoparticles and fabrication of nanocomposites. pp. 121–139. *In*: Synthesis of Inorganic Nanomaterials. Woodhead Publ. Ch. 5.

[64] Peralta-Videa, J.R., Y. Huang, J.G. Parsons, L. Zhao, L. Lopez-Moreno, J.A. Hernandez-Viezcas and J.L. Gardea-Torresdey. 2016. Plant-based green synthesis of metallic nanoparticles: scientific curiosity or a realistic alternative to chemical synthesis? Nanotechnol. Environ. Eng. 1: 4.

[65] Kachlicki, P., A. Piasecka, M. Stobiecki and L. Marczak. 2016. Structural characterization of flavonoid glycoconjugates and their derivatives with mass spectrometric techniques. Molecules 21: 1494.

[66] Winkel-Shirley, B. 2002. Biosynthesis of flavonoids and effects of stress. Current Opinion in Plant Biology 5: 218–223.

[67] Samsonowicz, M., E. Regulska and M. Kalinowska. 2017. Hydroxyflavone metal complexes - molecular structure, antioxidant activity and biological effects. Chemico-Biological Interactions 273: 245–256.

[68] Cherrak, S.A., N. Mokhtari-Soulimane, F. Berroukeche, B. Bensenane, A. Cherbonnel, H. Merzouk and M. Elhabiri. 2016. *In vitro* antioxidant versus metal ion chelating properties of flavonoids: a structure-activity investigation. PLoS ONE 11: e0165575.

[69] Kasthuri, J., S. Veerapandian and N. Rajendiran. 2009. Biological synthesis of silver and gold nanoparticles using apiin as reducing agent. Colloids and Surfaces B: Biointerfaces 68: 55–60.

[70] Halder, A., S. Das, T. Bera and A. Mukherjee. 2017. Rapid synthesis for monodispersed gold nanoparticles in kaempferol and anti-leishmanial efficacy against wild and drug resistant strains. RSC Adv. 7: 14159–14167.

[71] Govindaraju, S., A. Roshini, M.-H. Lee and K. Yun. 2019. Kaempferol conjugated gold nanoclusters enabled efficient for anticancer therapeutics to A549 lung cancer cells. Int. J. Nanomed. 14: 5147–5157.

[72] Dias, A.C.P., G. Marslin, R.K. Selvakesavan, G. Franklin and B. Sarmento. 2015. Antimicrobial activity of cream incorporated with silver nanoparticles biosynthesized from *Withania somnifera*. Int. J. Nanomed. 10: 5955–5963.

[73] Sahu, N., D. Soni, B. Chandrashekhar, D.B. Satpute, S. Saravanadevi, B.K. Sarangi and R.A. Pandey. 2016. Synthesis of silver nanoparticles using flavonoids: hesperidin, naringin and diosmin, and their antibacterial effects and cytotoxicity. Int. Nano Lett. 6: 173–181.

[74] Stephen, A. and S. Seethalakshmi. 2013. Phytochemical synthesis and preliminary characterization of silver nanoparticles using hesperidin. Journal of Nanoscience 6: 1–6.

[75] Sanna, V., N. Pala, G. Dessi, P. Manconi, A. Mariani, S. Dedola, M. Rassu, C. Crosio, C. Iaccarino and M. Sechi. 2014. Single-step green synthesis and characterization of gold-conjugated polyphenol nanoparticles with antioxidant and biological activities. Int. J. Nanomed. 9: 4935–4951.

[76] Nune, S.K., N. Chanda, R. Shukla, K. Katti, R.R. Kulkarni, S. Thilakavathy, S. Mekapothula, R. Kannan and K.V. Katti. 2009. Green nanotechnology from tea: phytochemicals in tea as building blocks for production of biocompatible gold nanoparticles. J. Mater. Chem. 19: 2912.

[77] Guo, Q., Q. Guo, J. Yuan and J. Zeng. 2014. Biosynthesis of gold nanoparticles using a kind of flavonol: Dihydromyricetin. Colloids and Surfaces A: Physicochemical and Engineering Aspects 441: 127–132.

[78] Borodina, V.G. and Yu.A. Mirgorod. 2014. Kinetics and mechanism of the interaction between $HAuCl_4$ and rutin. Kinet Catal. 55: 683–687.

[79] Mirgorod, Yu.A., V.G. Borodina and N.A. Borsch. 2013. Investigation of interaction between silver ions and rutin in water by physical methods. Biophysics 58: 743–747.

[80] Jeyaleela, G.D., J.R. Vimala, S.M. Sheela, A. Agila, M.S. Bharathy and M. Divya. 2020. Biofabrication of zinc oxide nanoparticles using the isolated flavonoid from *Combretum ovalifolium* and its anti-oxidative ability and catalytic degradation of methylene blue dye. Orient. J. Chem. 36: 655–664.

[81] Gokul, M., U.G. and A. Esakki. 2022. Green synthesis and characterization of isolated flavonoid mediated copper nanoparticles by using *Thespesia populnea* leaf extract and its evaluation of anti-oxidant and anti-cancer activity. Int. J. Chem. Res. 6: 15–32.

[82] Rajkumari, J., S. Busi, A.C. Vasu and P. Reddy. 2017. Facile green synthesis of baicalein fabricated gold nanoparticles and their antibiofilm activity against *Pseudomonas aeruginosa*. Microbial Pathogenesis 107: 261–269.

[83] Stolarczyk, E.U., K. Stolarczyk, M. Laszcz, M. Kubiszewski, W. Maruszak, W. Olejarz and D. Bryk. 2017. Synthesis and characterization of genistein conjugated with gold nanoparticles and the study of their cytotoxic properties. European Journal of Pharmaceutical Sciences 96: 176–185.

[84] Harris, A.T. and R. Bali. 2008. On the formation and extent of uptake of silver nanoparticles by live plants. J. Nanopart. Res. 10: 691–695.

[85] Marakov, V.V., A.J. Love, V. Sinitsyna, S.S. Marakova, I.V. Yaminsky, M.E. taliansky and N.O. Kalinina. 2014. 'Green' nanotechnologies: synthesis of metal nanoparticles using plants. Acta Naturae 6: 35–44.

[86] Erdogan, G., R. Karadag and A. Eler. 2010. Aluminium(III), Fe(II) Complexes and dyeing properties of apigenin (5,7,4' trihydroxy flavone). Reviews in Analytical Chemistry 29: 211–232.

[87] Pusz, J. and B. Nitka. 1997. Synthesis and physicochemical properties of the complexes of Co(II), Ni(II), and Cu(II) with chrysin. Microchemical Journal 56: 373–381.

[88] Dimitrić Marković, J.M., Z.S. Marković, T.P. Brdarić, V.M. Pavelkić and M.B. Jadranin. 2011. Iron complexes of dietary flavonoids: Combined spectroscopic and mechanistic study of their free radical scavenging activity. Food Chemistry 129: 1567–1577.

[89] Perez, C.A., Y. Wei and M. Guo. 2009. Iron-binding and anti-Fenton properties of baicalein and baicalin. Journal of Inorganic Biochemistry 103: 326–332.

[90] Rygula, A., T.P. Wrobel, J. Szklarzewicz and M. Baranska. 2013. Raman and UV–vis spectroscopy studies on luteolin–Al(III) complexes. Vibrational Spectroscopy 64: 21–26.

[91] Velmurugan, P., S-M. Lee, M. Iydroose, K-J. Lee and B-T. Oh. 2013. Pine cone-mediated green synthesis of silver nanoparticles and their antibacterial activity against agricultural pathogens. Appl. Microbiol. Biotechnol. 97: 361–368.

[92] Simon-Deckers, A., S. Loo, M. Mayne-L'hermite, N. Herlin-Biome, N. Menguy, C. Reynaud, B. Gouget and M. Carriere. 2009. Size-, composition- and shape-dependent toxicological impact of metal oxide nanoparticles and carbon nanotubes toward bacteria. Environ. Sci. Technol. 43: 8423–8429.

[93] Valodkar, M., R.N. Jadeja, M.C. Thounaojam, R.V. Devkar and S. Thakore. 2011. Biocompatible synthesis of peptide capped copper nanoparticles and their biological effect on tumor cells. Materials Chemistry and Physics 128: 83–89.

[94] Rajan, A., A.R. Rajan and D. Philip. 2017. *Elettaria cardamomum* seed mediated rapid synthesis of gold nanoparticles and its biological activities. OpenNano 2: 1–8.

[95] Ghosh, P., G. Han, M. De, C. Kim and V. Rotello. 2008. Gold nanoparticles in delivery applications. Advanced Drug Delivery Reviews 60: 1307–1315.

[96] Vimala, K., S. Sundarraj, M. Paulpandi, S. Vengatesan and S. Kannan. 2014. Green synthesized doxorubicin loaded zinc oxide nanoparticles regulates the Bax and Bcl-2 expression in breast and colon carcinoma. Process Biochemistry 49: 160–172.

[97] Sulaiman, G.M., H.M. Waheeb, M.S. Jabir, S.H. Khazaal, Y.H. Dewir and Y. Naidoo. 2020. Hesperidin loaded on gold nanoparticles as a drug delivery system for a successful biocompatible, anti-cancer, anti-inflammatory and phagocytosis inducer model. Sci. Rep. 10: 9362.

[98] Yeh, Y.-C., B. Creran and V.M. Rotello. 2012. Gold nanoparticles: preparation, properties, and applications in bionanotechnology. Nanoscale 4: 1871–1880.

[99] Ijaz, I., E. Gilani, A. Nazir and A. Bukhari. 2020. Detail review on chemical, physical and green synthesis, classification, characterizations and applications of nanoparticles. Green Chemistry Letters and Rev iews 13: 223–245.

14

Structural and Mechanical Aspects of Nanocomposite Hard Thin Films for Device Fabrication at Nanoscale

R. Dash,[1] R. P. Kumar,[3] A. K. Rajak,[1] A. Kumari[4] and
A.S. Bhattacharyya[1,2,*]

1. Introduction

The dimension, efficiency, and cost of N/MEMS-based devices are continuously been looked into for better performance [1–4]. Amongst these devices, piezoresistive pressure sensors are one of the most commonly used microsensors due to simple fabrication and circuits [5–13]. They are classified based on how the mechanical input (pressure) is transformed into electrical output; this includes piezoresistive, capacitive, piezoelectric, optical, and resonant pressure sensors. The properties of SiCN are also applicable to MEMS piezoresistive devices [14–17].

Nanocomposite hard films (e.g., SiN, SiC, TiN, and nanocomposites like SiCN, TiBCN, etc.) are used as protective coatings in industrial tools and nano/microelectromechanical systems (N/MEMS). The deposition of the nanocomposite films was carried out by RF and DC sputtering. The variation of

[1] Dept. of Nano Science and Technology, Central University of Jharkhand, Brambe, Ranchi: 835205.
[2] Centre of Excellence in Green and Efficient Energy Technology (CoE GEET), Central University of Jharkhand, Brambe, Ranchi: 835205.
[3] ICAR - CRIDA, Santhosh Nagar, Hyderabad. 5000593.
[4] Dept. of Materials Science and Engineering, Indian Institute of Technology Delhi, Hauz Khas, New Delhi 110016.
* Corresponding author: arnab.bhattacharya@cuj.ac.in; 2006asb@gmail.com

particle sizes and the nucleation and growth of different phases at different deposition conditions were observed. The mechanical properties like hardness and modulus were determined by nanoindentation. Scratch tests were done for adhesion studies of the films with the substrate. Failure studies performed by indentations showed the different cracking/failure phenomenon occurring, which were found to be dependent upon the coating thickness, hardness, and nature of the substrate. Radial and lateral cracks were mainly observed on coatings deposited on silicon substrates. This chapter provides an understanding of the mechanical properties of coatings at the nanoscale using nanoindentation which shall be useful in device fabrication [18–25]. Computational studies provide further insight into the aspects of the usage of these materials in devices at the nanoscale.

1.1 Si-C-N Based MEMS

Silicon-based MEMS sensors operate reliably only up to a temperature of about 150°C [26]. Therefore, high temperature, pressure, and vibrational domain applications such as automotive, gas turbine engines, and the oil industry, have induced the researchers to look for alternate materials to silicon in MEMS-based piezoresistive pressure sensors. In this connection, SiC stands out as one of the most promising candidates. An up-gradation to SiC comes in the form of SiCN which can withstand even higher temperatures than SiC. Phases like SiNx (including β-Si_3N_4) and CNx (including β-C_3N_4) are formed in the nanocomposite SiCN thin film providing good thermomechanical and conducting properties [27]. Silicon carbon nitride (Si-C-N) thin films have an application in aerospace and MEMS devices as high-temperature pressure sensors due to their piezoresistive properties [28].

Recently, other films like Cr_2O_3 have been also found as mechanically protective thin film applicable, for instance, in micro-electromechanical devices [29]. However, their high-temperature performance still needs to be studied. The variation of sputtering power during magnetron sputtering has been found to alter the piezoresistive properties of SiCN films and is an important consideration for the use as MEMS pressure sensors [30]. Other deposition parameters like ion acceleration voltages during ion beam assisted deposition also affect the mechanical properties. The percentage of carbon, which is the primary element in creating hard phases in the composite leads, to a lower friction coefficient being present in higher fractions [31]. Decreasing the power and temperature has been reported to increase the carbon content and lower the dielectric constant due to lower density in plasma-based atomic layer deposition of these films. The etch rate also got decreased due to high film density [32]. Hydrogenated SiCN:H and SiCN thin films have been synthesized from organosilicon compounds showing enhanced optical, thermal, dielectric, and mechanical properties [33]. Carbon Nanofiber (CNF)-SiCN nanocomposites with defect structure caused polarization [34] and polymer-derived SiCN are also used for electrochemical energy storage [35].

1.2 SiCN Based Memory Devices

The fabrication of CBRAM based transparent devices for non-volatile memory applications based on SiCN films has been reported [36]. Si-C-N films have the potential for futuristic nonvolatile memory application at high temperatures and harsh environments. Si-C-N thin films have also been shown to have switching properties applicable in resistive RAM (ReRAM) which are potential next-generation non-volatile memory devices having a fast operation, lower power consumption, higher stacking density, and higher scalability [37, 38].

1.3 SiCN in Transport and High-Frequency Applications

High electron mobility transistors (HEMTs) based upon heterojunctions are high-frequency devices used in satellite receivers and power amplifiers. They are mainly made of AlGaN/GaN layers. SiCN used as a cap layer in these HEMTs has been reported to cause a reduction in noise level [39]. SiCN cap layer used in AlGaN/GaN metal insulator semiconductor heterostructure field-effect transistors (MISHFETs) increased the 2D electron gas (2DEG) density, and also effectively passivated the surface of the AlGaN/GaN MISHFET leading to superior device performance [40].

1.4 Optoelectronic Properties of SiCN

Radio Frequency (RF)-magnetron sputtered SiCN films with controlled process parameters like pressure, substrate temperature and power have been used in optoelectronic devices by showing photoelectric and PL properties emitting light in the blue-violet region [41]. Annealing caused magnetron sputtered SiCN films to emit enhanced blue-violet light on excitation evident from the increase in PL intensity [42]. Photoemission studies in hydrogenated and non-hydrogenated SiCN using first principal MD simulations showed quenching in photoemission with an increase in hydrogen flow [43]. SiCN aids in low-cost photovoltaics by acting as a buffer layer in GaN/In$_x$Ga$_{1-x}$N-based solar cells [44].

1.5 SiCN in Electronic Packaging

The lower bonding temperature ($\sim 250°C$) in SiCN leads to its use in safer packaging in CMOS [45]. SiCN has application in wafer-level hybrid bonding [46]. Two Cu nano-pads on wafers were bonded with the help of SiCN. The adhesion between SiCN and ultralow K materials have been studied for better packaging to reduce signal processing delays [47, 48].

1.6 Microwave Absorption by SiCN

SiCN and CNT composites have shown improved dielectric and microwave absorption properties. The lightweight, thermal stability, oxidation resistance of SiCN makes it this capable. The addition of CNT improves its performance further in terms of conductivity and as an MW absorbing material in an alternating electric field [49]. Microwave absorption has also been reported by Fe doped SiCN composites where dielectric properties in terms of storage and transport properties on terms of the conductive network took place [50]. The addition of $\text{r-Fe}_2\text{O}_3$ in SiCN led to the formation of core-shell $\text{Fe@Si}_3\text{N}_4$ particles in SiCN composite fibers which affected the permittivity and permeability and aided in electromagnetic wave absorption [51]. Titanium Carbide (TiC) when added to SiCN caused the formation of microstructure containing nanocrystalline phases of TiC, SiC, as well as graphite and diamond. The composite showed goof impedance matching due to the formation of permittivity gradient between the nanodielectric loss phases. The EM absorbing properties were also seen [52]. The incorporation of graphitic carbon and SiC nanowires in SiCN improved the electrical conductivity and electromagnetic shielding abilities [53]. Polymer-derived SiCN ceramics were also subjected to 3D printing and 2D/3D micro-shaping. Honeycomb-shaped SiCN ceramic prepared by 3D printing has shown excellent MW absorbing properties [54–56]. SiCN has also shown catalytic and photocatalytic capabilities in harsh environments [57].

2. Sputter Deposition and Nanocrystalline Phases

The hard nanocrystalline phases formed in a nanocomposite film containing Ti, B, Si, C, and N justify their superiority over their monophasic forms. The restriction of crack growth and resistance to localized plastic deformation at hard operating conditions along with good electrical properties makes them lucrative towards N/MEMS devices. There are a lot of techniques by which these nanocomposite films may be produced, Magnetron sputtering is one of the highly acclaimed techniques which has the advantage of reactive sputtering based upon the choices of reactive gases and is also comparatively cleaner (high vacuum) and provides control over the stoichiometry. A 2-inch diameter sintered TiB_2 or SiC target which act as the cathode is placed in front of the magnetron which is a circular arrangement of magnets creating an $E \times B$ filed at the center (Fig. 1a, b). The ionized argon gas hitting the target produces adatoms by collision cascade. The magnetron helps in keeping the process localized over its dimension by controlling the charged species which also includes secondary electrons. A plasma is created during the process. These ad atoms produced travel along the line of sight and get deposited on the substrate placed at a certain distance and angle. The formation of nanocrystallites were observed under transmission electron microscope (Fig. 1c).

A representative SiCN thin film on a glass substrate in shown in Fig. 2. The formation of nanocrystallites in an amorphous matrix was evident from the TEM studies. The structural characterization showed the formation of phases of SiC Si_3N_4, CNx, nc-carbon (diamond), and graphite [18–25].

Both microstructural and structural characterization showed the formation of the highest fraction of hard phases at an optimum deposition condition for magnetron sputtered films. The nucleation of nanocrystalline phases on an amorphous matrix usually leads to an increase in hardness. However, coalescence of these crystalline phases may also reduce the hardness in the long run. The 3 stage Ferrari-Robertson model for carbon was modified into a 4-stage model for Si-C-N based upon the I_G and I_D bands and peak positions [20]. Whether DC or RF mode was used during sputtering was found to be also important showing variation in properties [24].

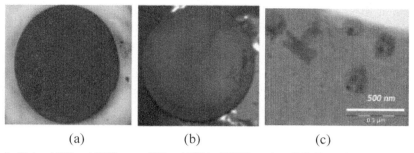

Glass (substrate)

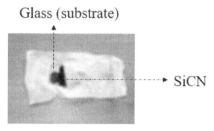

→ SiCN

3. Nanoindentation

Nanoindentation is a method to characterize material mechanical properties on a very small scale due to its high spatial and depth resolution of the measurement [58, 59]. Features less than 100 nm across, as well as thin films less than 50 nm thick, can be evaluated. The configuration of the nanoindentation setup. The nanoindentation is usually done with a 3-sided pyramidal Berkovich indenter, although spherical as well as 4-sided pyramidal cube-corner indenter are also available. The sample stage is in a floating condition attached with a spring to minimize any effect of vibration. The test methods include indentation for comparative and quantitative hardness determination and scratching for evaluation of wear resistance and thin-film adhesion. It has been also used to determine creep properties of materials based on time on the sample [60–62]. Analysis of time of interaction of the probe with the sample and deviation in mechanical parameters relating to microstructure has been given in this section [63]. Computational modeling relating to fitting parameters and physical properties have been shown here with an in-depth analysis of the experimental results.

For indentation, the probe is forced into the surface at a selected rate and to a selected maximum force. Nanoindentation studies were performed on the films by Nanoindenter XP (MTS, USA). Both bulk modulus (E) and hardness (H) are found from nanoindentation. The advantage lies in the possibility of very small indentation (~ 100 nm). Thus, it is useful in the case of thin films. During nanoindentation, a Berkovich indenter with 70.3°C effective cone angle is pushed into the material and withdrawn. The indentation load and displacement are recorded. The hardness and elastic modulus are determined with the depth of penetration after each 2 nm penetration [63]. The nanoindentation plots are shown in Fig. 3. The max load applied (P_{max}) corresponds to the maximum depth of penetration (h_{max}). Due to plastic deformation, a residual depth is observed (h_r) after full unloading which is after an elastic recovery denoted by the elastic depth (h_e). The depth h_c is the contact depth. The stiffness $S = dP/dh$ at maximum penetration, obtained from the unloading portion of the plot, is used in elastic modulus determination as given in eqn 1. The hardness is determined from eqn 2 where $A_{projected}$ in the projected area. The details are given in ref [88].

$$E_r = \frac{\sqrt{\pi}}{2} \cdot \frac{dP}{dh} \cdot \frac{1}{\sqrt{A}} .$$ (1)

$$H = \frac{P_{max}}{A_{projected}}$$ (2)

Nanoindentation has been used to characterize materials used for N/MEMS in terms of hardness, elastic modulus, creep and adhesion properties [64, 65]. Bending strength and fatigue properties of nanoscale Si beams were also studied using nanoindentation [66, 67]. Nanoindentation was also used to actuate a radio frequency micro switch [68]. Nanoindentation coupled with electrical measurements are useful in studying the contact resistance in metal contact switches [69].

Impulse plays an important role in nanoindentation, especially when dealing with a coating/substrate system. The time of contact of the indenter with the sample is also a major factor in determining the mechanical response of materials and is especially useful for N/MEMS based sensors. The time on sample and harmonic impulse plot for three different penetration depths is shown in Fig. 4 details of which are given in ref [63].

Piezoresistive MEMS used in pacemakers is based on impulse received from the heart's vibration for energy production proving a longer lifetime of the device. A silicon-based MEMS cantilever is used which uses CMOS compatible AlN as the piezoelectric layer and works on shock-induced vibration producing energy. SiCN having piezoelectric property can replace AlN [70]. The mechanical response of N/MEMs under impulse loading is a major criterion for device fabrication [71].

The features during unloading are usually different depicting interesting mechanical facts about the specimen at the nanoscale. As nanoindentation is based on continuous stiffness mode (CSM), the increase in slope indicates faster recovery as the material has been removed during unloading. A higher rate of change of slope will indicate higher elastic recovery. The effect of impulse is discussed in details in ref [72–77]. Deviation in mechanical properties due to indenter positioning and determination of fracture toughness of thin films by nanoindentation has also been

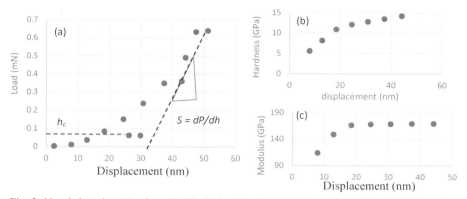

Fig. 3. Nanoindentation (a) schematic P-h (b) load-depth (c) hardness (d) modulus with penetration depth. Reproduced with permission from Elsevier [88].

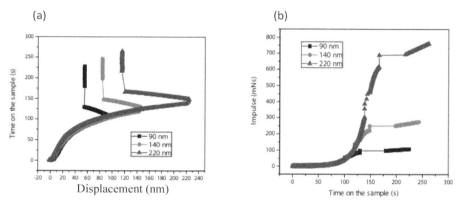

Fig. 4. (a) Time on sample and (b) Impulse for three different nanoindentation penetrations (Reproduced under CC BY License ⓒ ⓐ) [79].

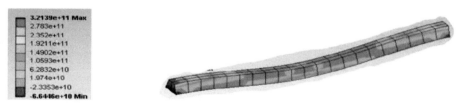

Fig. 5. Maximum principal stress distribution in a beam of trapezoidal cross-section (Reproduced with permission from Elsevier) [88].

reported [78–83]. Computational studies based on nanoindentation with molecular dynamics simulation and modeling for fracture analysis have been done [84–86]. Finite Element Modelling of cantilever N/MEMS resonators was done as shown in Fig. 5 indicating the stress distributions [87, 88].

4. Conclusions

Nanocrystalline phases of technologically important materials like SiC, Si_3N4, CNx, TiC, TiN and TiB_2 deposited by means of magnetron sputtering for N/MEMS based devices like piezoelectric sensors. Nanoindentation studies show the effect of impulse and the effect of microstructural features on the nanomechanical properties. FEM modelling was done to analyze the stress distribution on cantilever structures. All these studies are beneficial for the N/MEMS based devices.

Acknowledgements

The authors would like to thank Dr. S.K. Mishra, CSIR-National Metallurgical Laboratory, for experimental facilities.

Reference

[1] Yu, Xiaomo. Maalla, Allam and Moradi, Zohre. 2022. Electroelastic high-order computational continuum strategy for critical voltage and frequency of piezoelectric NEMS via modified multi-physical couple stress theory. Mechanical Systems and Signal Processing 165: 108373.

[2] Yadav, Shubham. Tripathy, Soumya and Sarkar, Deblina. 2022. NEMS sensors based on novel nanomaterials. Advanced MEMS/NEMS Fabrication and Sensors, 133–185. Springer.

[3] Pu, Dong and Hu, Huan. 2021. Tip-based nanofabrication for NEMS devices. Advanced MEMS/NEMS Fabrication and Sensors (2021): 1–18.

[4] Kim, Namjung. 2018. M/NEM devices and uncertainty quantification. Doctor of Philosophy in Theoretical and Applied Mechanics in the Graduate College of the University of Illinois at Urbana-Champaign.

[5] Fan, Xuge. Smith, Anderson D. Forsberg, Fredrik, Wagner, Stefan, Schröder, Stephan, Shirin, Sayedeh, Akbari et al. 2020. Manufacture and characterization of graphene membranes with suspended silicon proof masses for MEMS and NEMS applications. Microsystems & Nanoengineering 6: 17.

[6] Chang, Yuhua. Wei, Jingxuan and Lee, Chengkuo. 2020. Metamaterials—from fundamentals and MEMS tuning mechanisms to applications. Nanophotonics 9: 3049–3070.

[7] Zara, J.M., S. Yazdanfar, K.D. Rao, J.A. Izatt and S.W. Smith. 2003. Electro-static micromachine scanning mirror for optical coherence tomography. Opt. Lett. 28: 628–630.

[8] Patterson, Pamela Rae, Hah, Dooyoung, Fujino, Makoto, Piyawattanametha, Wibool and C. Wu, Ming. 2004. Scanning mirrors: an overview. Optomechatronic Micro/Nano Components, Devices, and Systems 5604: 1–13.

[9] Yalcinkaya, A.D., H. Urey, D. Brown, T. Montague and R. Sprague. 2006. Two-axis electromagnetic micro scanner for high resolution displays. Journal of Microelectromechanical Systems 15: 786–794.

[10] Hao, Z., B. Wingfield, M. Whiteley, J. Brooks and J.A. Hammer. 2003. A design methodology for a bulk-micromachined two-dimensional electrostatic torsion micromirror. Journal of Microelectromechanical Systems 12: 692–701.

[11] Bao, Minhang. 2005. Analysis and Design Principles of MEMS Devices. Elsevier.

[12] Bégot, Sylvie, Getie, Muluken Z. Diallo, Alpha, Lanzetta, François, Barthès, Magali and Labachelerie, Michel de. 2021. A novel model and design of a mems Stirling engine. International Journal of Heat and Technology 39: 1037–1046.

[13] Sadhukhan, Dhrubajyoti. Singh and Gajendra Prasad. 2020. Study of electrostatic actuated MEMS biaxial scanning micro-mirror with comb structure. AIP Conference Proceedings 2269: 030019.

[14] Karmarkar, Makarand. Singh, Gurpreet. Shah, Sandeep, Mahajan and Roop L. Priya, Shashank. 2009. Large piezoresistivity phenomenon in SiCN–(La, Sr) MnO_3 composites. Applied Physics Letters 94: 072902.

[15] Park, Nae-Man, Kim, Sang Hyeob and Sung, Gun Yong. 2003. Band gap engineering of SiCN film grown by pulsed laser deposition. Journal of Applied Physics 94: 2725.

[16] Lee, Jae-Hoon, Jeong, Jae-Hyun and Lee, Jung-Hee. 2012. Enhanced electrical characteristics of AlGaN-based SBD with *in situ* deposited silicon carbon nitride cap layer. IEEE Electron Device Letters 33: 492–494.

[17] Ting, Shyh-Fann, Fang, Yean-Kuen, Hsieh, Wen-Tse, Tsair, Yong-Shiuan, Chang, Cheng-Nan, Lin, Chun-Sheng, Hsieh, Ming-Chun, Chiang, Hsin-Che and Ho, Jyh-Jier. 2002. Heteroepitaxial silicon-carbide nitride films with different carbon sources on silicon substrates prepared by rapid-thermal chemical-vapor deposition. Journal of Electronic Materials 31: 1341–1346.

[18] Mishra, S.K. and A.S. Bhattacharyya. 2008. Effect of substrate temperature on the Adhesion properties of magnetron sputtered Nanocomposite Si–C–N thin films. Materials Letters 62: 98–402.

[19] Bhattacharyya, A.S., S.K. Mishra, S. Mukherjee and G.C. Das. 2009. A comparative study of Si–C–N films on different substrates grown by RF magnetron sputtering. Journal of Alloys and Compounds 478: 474–478.

[20] Bhattacharyya, A.S. and S.K. Mishra. 2010. Raman studies on nanocomposite silicon carbonitride thin film deposited by r.f. magnetron sputtering at different substrate temperatures. Journal of Raman Spectroscopy 41: 1234–1239.

[21] Bhattacharyya, A.S., S.K. Mishra and S. Mukherjee. 2010. Correlation of structure and hardness of rf magnetron sputtered silicon carbonitride films. Journal of Vacuum Science & Technology A 28: 505–509.

[22] Bhattacharyya, A.S. 2021. Sliding indentation: Failure modes with the study of velocity and loading rate. Surface Topography: Metrology and Properties 9: 035052.

[23] Bhattacharyya, A.S. and S.K. Mishra. 2010. Micro/nanomechanical behavior of magnetron sputtered Si–C–N coatings through nanoindentation and scratch tests. Journal of Micromechanics and Microengineering 21: 015011.

[24] Bhattacharyya, A.S., G.C. Das, S. Mukherjee and S.K. Mishra. 2009. Effect of radio frequency and direct current modes of deposition on protective metallurgical hard silicon carbon nitride coatings by magnetron sputtering. Vacuum 83: 1464–1469.

[25] Bhattacharyya, A.S., S.K. Mishra, G.C. Das and S. Mukherjee. 2009. SiCN:Hot properties. Eur. Coat. J. 3: 108–114.

[26] Yang, Jie. 2013. A harsh environment wireless pressure sensing solution utilizing high temperature electronics. Sensors 13: 2719–2734.

[27] Riedel, Ralf, Kleebe, Hans-Joachim, Schönfelder, Herbert and Aldinger, Fritz. 1995. A covalent micro/nano composite resistant to high temperature oxidation. Nature 374: 526–528.

[28] Jiang, Minming, Xu, Ke, Liao, Ningbo and Zheng, Beirong. 2022. Effect of sputtering power on piezoresistivity and interfacial strength of SiCN thin films prepared by magnetic sputtering. Ceramics International 48: 2112–2117.

[29] Jõgiaas, Taivo, Tarre, Aivar, Mändar, Hugo, Kozlova, Jekaterina and Tamm, Aile. 2021. Nanoindentation of chromium oxide possessing superior hardness among atomic-layer-deposited oxides. Nanomaterials 12: 82.

[30] Minming Jiang, Ke Xu, Ningbo Liao and Beirong Zheng. 2022. Effect of sputtering power on piezoresistivity and interfacial strength of SiCN thin films prepared by magnetic sputtering. Ceramics International 48: 2112–17.

[31] Tanaka, Ippei. Matuoka, Shinichiro and Harada, Yasunori. 2022. Mechanical properties of amorphous SiCN films deposited by ion-beam-assisted deposition. Diamond and Related Materials 121: 108732.

[32] Jung, Chanwon, Song, Seokhwi, Park, Hyunwoo, Kim, Youngjoon, Lee, Eun Jong, Lee, Sung Gwon and Jeon, Hyeongtag. 2021. Characteristics of carbon-containing low-k dielectric SiCN thin films deposited via remote plasma atomic layer deposition. Journal of Vacuum Science & Technology A 39: 042404.

[33] Ermakova, E. and M. Kosinova. 2022. Organosilicon compounds as single-source precursors for SiCN films production. Journal of Organometallic Chemistry 958: 122183.

[34] Liu, Xingmin, Li, Minghang, Liu, Heqiang, Duan, Wenyan, Fasel, Claudia, Chen, Yongchao, Qu, Fangmu, Xie, Wenjie et al. 2022. Nanocellulose-polysilazane single-source-precursor derived

defect-rich carbon nanofibers/SiCN nanocomposites with excellent electromagnetic absorption performance. Carbon 188: 349–359.

[35] Mujib, Shakir Bin and Singh, Gurpreet. 2021. Polymer derived SiOC and SiCN ceramics for electrochemical energy storage: A perspective. International Journal of Ceramic Engineering & Science 4: 4–9.

[36] Kumar, Dayanand, Aluguri, Rakesh, Chand, Umesh and Tseng, Tseung-Yuen. 2018. Conductive bridge random access memory characteristics of SiCN based transparent device due to indium diffusion. Nanotechnology 29: 125202.

[37] Singh, Narendra, Singh, Kirandeep and Kaur, Davinder. 2017. Bipolar resistive switching characteristics of silicon carbide nitride (SiCN)-based devices for nonvolatile memory applications. Ceramics International 43: 8970–74.

[38] Singh, Narendra and Kaur, Davinder. 2018. Origin of tri-state resistive switching characteristics in SiCN thin films for high-temperature ReRAM applications. Applied Physics Letters 113: 162103.

[39] Choi, Yeo-Jin, Lee, Jae-Hoon, Choi, Jin-Seok, An, Sung-Jin, Hwang, Young-Min, Roh, Jae-Seung and Im, Ki-Sik. 2021. Improved noise and device performances of AlGaN/GaN HEMTs with *in situ* silicon carbon nitride (SiCN) cap layer. Crystals 11: 489.

[40] Lee, Jae-Hoon, Im, Ki-Sik and Lee, Jung-Hee. 2021. Effect of *in-situ* silicon carbon nitride (SiCN) cap layer on performances of AlGaN/GaN MISHFETs. IEEE Journal of the Electron Devices Society 9: 728–734.

[41] Qiang Li, Cheng Chen, Mingge Wang, Yaohui Lv, Yulu Mao, Manzhang Xu, Yingnan Wang, Xuewen Wang, Zhiyong Zhang, Shouguo Wang, Wu Zhao and Johan Stiens. 2021. Study on photoelectricity properties of SiCN thin films prepared by magnetron sputtering, J. of Mater Res. and Technol. 15: 460–46.

[42] Qiang Li, Cheng Chen, Manzhang Xu, Yingnan Wang, Xuewen Wang, Zhiyong Zhang, Wu Zhao and Johan Stiens. 2021. Blue-violet emission of silicon carbonitride thin films prepared by sputtering and annealing treatment. Applied Surface Science 546: 149121.

[43] Ivashchenko, V.I., O.K. Porada, A.O. Kozak, V.S. Manzhara, O.K. Sinelnichenko, L.A. Ivashchenko and R.V. Shevchenko. 2022. An effect of hydrogenation on the photoemission of amorphous SiCN films. International Journal of Hydrogen Energy 47(11): 7263–73.

[44] Khan, A.N., K. Jena, G. Chatterjee et al. 2022. An approach towards low cost III-Nitride GaN/InGaN solar cell: the use of Si/SiCN substrate. Silicon 14: 2107–14.

[45] Xavier, F.B., C. Patrick and S. Ewald. 2021. Investigation of low stress and low temperature SiN and SiCN PVD films for advanced packaging applications. IEEE 71st Electronic Components and Technology Conference (ECTC) 2111–17.

[46] Iacovo, S. et al. 2021. Characterization of bonding activation sequences to enable ultra-low Cu/SiCN wafer level hybrid bonding. 2021 IEEE 71st Electronic Components and Technology Conference (ECTC) 2097–104.

[47] Kim, S.-W. et al. 2020. Novel Cu/SiCN surface topography control for 1 μm pitch hybrid wafer-to-wafer bonding. 2020 IEEE 70th Electronic Components and Technology Conference (ECTC) 216–22.

[48] Imbert, G., M. Neffati, C. Moutin, S. Chhun, D. Galpin, O. Kermarrec, E. Sabouret and D. Pinceau. 2012. Impact of Ultra Low K materials on flip chip copper pillar packaging. Minapad.

[49] Shan Wang, Hongyu Gong, Yujun Zhang and M. Zeeshan Ashfaq. 2021. Microwave absorption properties of polymer-derived SiCN(CNTs) composite ceramics. Ceramics International 47(1): 1294–302.

[50] Xiao Lin, Hongyu Gong, Yujun Zhang, Lu Zhang, Ma Li, Shan Wang and Saleem Adil. 2021. Targeted design and analysis of microwave absorbing properties in iron-doped SiCN/Si_3N_4 composite ceramics. Ceramics International 47(4): 4521–4530.

[51] Xue Guo, Feifei Xiao, Jiao Li, Hua Zhang, Qiangqiang Hu, Guochang Li and Haibin Sun. 2021. Fe-doped SiCN composite fibers for electromagnetic waves absorption. Ceramics International 47(1): 1184–1190,

[52] Liu, X., Z. Tang, J. Xue et al. 2021. Enhanced microwave absorption properties of polymer-derived SiC/SiCN composite ceramics modified by TiC. J Mater Sci: Mater Electron. 32: 25895–907.

[53] Xingmin Liu, Hailong Xu, Guoqiang Liu, Wenyan Duan, Yi Zhang, Xiaomeng Fan and Ralf Riedel. 2021. Electromagnetic shielding performance of SiC/graphitic carbon-SiCN porous ceramic nanocomposites derived from catalyst assisted single-source-precursors. Journal of the European Ceramic Society 41(9): 4806–14.

[54] Mahmoudi, Mohammadreza, Sungjin Kim, Arif M. Arifuzzaman, Tomonori Saito, Corson L. Cramer and Majid Minary-Jolandan. 2022. Processing and 3D printing of SiCN polymer-derived ceramics. International Journal of Applied Ceramic Technology 19(2): 939–948.

[55] Hagelüken, Lorenz, Sasikumar, Pradeep, Lee, Ho-Yun, Stadio, David Di, Chandorkar, Yashoda, Rottmar, Markus et al. 2022. Multiscale 2D/3D microshaping and property tuning of polymer-derived SiCN ceramics. Journal of the European Ceramic Society 42(5): 1963–1970.

[56] Pan, Zhenxue, Wang, Dan, Guo, Xiang, Li, Yongming, Zhang, Zongbo and Xu, Caihong. 2022. High strength and microwave-absorbing polymer-derived SiCN honeycomb ceramic prepared by 3D printing. Journal of the European Ceramic Society 42(4): 1322–31.

[57] Silva, Bernardo Araldi, Luiz Fernando Belchior Ribeiro, Sergio Yesid Gómez González, Dachamir Hotza, Regina de Fátima Peralta Muniz Moreira and Agenor De Noni Junior. 2021. SiOC and SiCN-based ceramic supports for catalysts and photocatalysts. Microporous and Mesoporous Materials 327: 111435.

[58] Oliver, W.C. and G.M. Pharr. 1992. An improved technique for determining hardness and elastic modulus using load and displacement sensing indentation experiments. Journal of Materials Research 7: 1564–83.

[59] Oliver, W.C. 2004. Measurement of hardness and elastic modulus by instrumented indentation: Advances in understanding and refinements to methodology. Journal of Materials Research 19: 3.

[60] He, L.H. and M.V. Swain. 2009. Nanoindentation creep behavior of human enamel. Journal of Biomedical Materials Research A 91(2): 352–59.

[61] Oyen, M.L. 2005. Spherical indentation creep following ramp loading. Journal of Materials Research 20(8): 2094–2100.

[62] Oyen, M.L. and C.C. Ko. 2007. Examination of local variations in viscous, elastic, and plastic indentation responses in healing bone. Journal of Materials Science Materials in Medicine 18(4): 623–628.

[63] Bhattacharyya, A., S. Kumar, P. Rajak, N. Kumar, R. Sharma, A. Acharya, G. V. Ranjan. 2016. Analyzing time on sample during nanoindentation. Material Science Research India 13(2): 74–79.

[64] Wu, Ziheng, Baker, Tyler A. Ovaert, Timothy C. Niebur and L. Glen. 2011. The effect of holding time on nanoindentation measurements of creep in bone. J. Biomech. 7; 44(6): 1066–1072.

[65] Tamin, Mohd Nasir. 2011. Damage and fracture of composite materials and structures. Advanced Structured Materials 17, Springer.

[66] Li, Xiaodong, Bhushan, Bharat, Takashima, Kazuki, Baek, Chang-Wook and Kim, Yong-Kweon. 2003. Mechanical characterization of micro/nanoscale structures for MEMS/NEMS applications using nanoindentation techniques. Ultramicroscopy 97(1–4): 481–494.

[67] Li, Xiaodong and Bhushan, Bharat. 2003. Fatigue studies of nanoscale structures for MEMS/NEMS applications using nanoindentation techniques. Surface and Coatings Technology 163–164: 521–526.

[68] Hyukjae Lee, Ronald A. Coutu Jr, Shankar Mall and Paul E. Kladitis. 2005. Nanoindentation technique for characterizing cantilever beam style RF microelectromechanical systems (MEMS) switches. J. Micromech. Microeng. 15: 1230.

[69] Broue, Adrien, Fourcade, Thibaut, Dhennin, Jérémie, Courtade, Frédéric, Charvet, Pierre–Louis, Pons, Patrick, Lafonta, Xavier and Plana, Robert. 2010. Validation of bending tests by nanoindentation for micro-contact analysis of MEMS switches. J. Micromech. Microeng. 20: 085025.

[70] Jackson, Nathan. Olszewski, Oskar Z. O'Murchu, Cian and Mathewson, Alan. 2017. Shock-induced aluminum nitride based MEMS energy harvester to power a leadless pacemaker. Sensors and Actuators A: Physical 264: 212–218.

[71] Kimberley, J., I. Chasiotis and J. Lambros. 2008. Failure of microelectromechanical systems subjected to impulse loads. International Journal of Solids and Structures 45(2): 497–512.

[72] Tamin, M.N. 2012. Damage and Fracture of Composite Materials and Structures. Springer Series Advanced Structured Materials Springer-Verlag Berlin Heidelberg.

[73] Burghard, Z. 2004. Behaviour of Glasses and Polymer-Derived Amorphous Ceramics Under Contact Stress. PhD-Thesis, Max-Planck Institute for Metals Research & University of Stuttgart Germany.

[74] Mishra, S.K. and A.S. Bhattacharyya. 2013. Silicon-based nanomaterials. Mishra, S.K. and A.S. Bhattacharyya (eds.). Springer Series in Materials Science, Vol. 187, Book Chapter 10.

[75] Bhattacharyya, A.S. and S.K. Mishra. 2011. Micro/nanomechanical behavior of magnetron sputtered Si–C–N coatings through nanoindentation and scratch tests. Journal of Micromechanics and Microengineering 21: 015011.

[76] Cuadrado, N., J. Seuba, D. Casellas, M. Anglada and E. Jiménez-Piqué. 2015. Geometry of nanoindentation cube-corner cracks observed by FIB tomography: Implication for fracture resistance estimation. J. Eur. Ceram. Soc. 35(10): 2949–55.

[77] Chen, Zhangwei, Bhakhri, Vineet, Giuliani, Finn and Atkinson, Alan. 2013. Nanoindentation of porous bulk and thin films of La0.6Sr0.4Co0.2Fe0.8O3−δ. Acta Mat. 61(15): 5720–5734.

[78] Moradkhani, Alireza, Baharvandi, Hamidreza, Tajdari, Mehdi, Latifi, Hamidreza and Martikainen, Jukka. 2013. Determination of fracture toughness using the area of micro-crack tracks left in brittle materials by Vickers indentation test. Journal of Advanced Ceramics 2(1): 87–102.

[79] Bhattacharyya, A.S. and R.P. Kumar. 2017. Deviation in nano-mechanical properties of ceramic nanocomposite thin films. Mat. Sci. Res. India 14(1): 1–4.

[80] Palmero, Paola. 2015. Structural ceramic nanocomposites: a review of properties and powders' synthesis methods. Nanomaterials 5: 656–696.

[81] Mishra, S.K., A.S. Bhattacharyya, P. Mahato and L.C. Pathak. 2012. Multicomponent TiSiBC superhard and tough composite coatings by magnetron sputtering. Surface Coat. Technol. 207: 19–23.

[82] Sha, Z.D., Q. Wan, Q.X.S.S. Pei, Z.S. Quek, Y. Liu et al. 2014. On the failure load and mechanism of polycrystalline graphene by nanoindentation. Scientific Reports 4: 7437.

[83] Sun, J. Ma, A. Jiang, J. Han, J. Han, Ying. 2016. Orientation-dependent mechanical behavior and phase transformation of mono-crystalline silicon. J. Appl. Phys. 119: 095904.

[84] Bhattacharyya, A.S., Kumar, Ramagiri. Priyadarshi, Shubham, Sonu, Shivam, Swetabh and S. Anshu. 2018. Nanoindentation stress-strain for fracture analysis and computational modeling for hardness and modulus. J. Mat. Engg. & Perform. 27: 2719–26.

[85] Du, Xiancheng, Hongwei, Zhao, Hongwei and Zhang, Lin. 2015. Molecular dynamics investigations of mechanical behaviours in monocrystalline silicon due to nanoindentation at cryogenic temperatures and room temperature. Scientific Reports 5: 16275.

[86] Bhattacharyya, A.S. 2015. Computational studies of the nanoindentation load depth curves. J. Sc. & Ind. Res. 74(4): 223–224.

[87] Bhushan, Bharat and Agarwal, B. Gaurav. 2002. Stress analysis of nanostructures using a finite element method. Nanotechnology 13: 515–23.

[88] Dash, Ritambhara and A.S. Bhattacharyya. 2022. Nanoindentation and stress analysis of Si-based N/MEMS. Materials Today: Proceedings. Article in Press.

15

Nanocrystalline Diamond Films as Solid Lubricant Coatings for Extreme Tribological Environments

Vikash Kumar,[1] *Rishi Sharma*[1,]* and *Manish Roy*[2]

1. Introduction

Solid lubricants are those materials that are used to lubricate mainly in dry circumstances. Its main role is similar to that of oils and greases, which is used to create a continuous and adherent lubricant film on the tribological pair surfaces for minimising friction and wear [1]. These coatings are typically employed in situations where liquid lubricants cannot be used or do not offer expected lubrication, such as in high or cryogenic temperatures, high vacuum, ultrahigh-radiation, reactive environments and in extreme contact pressure conditions [2]. Different types of solid lubricants, including graphite, have been extensively used since the middle of the 20th century [3]. From 1950 onwards, development in aeronautics industries emphasised the research and development of advanced solid lubricants. They can be classed based on their crystalline structure, features, properties, or functions, among other things. Different types of solid lubricant coating are shown in Fig. 1 [1].

The research and development of carbon-based solid lubricant films, such as diamond-like carbon (DLC), has received a lot of interest in the last two decades. These films have a crystalline structure identical to diamond, except they are amorphous. Commonly, a-C has a hardness between 12 to 25 GPa and sp³ bonds up

[1] Department of Physics Birla Institute of Technology, Mesra, Ranchi-835215, India.
[2] Defence Metallurgical Research Laboratory, Kanchanbagh, Hyderabad-500058, India.
* Corresponding author: rsharma@bitmesra.ac.in; rishisharmabit@hotmail.com

to 50%, whereas the hardness of ta-C lies in the range of 30 to 70 GPa and has 50 to 85% sp^3 bonds [4]. DLC coatings, which are generally characterized by large residual stresses and limited toughness, are favoured because of their superior wear resistance. These coatings would be susceptible to cracking failure at low loads, regardless of their enhanced hardness. Another widely used solid lubricant is MoS_2 (molybdenum disulphide), alloys of MoS_2 [5] or other transition metal dichalcogenide [6, 7], which have been used in many applications such as aerospace and automobile industries [8]. Its thermal stability in non-oxidizing conditions is adequate up to 1373 K. However, oxidation can restrict the temperature limit of these films in the air to a range of 623 K to 673 K. Adsorbed water vapours and oxidizing conditions can also cause a small but significant increase in friction and wear [1].

Since all the solid lubricants discussed above have certain limitations, that is why the development of new and advanced solid lubricant coating material is one of the challenging tasks for researchers till date. Solid lubricant should have some of the properties as shown in Fig. 2 [1].

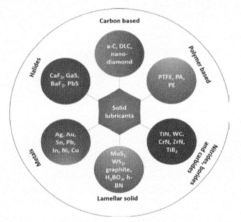

Fig. 1. Types of solid lubricants [1].

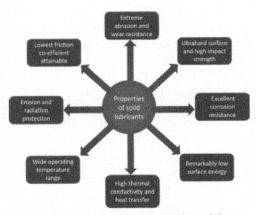

Fig. 2. Properties of the solid lubricants [1].

Diamond is the hardest known natural material, which provides a wide range of possibilities for protecting wear and friction even in the most challenging circumstances. Diamond generally has a coefficient of friction against many engineering materials of less than 0.1 [9]. It may exhibit oxidative wear at high temperatures, especially when sliding against ferrous-based surfaces. Diamonds have the highest heat conductivity of all known materials. At room temperature, a highly-pure, single-crystal CVD diamond has a thermal conductivity of more than 2000 $Wm^{-1}K^{-1}$, decreasing to around 700 $Wm^{-1}K^{-1}$ at 773 K [10]. Its optical characteristics, including transmission from ultraviolet to microwave wavelengths, coupled with its highest thermal conductivity and low thermal expansion coefficient, makes it an excellent window material [11]. The chemical inertness of diamond guarantees extreme resistance to corrosion in acidic medium or other forms of chemical attack [12]. Natural diamond, however, cannot be employed in many tribological applications due to its high cost. Synthetic diamond films have been grown using CVD techniques for tribological applications during the past three decades. Nano-crystalline diamond (NCD) film, which can be directly grown on a substrate, and composed of nanosized grains, is desirable in application fields of tribology. Because of the small crystal size, tunable thermal conductivity, chemical inertness, high hardness, smooth surfaces, flexibility to deposit on various substrates, NCD can function extremely well in tribological applications [2, 13]. Because of the superlative tribological and mechanical properties, these films may be used to coat the majority of mechanical tools and components to enhance their durability and performance; however, the development of these coatings is still at the stage of infancy [8]. Due to the atomic level surface smoothness and tunable properties of the NCD films, superlubricity may be achieved with these films.

The present chapter concerns the self-lubricating characteristics of NCD films keeping in mind its application in a demanding environment. An attempt will be made to outline a brief review of development in NCD films for such application in the recent past. After the introduction, this chapter discusses advances in deposition techniques of NCD films and pre-treatment of substrate materials to increase the density of nucleation of the diamond. This was followed by characterisation techniques, mechanical properties and tribological performances of these films. Finally, the chapter is concluded along with a brief write up on the direction of future research.

2. Advances in Deposition Techniques for NCD Coatings

Unlike various carbon films [14] or carbon-containing other self-lubricating films [15], chemical vapour deposition (CVD) is the most popularly used approach for the deposition of nanocrystalline diamond films [16]. This process involves the gas phase decomposition of a gas mixture containing hydrocarbon, argon and hydrogen. Several methods, including microwave plasma, radio frequency plasma, and hot filament, are available for activating the gas combination [17–21]. Since the gas-phase chemistry is so identical, the appearance and characteristics of the nanocrystalline diamond films synthesized by each process are almost identical.

Table 1. Advantages and disadvantages of Microwave PECVD and Hot-filament CVD techniques.

S. No.	Deposition technique	Advantages	Disadvantages
1	MPECVD	1. High-quality diamond film deposition. 2. No use of electrodes or filament in the system. 3. Tuneable control over the chemical composition of deposited NCD film. 4. Faster deposition rate as compared to other CVD techniques.	1. Sophisticated system design and operation. 2. High power consumption. 3. Substrate size limitation. 4. Difficulty in handling of the microwave plasma device and relatively higher cost. 5. Not suitable for many applications, including large area substrate coating.
2	HFCVD	1. Simple system design and easy handling. 2. Low cost of the equipment. 3. Suitable for diamond deposition on three-dimensional substrates. 4. The thick dense coating on large surfaces area with a dense layer. 5. Coatings can be applied to a variety of substrates, such as metals and alloys. 6. Temperature uniformity throughout the surface of the substrate.	1. Low chemical stability of the filaments. 2. High substrate temperature is required for the deposition of NCD film. 3. Optimization of process parameters such as gas flow, filament temperature and pressure inside the chamber is a tedious task 4. Contamination of the growing diamond film by the filaments.

Hot Filament CVD (HFCVD) and Microwave PECVD (MPECVD) are the commonly used techniques for the deposition of NCD films. In addition to these techniques, direct current (dc) discharge [22], magnetron sputtering [23] and radio frequency (rf) plasma [20,24,25] have been utilized for NCD film deposition. Diamond films can be deposited below 1 torr using ECR plasma [26–28]. Bozeman et al. in 1995 reported diamond deposition at 4 Torr using planar inductively coupled plasma [29]. Okada and co-workers also reported the deposition of NCD films at low-pressure $CH_4/CO/H_2$, followed by Teii and Yoshida using the identical gas composition [30, 31]. A detailed description of MPECVD and HFCVD techniques is given below. The advantages and disadvantages of these two techniques are also listed in Table 1.

2.1 Microwave Plasma-Enhanced CVD (MPECVD)

A microwave plasma-enhanced chemical vapour deposition (microwave PECVD) is a commonly employed technique for the deposition of diamond films. In this technique, the operating pressure is kept between 20–50 Torr [32]. A CH_4/H_2 mixture (with 5% CH_4) leads to polycrystalline diamond films of micrometer size. NCD film can be synthesized by increasing CH_4 content up to 10% while keeping the other parameters constant [19, 33]. NCD can also be grown by substituting hydrogen with a noble gas while keeping the CH_4 content the same. Gruen and co-workers showed the synthesis of NCD films in a CH_4/Ar or C_{60}/Ar microwave discharge without

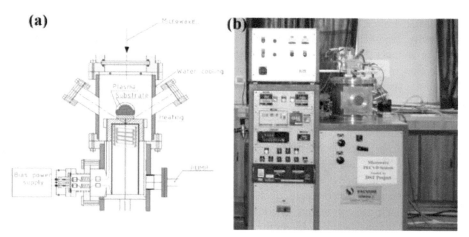

Fig. 3. (a) Schematic diagram of a microwave PECVD system and (b) MPECVD system available at Plasma Lab, Department of Physics, Birla Institute of Technology, Mesra, Ranchi, India.

hydrogen [34, 35]. The deposition of diamond films with micrometre-sized crystals was reported by Philip et al. under conventional deposition conditions [36].

The MPECVD system has several advantages, including the avoidance of diamond film contamination due to hot wire evaporation with a variety of reactive gases. In this method, no electrode or filament is used in the reactor. This ensures that diamonds grow in a clean environment. Because of the prominent input power and the substrate kept in the plasma, the diamond deposition rate is also relatively faster. Thin films with the necessary microstructure and mechanical properties can be consistently produced by controlling operating parameters such as gas flow rate and its constituents, chamber pressure, substrate temperature, and microwave power. The microwave power can be changed continuously and smoothly, allowing the deposition temperature to change steadily. Furthermore, a large-area and sustained plasma sphere may be produced by adjusting the MPECVD reaction chamber geometry. MPECVD systems are usually expensive, and the handling and operation of these systems are complicated. The research group at Plasma Lab in BIT Mesra, Ranchi, has indigenously developed a modest, safe and sparing microwave deposition instrument for developing good quality ultra nanocrystalline diamond (UNCD) films. This microwave PECVD system works at 2.45 GHz, 3 kW, which is powered by a magnetron operating at 50 Hz. The schematic diagram and photograph of the MPECVD system are shown in Figs. 3(a) and 3(b). The substrate holder is equipped with an additional heating system that allows us to regulate the temperature of the substrate. The height of the sample holder can be shifted to fit the plasma ball location, which is determined by the microwave power and chamber pressure [37].

2.2 The Hot-Filament Chemical Vapour Deposition

The microwave PECVD, discussed above, is a commonly used technique for the deposition of diamond films; however, substrate size limitation, difficulty in handling the microwave plasma device and relatively higher cost makes it unsuitable for many applications, including large-area substrate coating. In comparison to plasma-enhanced CVD, the hot-filament CVD method is mainly capable of deposition of diamond films over the substrate of various shapes and sizes. Since the first experimental demonstration of CVD diamond with heated filaments by Matsumoto et al. in the past 1980s, the hot-filament CVD method has been used for the deposition of polycrystalline diamond coatings at the industrial scale [38–40]. High film uniformity, low cost of the equipment, the probability of depositing dense layers on larger areas, uniformity of temperature over the substrate surface, coating on different types of substrates, including metals, make HFCVD the first choice for the deposition of NCD films. Hirose and Terasawa [41] claimed that diamond films may be deposited onto silicon substrates at faster growth rates (8–10 μm/h) by employing organic compounds with high methyl concentrations, such as acetylene, ethanol, methanol, acetone, tri-methylamine, etc., instead of methane (CH_4). Chen et al. [42] reported that the accumulation of oxygen-rich gases such as CO, CO_2, and H_2O to CH_4-H_2 could influence the diamond's growth rates and crystallization.

The hot-filament chemical vapour deposition technology uses a hot coiled wire to break down the precursor reactants in the gas mixture and deposit a coating on the substrate surface, which is placed near the filament. For the deposition of nanocrystalline diamond films, the filament is resistively heated, the temperature between 1800–2300°C is maintained and a gas mixture composed of a hydrocarbon like CH_4 or C_2H_2 in hydrogen or argon is decomposed at that temperature. The decomposition of hydrocarbon gases takes place via heterogeneous reactions at the heated substrate surface, which initiates the chemical vapour deposition process. Metals like tungsten (W), tantalum (Ta), rhenium (Re), etc., are being used for making the filament. The filament temperature is vital in deciding the type and quality of the diamond films. No diamond film got deposited for filament temperatures lower than 1800°C, whereas higher filament temperatures, around 2300°C, result in a significant growth rate and superior polycrystalline diamond quality. The substrate holder of the hot-filament CVD system is heated up to 850°C, in general [9].

Figure 4(a) and 4(b) show the photograph and filament assembly of the HFCVD system available at Plasma Lab, Department of Physics, Birla Institute of Technology, Mesra, Ranchi, India. The system typically consists of a stainless-steel chamber. The substrate holder is placed over the top of the substrate heater at the centre of the chamber, and the filament assembly is held at 5–10 mm above the substrate holder. Spring-shaped filaments are frequently used because of the large surface area; however, these filaments possess a bending tendency over the time during film growth, resulting in unsteady growth conditions. The multiple parallel wire filament system, on the other hand, improves the homogeneity and overall area of the resultant films; however, they need a high-current power supply.

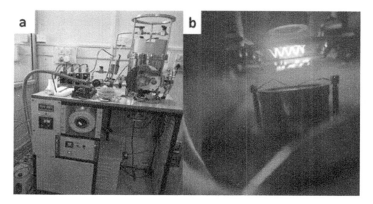

Fig. 4. (a) HFCVD system at Plasma Lab, Department of Physics, Birla Institute of Technology, Mesra, Ranchi, India (b) Photograph of the filament assembly.

3. Pre-Treatment Process to Enhance the Nucleation Density of NCD Films

Pre-treatment process plays an important role in diamond nucleation. The properties of diamond such as orientation, transparency, grain size, adhesion and roughness that are necessary for targeted applications can be optimized by controlling the nucleation. Two separate phases of film deposition, nucleation and growth, are subject to various criteria. The initial nucleation step in the CVD deposition of NCD films significantly affects the properties of the deposited film. A detailed study on pre-treatment method and growth has been discussed by Lee et al. and Sharma et al. [43, 44]. Nowadays, various pre-treatment methods are being used to enhance nucleation; a few of them are discussed below.

3.1 Mechanical Abrasion of the Substrate

The diamond powder can be used to scratch the substrate surface to enhance the nucleation density [45]. Nowadays, scratching the substrates is being used popularly for diamond growth. While not as effective as diamond powder, scratching with silicon carbide, cubic boron nitride, copper, stainless steel, ZrB_2, and Al_2O_3 also increases nucleation. According to some reports, using diamond grit to scratch substrates can increase the nucleation density by about three orders of magnitude compared to substrates that aren't scratched. A compilation of various diamond powders used for scratching is made in Table 2.

3.2 Bias-Enhanced Nucleation

Surface free energies and lattice constants of the silicon and silicon carbide substrates are much distinct from that of diamond; hence, it is hard for the diamond to nucleate on these substrates. By using a negative substrate bias voltage in a microwave PECVD system, Yugo et al. were able to achieve a nucleation density of approximately 10^9–10^{10} cm^{-2} on a mirror-polished silicon substrate [46]. Using

Table 2. Diamond powders used for nucleation experiments [43].

1	Graphite and Diamond Nano-mixture, raw > 16% diamond phase (Cat. No. PL-GD-5g)
2	Graphite and Diamond Nano-mixture, purified, > 16% diamond phase (Cat. No. PL-GDMOF-5g)
3	Nano-diamonds, > 97% grade G nano-diamonds powder (Cat. No. PL-D-G-5g)
4	Nanopure, Aqueous suspension of 4% Nano-diamonds (Cat. No. PL-Nano)
5	Nano-diamonds, > 97% grade G01 nano-diamonds powder (Cat. No. PL-D-G01-5g)
6	NanoPure, Aqueous suspension of 4% Nano-diamonds (Cat. No. PL-Nanopure-G01- 50m)
7	Nano-diamonds, Agglomerate free, positively charged and 10% aqueous suspension
8	Sufipol BG and Nano-diamonds Super-Finish Polishing Paste

this method, mirror-polished silicon has witnessed the maximum nucleation density, which has been measured at 10^{10}–10^{11} cm^{-2}. When a negative bias is applied to the substrate in the HFCVD system, Stubhan et al. demonstrated, diamond nucleation enhancement is also possible [47]. The highest nucleation density can reach up to 10^{9}–10^{10} cm^{-2} on mirror-polished silicon.

3.3 Diamond Nucleation at a Low Gas Pressure

Using either HFCVD or ECR plasma CVD without the use of surface scratching or a substrate bias, a high density of diamond nucleation (10^{9}–10^{11} cm^{-2}) has been attained on mirror-polished silicon surfaces at low pressures (0.1–1 Torr) [44]. On Titanium substrates, similar outcomes have also been obtained. This technique enables the development of diamond grains with a density > 10^{10} cm^{-2}.

3.4 Ion Implantation Enhanced Nucleation

Ion implantation can also be used to produce diamonds with a high nucleation density using CVD techniques [48]. Silicon ions (Si^{+}) are implanted into a mirror-polished silicon wafer. Only the surface structure, not the composition of silicon, is altered by the implantation of Si^{+}. The diamond may easily nucleate and grow on a silicon wafer after treatment with Si^{+} (25 keV) with an implantation dose of 2×10^{17} cm^{-2}, and a continuous diamond layer can be produced.

Sharma et al. [43] has investigated the impact of various pre-treatment procedures and specified plasma properties. Eight different diamond powders were selected for pre-treatment in order to examine the effects of pre-treatment techniques on the nucleation of nanocrystalline diamond. All types of used diamond powder have been shown in Table 2. SEM image of the diamond nucleation on silicon is shown in Fig. 5(a), and Fig. 5(b) shows the growth of the individual nuclei in 5 hours. A comparison of different pre-treatment methods is listed in Table 3.

Table 3. Compilation of different pre-treatment methods.

S. No.	Nucleation techniques	Investigators	Remark
1	Mechanical abrasion of substrate	Mitsuda et al. [45]	Nucleation density is enhanced by roughly three order of magnitude compared with non-scratched silicon (up to 10^7 cm^{-2}).
2	Bias-enhanced nucleation (BEN)	Yugo et al. and Stubhan et al. [46, 47]	Nucleation density of about 10^9–10^{10} cm^{-2} on a mirror-polished silicon.
3	Nucleation at low gas pressure	Lee, Lin and Jiang [44]	High nucleation density (10^9–10^{11} cm^{-2}) has been achieved under low pressures (0.1–1 Torr).
4	Ion implantation enhanced nucleation	Yang et al. [48]	Diamond can easily nucleate and grow on a silicon wafer after treating substrate with Si$^+$ (25 keV) and an implantation dose of 2×10^{17} cm^{-2}.

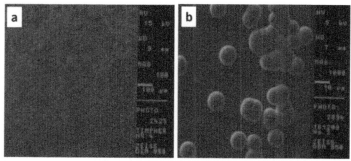

Fig. 5. (a) SEM image of diamond nucleation on silicon and (b) SEM image of growth of nuclei after 5 hours [43].

4. Characterization of Nanocrystalline Diamond Films

To study the various properties of nanocrystalline diamond films, different characterization techniques are used. A few important characterization techniques have been discussed below.

4.1 Raman Spectroscopy

Not long after C. V. Raman discovered the Raman Effect in 1928, Raman spectroscopy was utilized to characterize various carbon species. Also, it is one of the most reliable tools used to validate the growth of NCD films. Raman spectra of the NCD films deposited with the variation of microwave power are shown in Fig. 6. Raman spectra of the NCD films, which are predominated by the G peak and D peak, can contribute a view of sp^3 and sp^2 bonded carbon atom content at the grain boundaries by observing both G peak position and ratio of I(D) and I(G). In each spectrum, four broad peaks are identified. The peak at 1550 cm^{-1} (G peak) is caused by sp^2 bonded graphite, while the peak at 1345 cm^{-1} (D peak) is caused by graphite disorder. Peaks centred at 1140 cm^{-1} and 1470 cm^{-1} are common in NCD films and are related to the v_1 and

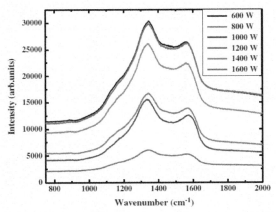

Fig. 6. RAMAN spectra of NCD films [Reprinted with permission from Elsevier [21]].

v_3 vibration modes of transpolyacetylene developed with the diamond phase at the grain boundaries. Diamond is represented by a strong peak around 1332 cm^{-1} located on the right side of the D peak. The Raman spectra of NCD films are significantly different from those of single-crystal diamonds. The diamond peak at 1332 cm^{-1} is much diminished, and the spectra are dominated by D and G peaks produced by sp^2 bonded carbon located at the grain boundaries of the NCD films [43].

4.2 X-ray Diffractometer (XRD)

XRD is a technique used in materials science to investigate crystallographic structure. This technique works by irradiating a material with X-rays and then measuring the intensities and scattering angles. An XRD scan of a few μm thick NCD film deposited on silicon substrate is shown in Fig. 7 [21]. Constructive interference between the (111) lattice planes of the crystalline diamond are shown by the peak at scattering angle of 44°. As a result, the only crystalline phase present within these NCD films

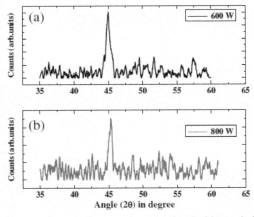

Fig. 7. XRD pattern of the NCD films grown on silicon [Reprinted with permission from Elsevier [21]].

is polycrystalline diamond. The width of diffraction peaks is further investigated to determine the average crystallite size. The width of a diffraction peak in a perfect infinite crystal is solely limited by the X-ray diffractometer's resolution [49]. The peak broadening of XRD is mainly induced by finite crystallite size and hence used to find the crystal size of the investigated particles.

4.3 Atomic Force Microscopy (AFM)

An AFM produces topographic images by scanning a tiny cantilever across a sample's surface. The cantilever's pointed tip makes contact with the surface, bending it and altering the quantity of laser light reflected into the photodiode. The response signal is then restored by adjusting the height of the cantilever, resulting in the recorded cantilever height following the surface. The AFM studies of nanocrystalline diamond film by many authors clearly shows that the topology of the sample varies significantly with the process parameters. AFM micrograph of the NCD films is shown in Fig. 8 [21]. The formation of nanograins, elongated along one direction, separated by sharp grain boundaries, has clearly been observed in the image.

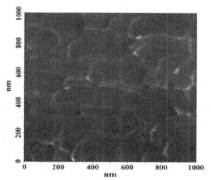

Fig. 8. AFM (Lateral force images) of the nanocrystalline diamond films [Reprinted with permission from Elsevier [21]].

4.4 Field Emission Scanning Electron Microscope (FESEM)/Scanning Electron Microscope (SEM)

FESEM and SEM are the advanced techniques that are used to capture the microstructure images of different materials. It is used to study the micrographs and cross-sectional images of nanocrystalline diamond film to study the surface morphology and the thickness of NCD films by many research groups. The surface topography of the NCD films obtained by SEM is shown in Fig. 9 [21]. The fine grain structure of the NCD film is clearly visible in the morphology.

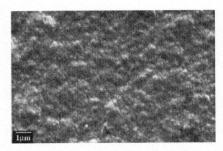

Fig. 9. SEM image of an NCD film [Reprinted with permission from Elsevier [21]].

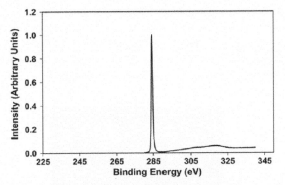

Fig. 10. XPS spectra of an NCD film [Reprinted with permission from Elsevier [50]].

4.5 X-ray Induced Photoelectron Spectroscopy (XPS)

XPS is a powerful tool for detecting contaminants and analysing binding relationships. XPS is primarily used to explore the chemical bonding states, namely the sp^2 and sp^3 fractions, present in the nanocrystalline diamond films. It is also used to track chemical changes in the diamond films' near-surface region. The XPS spectra of the NCD are shown in Fig. 10. The C1s core level is concentrated on 284 eV [50].

4.6 Fourier-transform Infrared Spectroscopy (FTIR)

The IR spectrum of absorbance or emission of a solid, liquid, or gas is obtained using the Fourier-transform infrared spectroscopy technique. It is the most extensively used method for determining the material's bonding and chemical bondings. Various research groups have investigated FTIR spectroscopy of nanocrystalline diamond film, which provides information about different bending and stretching modes between carbon and hydrogen atoms. FTIR spectra of NCD films investigated by Sharma et al. is shown in Fig. 11, which shows bending and stretching of different peaks [21]. Peaks lying between 2800 and 3300 cm^{-1} are due to C-H stretching modes.

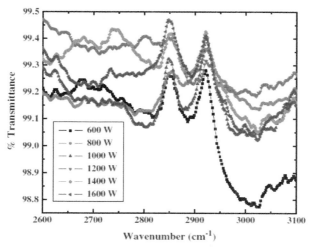

Fig. 11. FTIR spectra of NCD films [Reprinted with permission from Elsevier [21]].

5. Mechanical Properties of Nanocrystalline Diamond (NCD) Films

Hardness and elastic modulus of naocrystalline diamond film is the most widely investigated mechanical properties. A representative load vs. displacement curves along with load vs. square of displacement curves of H terminated and O terminated NCD films are provided in Fig. 12 and Fig. 13 [51, 52]. An important feature of load vs. displacement curves of diamond film is absence of indentation creep [53]. That means there is no increase of displacement even though the load is held constant at highest load. However, such phenomenon is highly conspicuous in carbon films [54, 55]. According to the contact mechanics' theories of plasticity, the load varies with the square of depth of penetration. It is clear from Fig. 13 that all the curves exhibit a straight line without any step and with a turning point during loading. This indicates the high cohesive strength and high fracture toughness of these NCDs [56]. No cracking in these films can be observed in the applied load range. Further, the maximum Hertz-like shear stresses experienced by these films are not enough to make the substrate yield, although these films deform substantially.

A compilation of mechanical properties of various NCD films available in literature is made in Table 4. Both hardness and elastic modulus of NCD films vary over a wide range. The highest hardness of 121 GPa is shown by the film deposited by hot wire CVD technique at very low temperature 635°C and the hardness was measured at a very low load of 47 mN by Cicala et al. [57]. In contrast, the lowest hardness pertains to UNCD deposited in argon free environment employing PVD technique by Shen et al. [58]. All the cases films with higher hardness possess lower elastic modulus and vice versa.

Off late, the ratio of hardness to elastic modulus (H/E) is found to be a very important material parameter [59, 60]. When this ratio is multiplied by the ratio of the diameter of plastic zone to the diameter of the total deformed zone, it gives

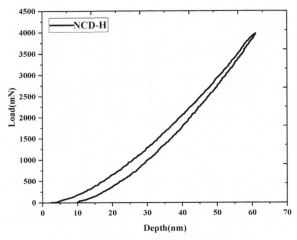

Fig. 12. Load vs. displacement curves for H-terminated and O-terminated NCD films.

an index known as plasticity index which, in turn, governs deformation behaviour of contacting surfaces. This parameter is also an important part of expressions for fracture toughness [61]. In addition to this parameter, the ratio of the hardness to the power three to square of elastic modulus, i.e., the ration H^3/E^2 is also another important parameter referred as elasticity of the film [62]. These two parameters are also listed in Table 4. Both these parameters play an important role on the wear behaviour governed by deformation behaviour of materials. It is interesting to note that the increasing or decreasing trend of these two parameters are not related to increase or decrease of hardness or elastic modulus of the investigated films. The highest H/E and H^3/E^2 values are indicated by highly transparent NCD film deposited using PVD technique by You et al. [63] signifying the fact that this film has the maximum fracture toughness and elasticity.

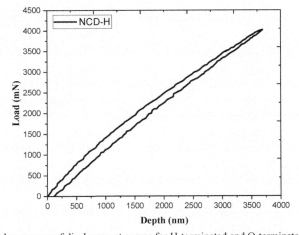

Fig. 13. Load vs. square of displacement curves for H-terminated and O-terminated NCD films.

Table 4. Compilation of various mechanical properties NCD reported in literature.

Si No	Investigators	H (GPa)	E (GPa)	H/E	H^3/E^2 (GPa)	Remark
1	Roy et al. [50]	58.7 ± 9.4	419 ± 40	0.14	1.15	O terminated NCD
2	Kumar et al. [13]	36.2	492.8	0.07	0.19	NCD with grain size between 80–100 nm.
3	You et al. [63]	64 ± 1	395 ± 5	0.16	1.71	Highly transparent NCD film
4	Cicala et al. [57]	121 ± 25	1036 ± 163	0.11	1.65	Low deposition temperature 653°C and 47 mN load
5	Gu et al. [64]	38	315	0.12	0.55	Low pressure deposition (0.3 mbar)
6	Shen et al. [58]	28.8	225	0.13	0.47	UNCD deposited in argon free environment
7	Gruber et al. [65]	46.5 ± 1.7	903 ± 35.3	0.05	0.12	Hardness of NCD sub-layer evaluated by bending experiment
8	Yan et al. [66]	94.01	936.26	0.10	0.95	NCD deposited on cobalt-cemented tungsten carbide (WC-Co)
9	Wiora et al. [18]	96	1050	0.09	0.80	Young's modulus and hardness as a function of grain size.
10	Yang et al. [67]	91	721	0.12	1.44	NCD film deposited by Laser MPCVD

6. Tribological Properties of Nanocrystalline Diamond (NCD) Films

Tribology is the study of interacting surfaces which are in relative motion. It involves the study and application of friction, wear and lubrication. Lubricants are materials which reduce friction between surfaces and keep wear under control [68]. It is generally assumed that for better tribological performance, a material should have high hardness as well as very smooth surface morphology. A lot of studies have been done to investigate the tribological properties of NCD film. Some of the important factors that influence the tribological properties such as wear and friction coefficient are microstructure, hardness and elastic modulus of a material. Kumar et al. [9] deposited nanocrystalline diamond film using hot-filament CVD and showed that NCD film deposited at higher substrate temperature has high hardness and elastic modulus due to increase in grain size from 30 nm at 600°C to 80 nm at 870°C. Researchers report that the results of sliding friction studies on NCD films are encouraging [69, 70]. Coefficient of friction between 0.1–0.15 and wear rates $\sim 3 \times 10^{-7}$ mm³/Nm of the diamond films have been observed for large-duration test ($> 5 \times 10^4$ s) opposite to Si_3N_4 balls in the air. These wear rates seem to reflect initial wear asperities. After wear track flatening, wear rates become essentially immeasurable [69, 71, 72]. Recently, tribological and corrosion resistance behaviour of the NCD coated on Ti alloy has been studied [73]. It has been shown that the NCD coated samples show a mixed response in both electrochemical and tribo-electrochemical environments.

The tribological properties of the NCD films are measured using a tribometer. This system measures tribology between counteracting surfaces, such as coefficient of friction, frictional force, and wear volume. One of the most widely used tribometers is the pin on disc tribometer, which consists of a stationary pin that is generally loaded against a rotating disc. To simulate a specific contact, the pin can be any form, but cylindrical tips are widely employed to optimize the contact geometry. The ratio of the frictional force to the loading force on the pin determines the coefficient of friction. The total volume of material lost during sliding (the wear volume), V, is proportional to the actual area of contact multiplied by the sliding distance by a wear factor, K, which is a unitless proportionality constant. The wear factor can be modified to determine the specific wear rate K, which is generally measured in mm^3/Nm and is often more practical and physically direct. As demonstrated, the specific wear rate is calculated using the formula below.

$$K = \frac{V}{F_n d}$$

A few tribological properties of the NCD films are discussed below.

6.1 *Friction Coefficient of NCD*

Friction force is a physical quantity, which acts between two surfaces when one surface moves or tries to move over another surface. The ratio between friction force and normal force is a constant known as coefficient of friction (COF) which is a dimensionless number denoted by μ. COF is a measure of the quantity of friction between two surfaces, i.e., if the coefficient of friction value is low, then it specifies that the force needed for sliding to start is less than the force needed when the quantity of coefficient of friction is high. For lubricious materials, it is estimated that COF should be lower than 0.1. COF depends upon the nature of the materials and roughness of the surface. Hence, for better tribological properties, the surface must be very smooth because in case of rough surface, the friction coefficient increases which leads to wastage of energy in form of generation of heat.

Investigation indicates [74] that friction coefficient of NCD films is not influenced much by roughness of the film. Further, it is also observed that friction coefficient is not altered much with change of lubrication signifying the fact that cheap lubricant can be used instead of expensive lubricant. Bar diagram showing the friction coefficient of oxygen terminated and hydrogen terminated NCD films in various synthetic lubricant as noted by Schneider et al. is given in Fig. 14. The figure is in conformity with above statements. Schneider et al. also reported a significant change in friction coefficient of NCD films depending on geometry, direction of movement and counter body materials.

Roy et al. investigated friction behaviour of oxygen terminated (O-terminated) and hydrogen terminated (H-terminated) nanocrystalline diamond film [50] at very low load to explore possible application of this film as self-lubricating film in micro

[22] Konov, V.I., A.A. Smolin, V.G. Ralchenko, S.M. Pimenov, E.D. Obraztsova, E.N. Loubnin, S.M. Metev and G. Sepold. 1995. Dc arc plasma deposition of smooth nanocrystalline diamond films. Diamond and Related Materials 4: 1073–1078.

[23] Kundu, S.N., M. Basu, A.B. Maity, S. Chaudhuri and A.K. Pal. 1997. Nanocrystalline diamond films deposited by high pressure sputtering of vitreous carbon. Materials Letters 31: 303–309.

[24] Amaratunga, G.A.J., S.R.P. Silva and D.R. McKenzie. 1991. Influence of dc bias voltage on the refractive index and stress of carbon-diamond films deposited from a CH_4/Ar RF plasma. Journal of Applied Physics 70: 5374.

[25] Fedoseev, D.V., V.P. Varnin and B.V. Deryagin. 1984. Synthesis of diamond in its thermodynamic metastability region. Russian Chemical Reviews 53: 435–444.

[26] Eddy, C.R., D.L. Youchison, B.D. Sartwell and K.S. Grabowski. 1992. Deposition of diamond onto aluminum by electron cyclotron resonance microwave plasma-assisted CVD. Journal of Materials Research 7: 3255–3259.

[27] Wei, J., H. Kawarada, J. ichi Suzuki and A. Hiraki. 1990. Growth of diamond films at low pressure using magneto-microwave plasma CVD. Journal of Crystal Growth 99: 1201–1205.

[28] Zarrabian, M., N. Fourches-Coulon, G. Turban, C. Marhic and M. Lancin. 1997. Observation of nanocrystalline diamond in diamondlike carbon films deposited at room temperature in electron cyclotron resonance plasma. Applied Physics Letters 70: 2535.

[29] Bozeman, S.P., D.A. Tucker, B.R. Stoner, J.T. Glass and W.M. Hooke. 1995. Diamond deposition using a planar radio frequency inductively coupled plasma. Applied PhysicsnLetters 66: 3579.

[30] Okada, K., S. Komatsu and S. Matsumoto. 1999. Preparation of microcrystalline diamond in a low pressure inductively coupled plasma. Journal of Materials Research 14: 578–583.

[31] Teii, K., H. Ito, M. Hori, T. Takeo and T. Goto. 2000. Kinetics and role of C, O, and OH in low-pressure nanocrystalline diamond growth. Journal of Applied Physics 87: 4572.

[32] Kamo, M., Y. Sato, S. Matsumoto and N. Setaka. 1983. Diamond synthesis from gas phase in microwave plasma. Journal of Crystal Growth 62: 642–644.

[33] Erz, R., W. Dötter, K. Jung and H. Ehrhardt. 1993. Preparation of smooth and nanocrystalline diamond films. Diamond and Related Materials 2: 449–453.

[34] Gruen, D.M., S. Liu, A.R. Krauss, J. Luo and X. Pan. 1994. Fullerenes as precursors for diamond film growth without hydrogen or oxygen additions. Applied Physics Letters 64: 1502.

[35] Zhou, D., T.G. McCauley, L.C. Qin, A.R. Krauss and D.M. Gruen. 1998. Synthesis of nanocrystalline diamond thin films from an Ar–CH_4 microwave plasma. Journal of Applied Physics 83: 540-543.

[36] Philip, J., P. Hess, T. Feygelson, J.E. Butler, S. Chattopadhyay, K.H. Chen and L.C. Chen. 2003. Elastic, mechanical, and thermal properties of nanocrystalline diamond films. Journal of Applied Physics 93: 2164-2171.

[37] Chatterjee, V., R. Sharma and P.K. Barhai. 2014. Effect of process parameters on the properties of ultrananocrystalline diamond films deposited using microwave plasma enhanced chemical vapor deposition. Advanced Materials Letters 5: 172–179.

[38] Matsumoto, S., Y. Sato, M. Kamo and N. Setaka. 1982. Vapor deposition of diamond particles from methane. Japanese Journal of Applied Physics 21: L183–L185.

[39] Herlinger, J. 2006. sp³'s experience using hot filament CVD reactors to grow diamond for an expanding set of applications. Thin Solid Films 501: 65–69.

[40] Zhang, J. J.W. Zimmer, R.T. Howe and R. Maboudian. 2008. Characterization of boron-doped micro-and nanocrystalline diamond films deposited by wafer-scale hot filament chemical vapor deposition for MEMS applications. Diamond and Related Materials 17: 23–28.

[41] Hirose, Y. and Y. Terasawa. 1986. Synthesis of diamond thin films by thermal CVD using organic compounds. Japanese Journal of Applied Physics 25(6A): L519.

[42] Huang, C., X. Peng, B. Yang, X. Chen, Q. Li, D. Yin and T. Fu. 2018. Effects of strain rate and annealing temperature on tensile properties of nanocrystalline diamond. Carbon 136: 320–328.

[43] Sharma, R., N. Woehrl, P.K. Barhai and V. Buck. 2010. Nucleation density enhancement for nanocrystalline diamond films. Journal of Optoelectronics and Advanced Materials 12: 1915–1920.

[44] Lee, S.T., Z. Lin and X. Jiang. 1999. CVD diamond films: nucleation and growth. Materials Science and Engineering: R: Reports 25: 123–154.

[45] Mitsuda, Y., Y. Kojima, T. Yoshida and K. Akashi. 1987. The growth of diamond in microwave plasma under low pressure. Journal of Materials Science 22: 1557–1562.

[46] Yugo, S., T. Kanai, T. Kimura and T. Muto. 1991. Generation of diamond nuclei by electric field in plasma chemical vapor deposition. Applied Physics Letters 58: 1036.

[47] Stubhan, F., M. Ferguson, H.J. Füsser and R.J. Behm. 1995. Heteroepitaxial nucleation of diamond on Si (001) in hot filament chemical vapor deposition. Applied Physics Letters 66: 1900.

[48] Yang, J., X. Su, Q. Chen and Z. Lin. 1995. Si$^+$ implantation: A pretreatment method for diamond nucleation on a Si wafer. Applied Physics Letters 66: 3284.

[49] Steinmüller-Nethl, D., F.R. Kloss, M. Najam-Ul-Haq, M. Rainer, K. Larsson, C. Linsmeier and G. Bonn. 2006. Strong binding of bioactive BMP-2 to nanocrystalline diamond by physisorption. Biomaterials 27(26): 4547–4556.

[50] Roy, M., S. Ghodbane, T. Koch, A. Pauschitz, D. Steinmüller-Nethl, A. Tomala, C. Tomastik and F. Franek. 2011. Tribological investigation of nanocrystalline diamond films at low load under different tribosystems. Diamond and Related Materials 20: 573–583.

[51] Roy, M. and R. Haubner. 2013. Diamond Films and Their Tribological Performances. Springer Vienna 79–110.

[52] Koch, T., M. Evaristo, A. Pauschitz, M. Roy and A. Cavaleiro. 2009. Nanoindentation and nanoscratch behaviour of reactive sputtered deposited W–S–C film. Thin Solid Films 518: 185–193.

[53] Bogus, A., I.C. Gebeshuber, A. Pauschitz, M. Roy and R. Haubner. 2008. Micro-and nanomechanical properties of diamond film with various surface morphologies. Diamond and Related Materials 17: 1998–2004.

[54] Kvasnica, S., J. Schalko, C. Eisenmenger-Sittner, J. Benardi, G. Vorlaufer, A. Pauschitz and M. Roy. 2006. Nanotribological study of PECVD DLC and reactively sputtered Ti containing carbon films. Diamond and Related Materials 15: 1743–1752.

[55] Tomastik, C., J.M. Lackner, A. Pauschitz and M. Roy. 2016. Structural, chemical and nanomechanical investigations of SiC/polymeric a-C: H films deposited by reactive RF unbalanced magnetron sputtering. Solid State Sciences 53: 1–8.

[56] Ding, J., Y. Meng and S. Wen. 2000. Mechanical properties and fracture toughness of multilayer hard coatings using nanoindentation. Thin Solid Films 371: 178–182.

[57] Cicala, G., V. Magaletti, G. Carbone and G.S. Senesi. 2020. Load sensitive super-hardness of nanocrystalline diamond coatings. Diamond and Related Materials 101: 107653.

[58] Shen, B., Q. Lin, S. Chen, Z. Ji, Z. Huang and Z. Zhang. 2019. High-rate synthesis of ultra-nanocrystalline diamond in an argon-free hot filament chemical vapor deposition atmosphere for tribological films. Surface and Coatings Technology 378:124999.

[59] Musil, J. and M. Jirout. 2007. Toughness of hard nanostructured ceramic thin films. Surface and Coatings Technology 201: 5148–5152.

[60] Roy, M., T. Koch and A. Pauschitz. 2010. The influence of sputtering procedure on nanoindentation and nanoscratch behaviour of W–S–C film. Applied Surface Science 256: 6850–6858.

[61] Sapate, S.G., N. Tangselwar, S.N. Paul, R.C. Rathod, S. Mehar, D.S. Gowtam and M. Roy. 2021. Effect of coating thickness on the slurry erosion resistance of HVOF-sprayed WC-10Co-4Cr coatings. Journal of Thermal Spray Technology 30: 1365–1379.

[62] Charitidis, C.A. and S. Logothetidis. 2005. Effects of normal load on nanotribological properties of sputtered carbon nitride films. Diamond and Related Materials 14: 98–108.

[63] You, M.S., F.C.N. Hong, Y.R. Jeng and S.M. Huang. 2009. Low temperature growth of highly transparent nanocrystalline diamond films on quartz glass by hot filament chemical vapor deposition. Diamond and Related Materials 18:155–159.

[64] Gu, J., Z. Chen, R. Li, X. Zhao, C. Das, V. Sahmuganathan, J. Sudijono, M. Lin and K.P. Loh. 2021. Nanocrystalline diamond film grown by pulsed linear antenna microwave CVD. Diamond and Related Materials 119: 108576.

[65] Gruber, D.P., J. Todt, N. Wöhrl, J. Zalesak, M. Tkadletz, A. Kubec, S. Niese, M. Burghammer, M. Rosenthal, H. Sternschulte, M.J. Pfeifenberger, B. Sartory and J. Keckes. 2019. Gradients of microstructure, stresses and mechanical properties in a multi-layered diamond thin film revealed by correlative cross-sectional nano-analytics. Carbon 144:666–674.

[66] Yan, G., Y. Wu, D. Cristea, L. Liu, M. Tierean, Y. Wang, F. Lu, H. Wang, Z. Yuan, D. Munteanu and D. Zhao. 2019. Mechanical properties and wear behavior of multi-layer diamond films deposited by hot-filament chemical vapor deposition. Applied Surface Science 494: 401–411.

[67] Yang, M., S. Bai, Q. Xu, J. Li, T. Shimada, Q. Li, T. Goto, R. Tu and S. Zhang. 2020. Mechanical properties of high-crystalline diamond films grown via laser MPCVD. Diamond and Related Materials 109: 108094.

[68] Szeri, A. 2010. Fluid Film Lubrication. Cambridge University Press, 2010.

[69] Erdemir, A., C. Bindal, G.R. Fenske, C. Zuiker, A.R. Krauss and D.M. Gruen. 1996. Friction and wear properties of smooth diamond films grown in fullerene + argon plasmas. Diamond and Related Materials 5: 923–931.

[70] Erdemir, A., M. Halter, G.R. Fenske, C. Zuiker, R. Csencsits, A.R. Krauss and D.M. Gruen. 2008. Friction and wear mechanisms of smooth diamond films during sliding in air and dry nitrogen. Tribology Transactions 40: 667–675.

[71] Erdemir, A., G.R. Fenske, A.R. Krauss, D.M. Gruen, T. McCauley and R.T. Csencsits. 1999. Tribological properties of nanocrystalline diamond films. Surface and Coatings Technology 120–121: 565–572.

[72] Erdemir, A., M. Halter, G.R. Fenske, A. Krauss, D.M. Gruen, S.M. Pimenov and V.I. Konov. 1997. Durability and tribological performance of smooth diamond films produced by Ar-C_{60} microwave plasmas and by laser polishing. Surface and Coatings Technology 94: 537–542.

[73] Gopal, V., M. Chandran, M.S.R. Rao, S. Mischler, S. Cao and G. Manivasagam. 2017. Tribocorrosion and electrochemical behaviour of nanocrystalline diamond coated Ti based alloys for orthopaedic application. Tribology International 106: 88–100.

[74] Schneider, A., D. Steinmueller-Nethl, M. Roy and F. Franek. 2010. Enhanced tribological performances of nanocrystalline diamond film. International Journal of Refractory Metals and Hard Materials 28: 40–50.

[75] Schneider, A., J. Brenner, D. Steinmüller-Nethl, M. Roy and F. Franek. 2009. Tribological properties of lubricated nanocrystalline diamond surfaces for various loads and geometries. Tribology-Materials, Surfaces & Interfaces 3(4): 175–181.

Index